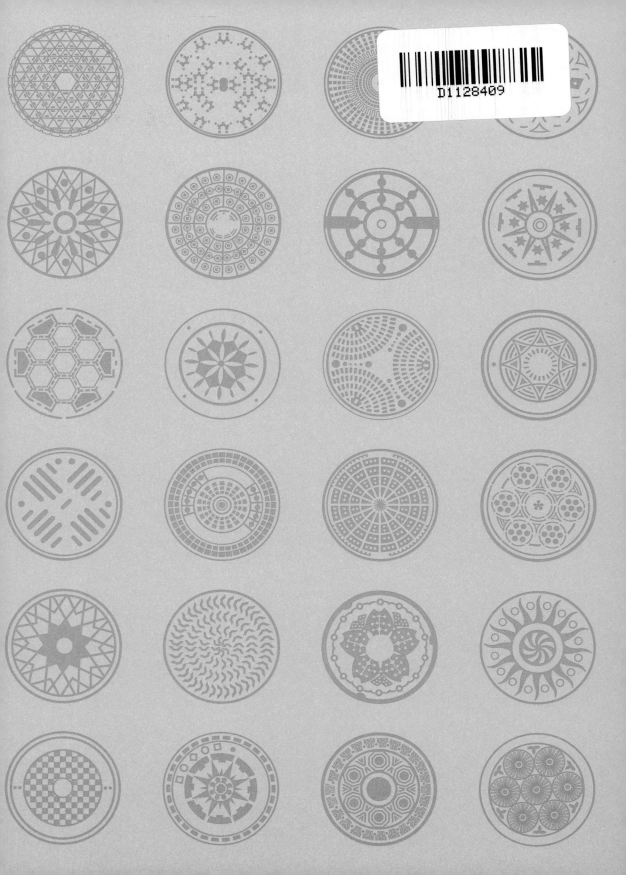

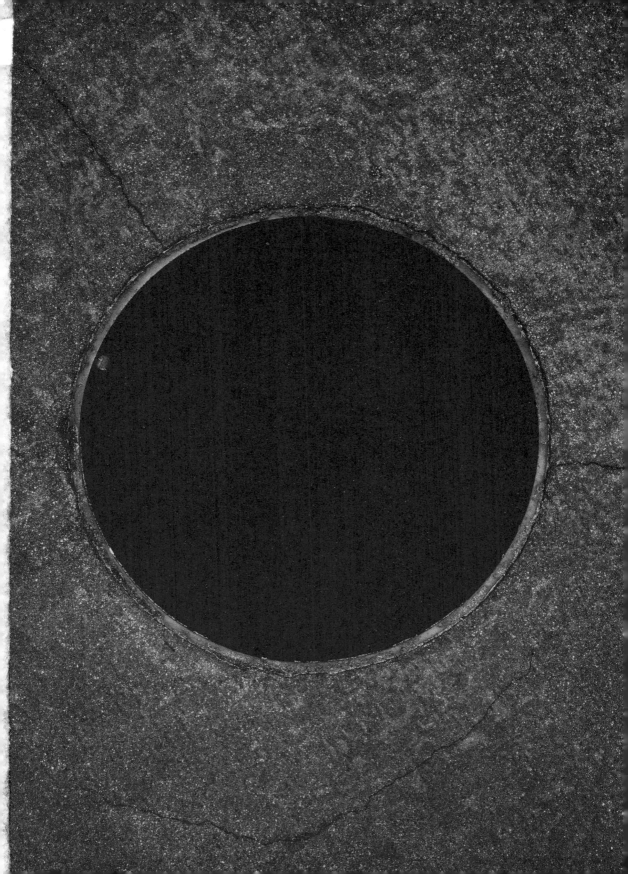

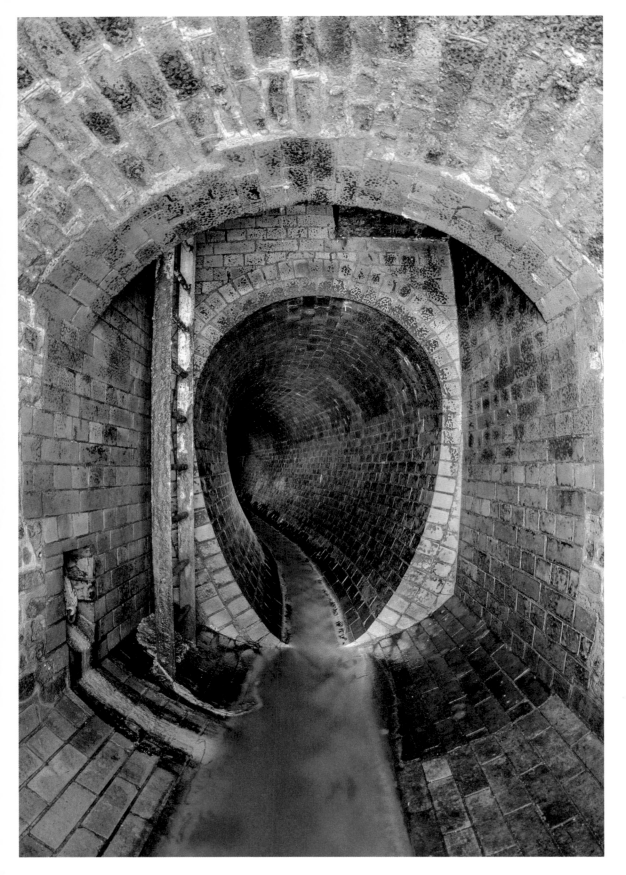

AN UNDERGROUND GUIDE

TO

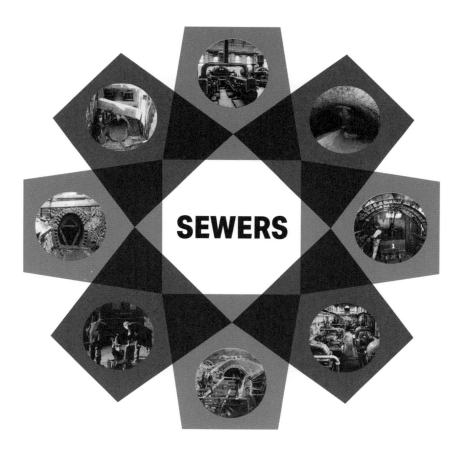

SEWERS

OR:
DOWN, THROUGH & OUT IN PARIS, LONDON, NEW YORK &c.

STEPHEN HALLIDAY

The MIT Press | Cambridge, Massachusetts

FOREWORD BY SIR PETER BAZALGETTE

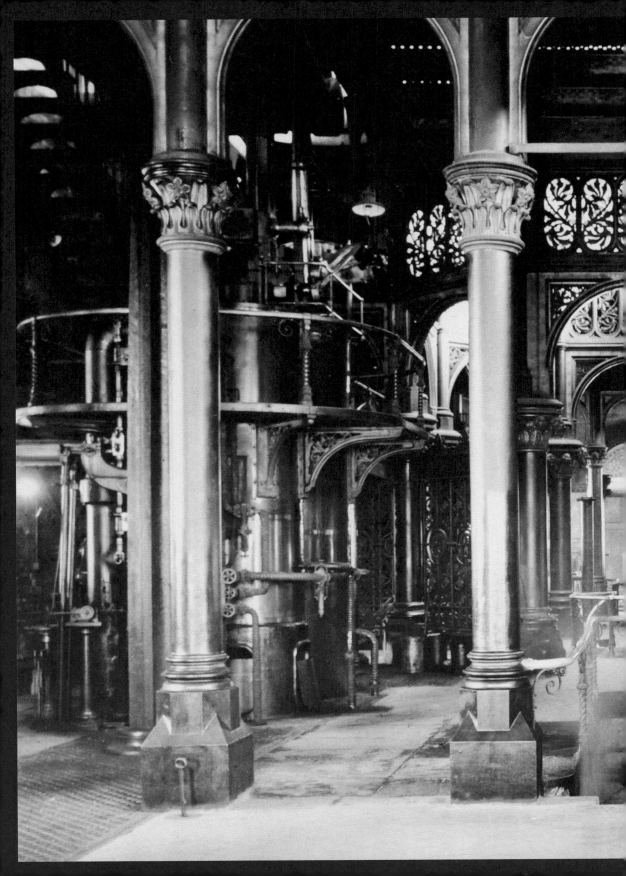

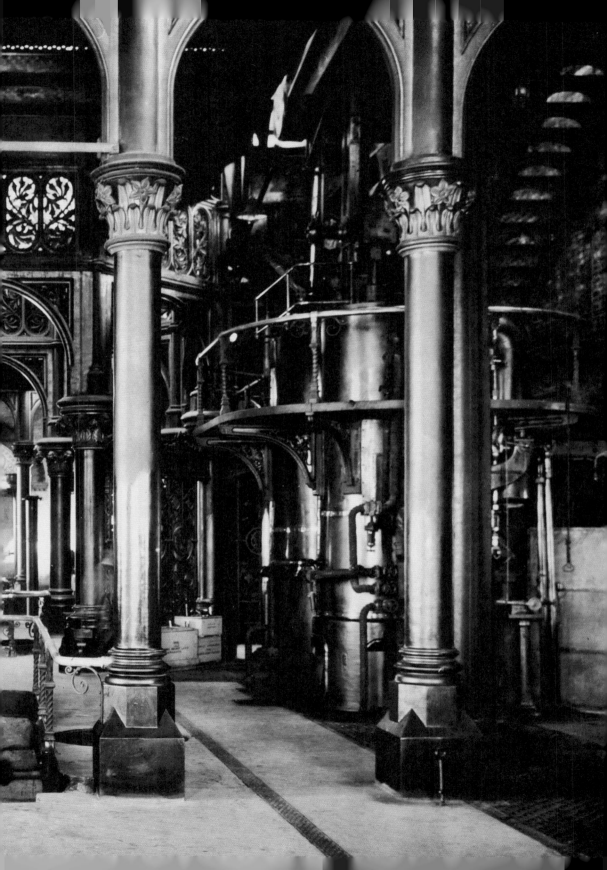

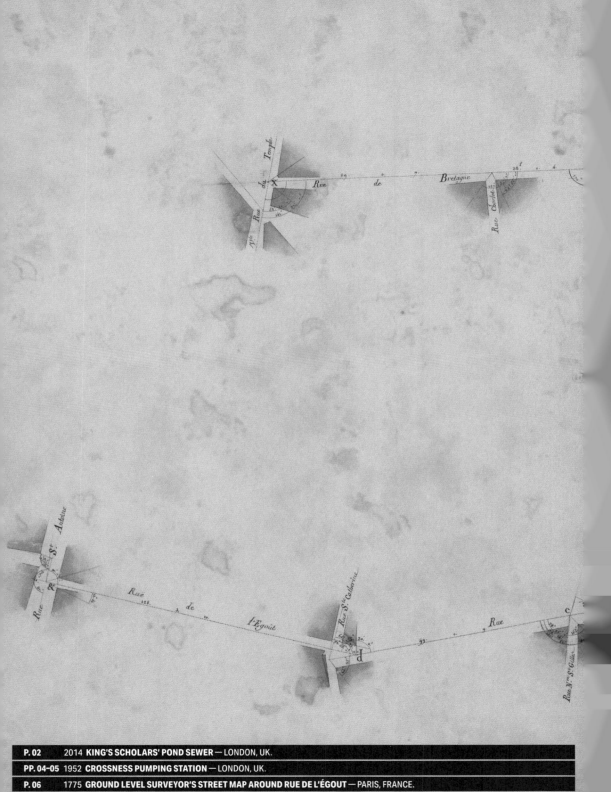

P. 02   2014 **KING'S SCHOLARS' POND SEWER** — LONDON, UK.

PP. 04–05   1952 **CROSSNESS PUMPING STATION** — LONDON, UK.

P. 06   1775 **GROUND LEVEL SURVEYOR'S STREET MAP AROUND RUE DE L'ÉGOUT** — PARIS, FRANCE.

P. 08   1862 **BAZALGETTE'S CONTRACT DRAWING OF THE ENTRANCE TO CROSSNESS** — LONDON, UK.

CONTENTS

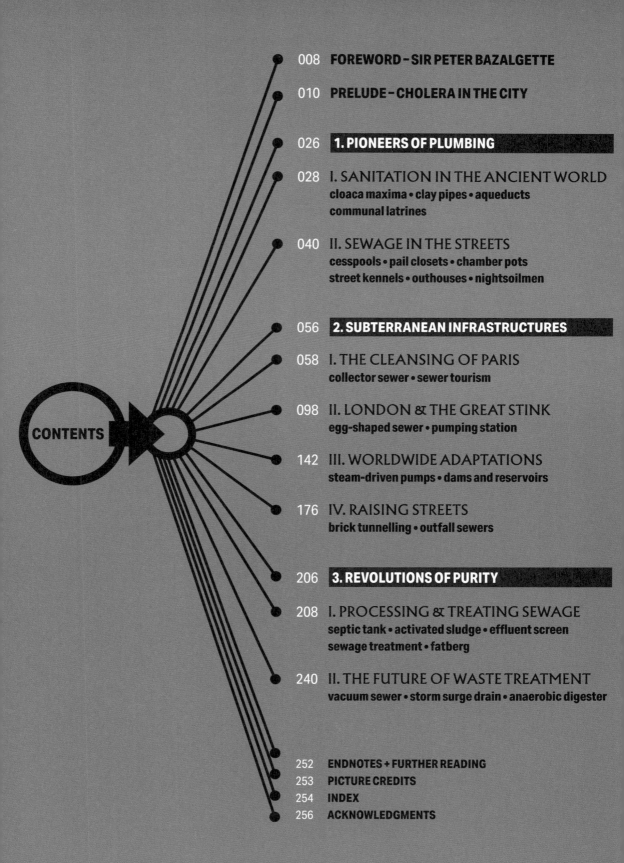

008 **FOREWORD – SIR PETER BAZALGETTE**

010 **PRELUDE – CHOLERA IN THE CITY**

026 **1. PIONEERS OF PLUMBING**

028 I. SANITATION IN THE ANCIENT WORLD
**cloaca maxima • clay pipes • aqueducts
communal latrines**

040 II. SEWAGE IN THE STREETS
**cesspools • pail closets • chamber pots
street kennels • outhouses • nightsoilmen**

056 **2. SUBTERRANEAN INFRASTRUCTURES**

058 I. THE CLEANSING OF PARIS
collector sewer • sewer tourism

098 II. LONDON & THE GREAT STINK
egg-shaped sewer • pumping station

142 III. WORLDWIDE ADAPTATIONS
steam-driven pumps • dams and reservoirs

176 IV. RAISING STREETS
brick tunnelling • outfall sewers

206 **3. REVOLUTIONS OF PURITY**

208 I. PROCESSING & TREATING SEWAGE
**septic tank • activated sludge • effluent screen
sewage treatment • fatberg**

240 II. THE FUTURE OF WASTE TREATMENT
vacuum sewer • storm surge drain • anaerobic digester

252 **ENDNOTES + FURTHER READING**
253 **PICTURE CREDITS**
254 **INDEX**
256 **ACKNOWLEDGMENTS**

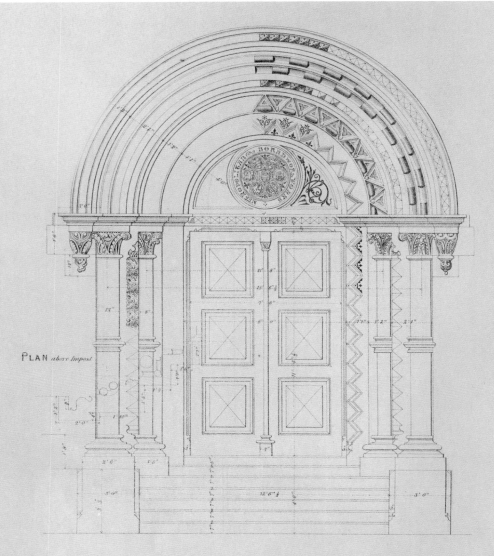

PLAN *above Impost*

ELEVATION

FRONT ENTRANCE

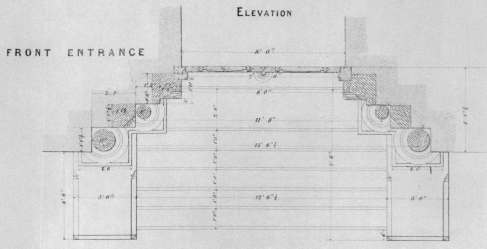

PLAN

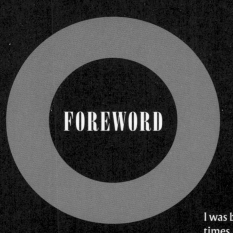

FOREWORD

SIR PETER BAZALGETTE

I was born with an unusual medical condition: sewage in the blood. In Victorian times, my great great grandfather designed and executed a modern sewerage system for London. In the family we like to think of Sir Joseph Bazalgette as the 'Drain Brain'. Now here comes a book that puts good old Sir Joe in the context of history – from the ancient Romans and their Cloaca Maxima to London's new Thames Tideway Tunnel, with several civilizations in between, including the genius of the 8th-century Mexicans.

An Underground Guide To Sewers tells the revealing and entertaining tale of how we've dealt with our ordure over the centuries. But it's about so much more: health, wealth and also beauty. Without sanitation there is death and degradation. But without it cities, the engine of our economies, cannot function or grow either. It's their growth which delivers the wealth. And in the process engineers have constructed, through the centuries, wondrous infrastructures which are not only functional but often beautiful to behold. This generously illustrated work makes the last point eloquently. And it's packed with heroes and heroines – engineers, scientists, environmentalists and social reformers. These are the people who advanced civilization by elevating humankind above its own detritus. A heady story, indeed.

In this rich history, narrated with gusto by Stephen Halliday, we learn how engineers of common sense had to come up with practical solutions prior to any clear scientific proof. James Simpson filtered water for the Victorian householders of Chelsea long before the definitive clinical purification experiments of Lockett and Ardern in the 20th century. Doctor John Snow first proposed cholera was water borne in 1849, contradicting the belief that it was an airborne contagion, a 'miasma'. Many life-saving schemes, such as Bazalgette's, had been constructed by the time Robert Koch actually identified waterborne bacteria in 1883. In fact, the ferocious Florence Nightingale died in 1910 still believing in miasma. Hence Lytton Strachey's description of the great sanitary reformer's immovable faith in eminent Victorians: 'She felt toward (God) as she might have felt towards a glorified sanitary engineer... She seems hardly to distinguish between the Deity and the Drains.'

So what you're about to read is a work of scholarship which entertains. A sort of *Around the World In Eighty Toilets*...how could that fail to provoke a smile? I was particularly taken with Georges-Eugène Haussmann, who masterminded Paris's system in the 1850s. He was so proud of the result that he conducted candlelit tours 'in which ladies need have no hesitation in taking part'. Pride is one thing, fastidiousness quite another. He apparently would accept the passage of storm water and urine, but not faeces. His sewers were too good for that. This reminded me of the answer I once got when I asked an extravagant maker of gold baths whether they were not a bit too much for a simple wash: 'Wash? Wash?' he exploded, 'people should wash before they get in my baths!'

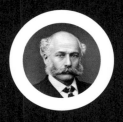

SIR JOSEPH WILLIAM BAZALGETTE
[1819–1891]

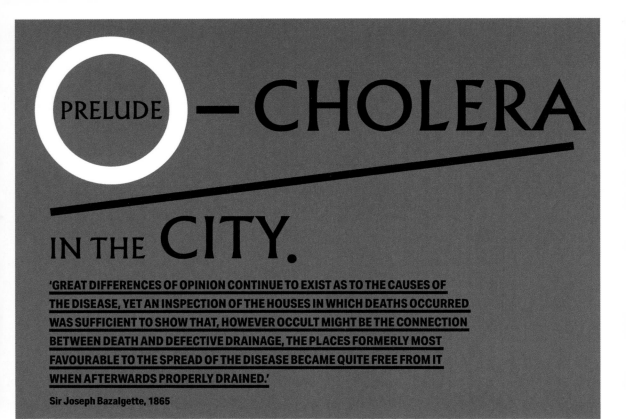

PRELUDE O – CHOLERA IN THE CITY.

'GREAT DIFFERENCES OF OPINION CONTINUE TO EXIST AS TO THE CAUSES OF THE DISEASE, YET AN INSPECTION OF THE HOUSES IN WHICH DEATHS OCCURRED WAS SUFFICIENT TO SHOW THAT, HOWEVER OCCULT MIGHT BE THE CONNECTION BETWEEN DEATH AND DEFECTIVE DRAINAGE, THE PLACES FORMERLY MOST FAVOURABLE TO THE SPREAD OF THE DISEASE BECAME QUITE FREE FROM IT WHEN AFTERWARDS PROPERLY DRAINED.'

Sir Joseph Bazalgette, 1865

In the 1820s, a new and terrifying epidemic disease was making its way from the delta of the Ganges across Asia towards Europe. It was facilitated by the movement of people associated with trade between the East and Europe, which accompanied the Industrial Revolution. The terrible sickness was characterized by acute diarrhoea that emptied the body of nutrients and for most brought on a swift and undignified death, sometimes in hours. The malady was compared with the bubonic plague (or 'Black Death') that had devastated Europe during the Middle Ages and intermittently since then: it had killed 50,000 people in Marseilles in one outbreak during the previous century. As epidemics of this alarming new plague approached Western Europe in a relentless northern and westward march, the pages of national newspapers and medical journals such as *The Lancet* were filled with fearful speculation as to its cause and possible consequences. When the plague came ashore in Sunderland in 1831, *The Lancet* reported from Vienna that a community of Jews had escaped its effects by rubbing their bodies with a liniment consisting of wine, vinegar, camphor powder, pepper, garlic and ground beetles. The journal also speculated as to the nature of the disease: 'Is it a fungus, an insect, a miasma, an electrical disturbance, a deficiency of ozone, a morbid off-scouring of the intestinal canal? We know nothing; we are at sea in a whirl of conjecture.'

It was not only Londoners who worried about the horrific epidemic – which, unlike many diseases associated with dirty living conditions, made its way into the homes of all classes of society. A particularly horrifying story comes from a masked ball held in Paris in March 1832 as cholera ravaged the city. The German poet Heinrich Heine (1797–1856) attended and recorded the event. Some participants appeared in cholera-themed costumes. Around midnight, 'suddenly...one dancer

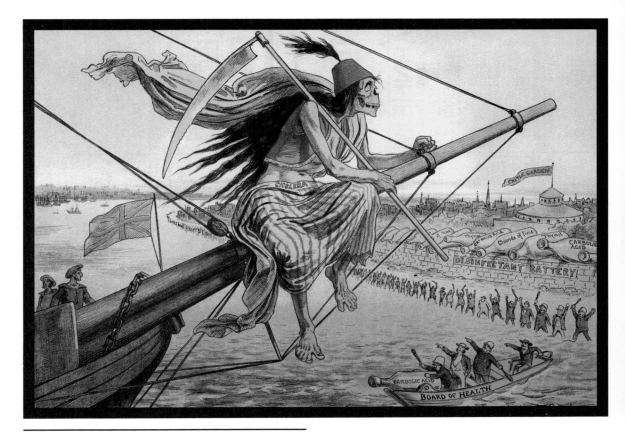

FIG. 1 1883 **THE THREAT OF CHOLERA.** CHOLERA (WEARING A FEZ AS THE DISEASE WAS BELIEVED TO ORIGINATE IN EGYPT) APPROACHES A NEW YORK SHORE IN 1883. THE 'BOARD OF HEALTH' MEETS THE BRITISH SHIP, READY TO DEFEAT CHOLERA WITH THE DISINFECTANT CARBOLIC ACID. IN FACT, BAZALGETTE'S SEWERS HAD ALREADY BANISHED THE DISEASE FROM LONDON.

after the other fell to the ground with shrieks' and, shortly thereafter, fifty victims were carried to Paris's Hôtel Dieu Hospital where, a few hours later, many 'were buried in their masquerade clothes'. A newspaper described how 'the grave diggers of Montmartre cannot dig graves enough...The funerals all take place by night and it is not uncommon to see layers of carcasses which the grave diggers have no time to cover.' It is estimated that 20,000 people died in Paris in this first cholera epidemic of 1831–32. Soon it had spread to Germany, and by the 1840s it had reached New York. London would eventually suffer four cholera epidemics, which between them claimed the lives of almost 40,000 citizens.

Successive pandemics swept the globe during the 19th century. Russia was particularly devastated. The panic and fear induced by the disease led to riots in multiple cities across the country in 1831 as rumours quickly spread that anti-cholera measures such as quarantines and cordons were in fact designed for the deliberate contamination of ordinary people. The third cholera pandemic in 1852 was even more deadly, bringing the death toll in Russia to 1 million, and killing 5,000 people in Copenhagen, Denmark, in less than three months. In 1865 the Mecca Pilgrimage also became the scene of a major outbreak, as around 30,000 pilgrims died out of a total of 90,000.

o———————> 16

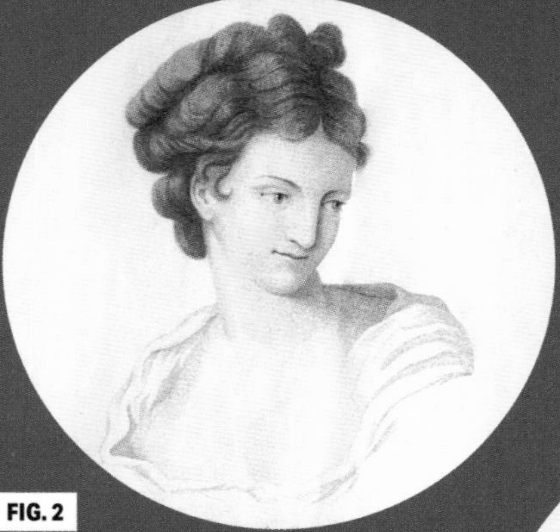

FIG. 2

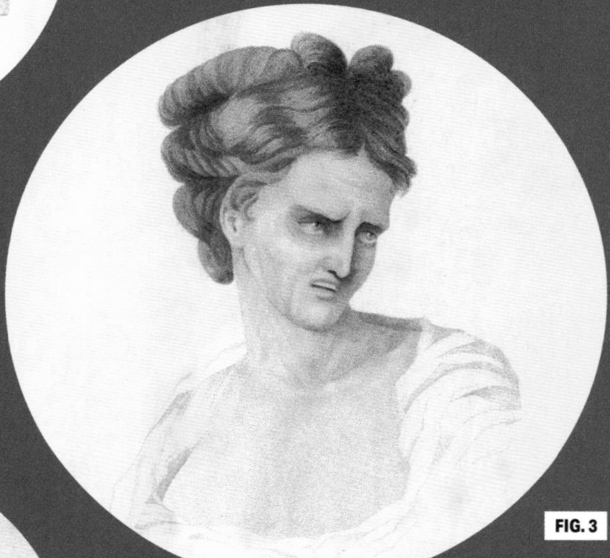

FIG. 3

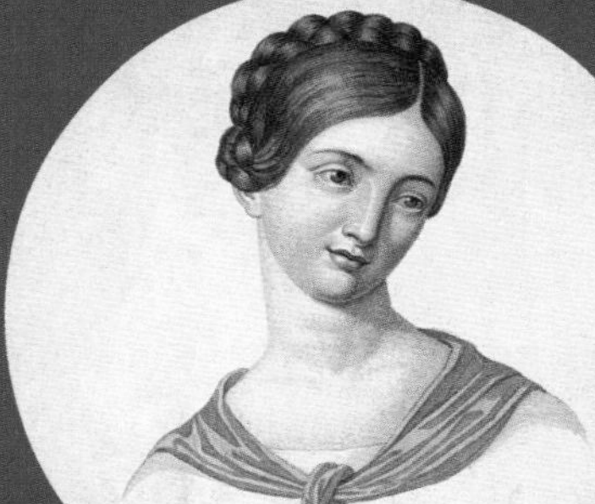

FIG. 4

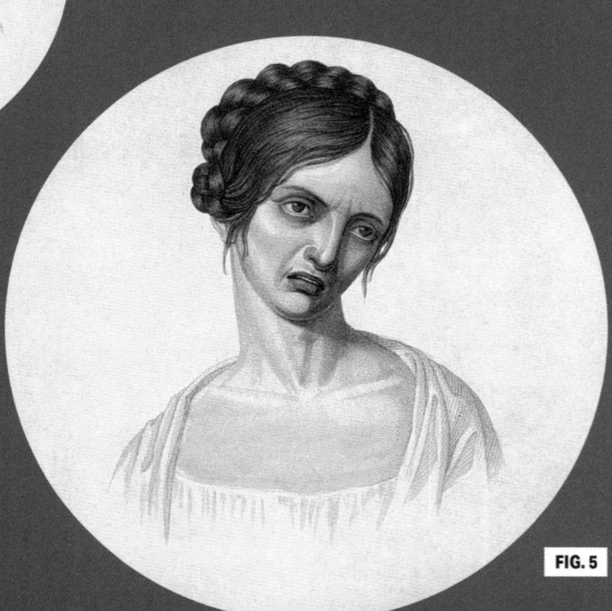

FIG. 5

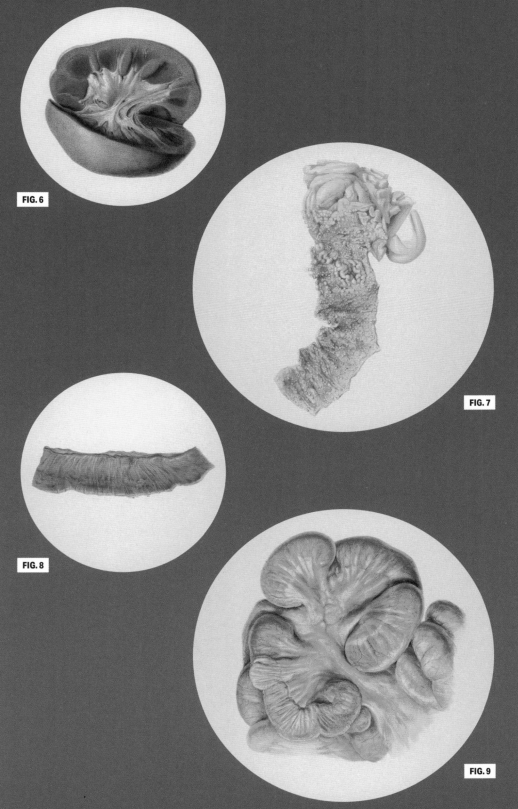

FIG. 6

FIG. 7

FIG. 8

FIG. 9

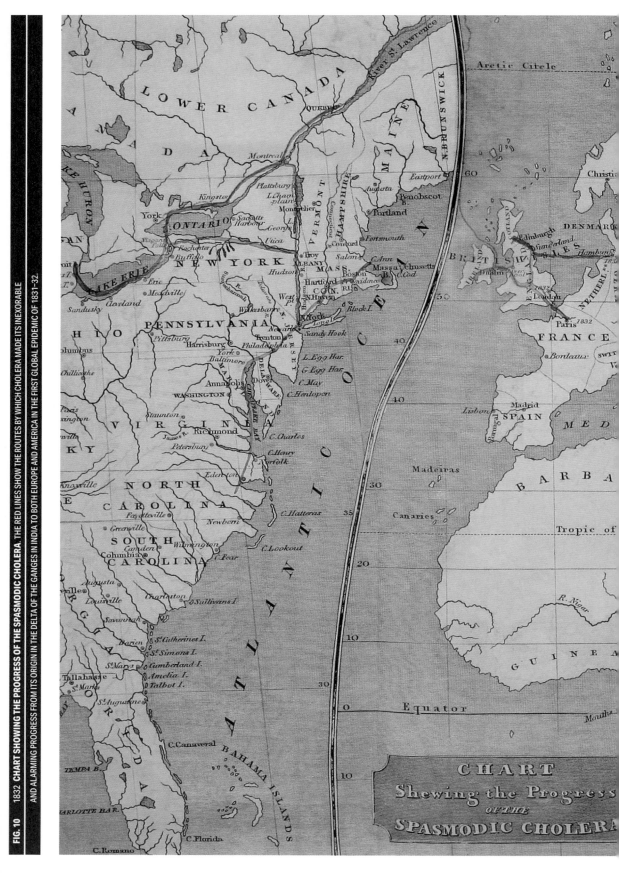

CHART
Shewing the Progress
OF THE
SPASMODIC CHOLERA

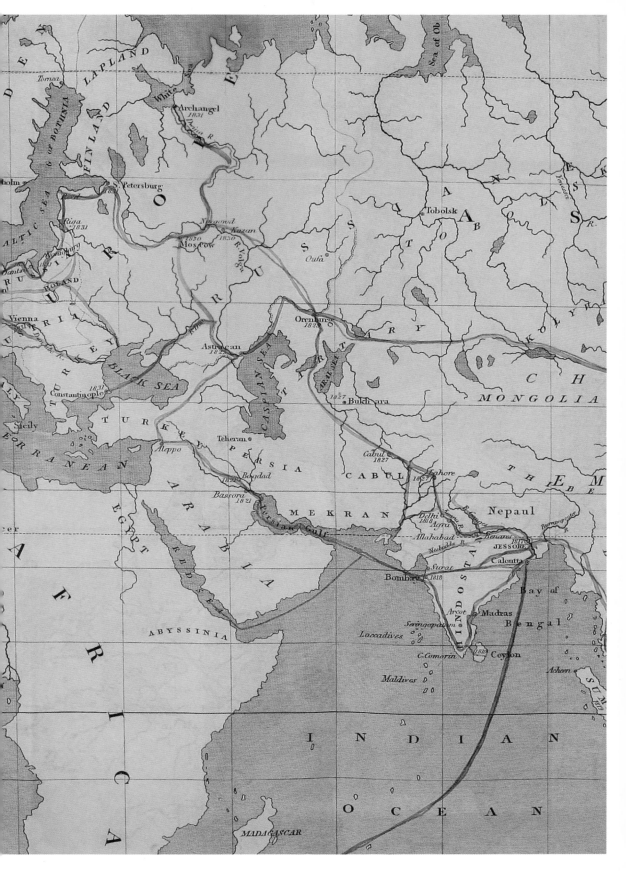

In the same year cholera arrived in America, where conditions similar to those in Europe meant that the disease spread quickly. By 1881 a pandemic reached South America, and in the 1890s outbreaks began in Japan, in cities such as Tokyo and Osaka. This was a global crisis of unparalleled proportion.

A particularly horrifying outbreak of cholera struck Hamburg with devastating force in 1892. In all, 8,605 people were killed in a city whose population was one-seventh that of London, more than had died in all the previous epidemics to strike the city. English newspapers carried stories of Hamburg's epidemic, with Londoners fearful that the cholera would soon be brought to their own city by ships from Hamburg. The weather was exceptionally dry and hot and the tide high, a combination of factors that encouraged the cholera bacillus to multiply quickly and the infected water to penetrate farther upstream along the Elbe than usual. Initially, the authorities in Hamburg (like those in London thirty years earlier) were reluctant to acknowledge that the cholera was carried in the drinking water, even though it was observed that occupants of the central prison and of the Attendorfer lunatic asylum were completely unaffected by the epidemic, their drinking water being drawn from sources separate from those of Hamburg's system. And in the adjoining town of Altona, whose drinking water was also drawn from the Elbe – but through

FIGS. 11–18 ENGRAVINGS SHOWING THE IMPACT OF CHOLERA ON CITIES IN EUROPE AND AMERICA. ACROSS THE WORLD THE HORRIFIC SCENES THAT FOLLOWED AN OUTBREAK OF CHOLERA – WHETHER IN THE STREETS OR IN HOSPITALS – WERE RECORDED.

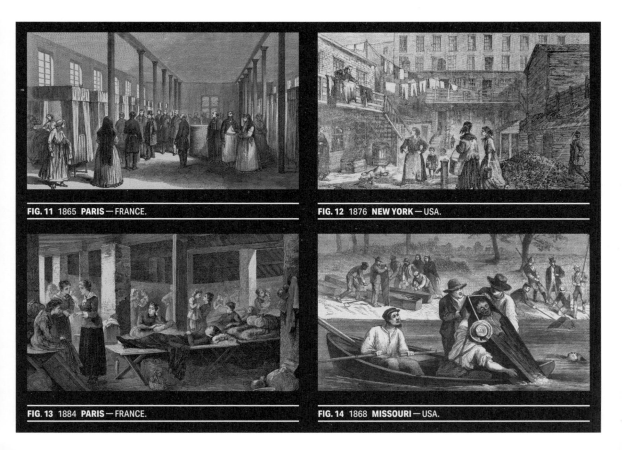

FIG. 11 1865 **PARIS** — FRANCE.

FIG. 12 1876 **NEW YORK** — USA.

FIG. 13 1884 **PARIS** — FRANCE.

FIG. 14 1868 **MISSOURI** — USA.

a sand filter bed – the fatalities were much lower. The cause of science and health received a setback at the hands of the eminent chemist Max Joseph von Pettenkofer (1818–1901) who despite a long and distinguished career as a campaigner for public health and hygiene, was so convinced that water containing the cholera bacillus was safe to drink that he publicly swallowed water that was known to contain it. A bout of severe diarrhoea was followed by his complete recovery. He had probably previously had a mild dose of cholera and had developed resistance to it. Ultimately, it would take a Nobel Prize winner to overturn his convictions.

We now know that cholera (its name based on the Greek word for 'bile') is carried in infected water. A victim of the infection passes it on in faeces, which, when it finds its way into drinking water, claims further victims. So *The Lancet* was close to the truth by referring to 'a morbid off-scouring of the intestinal canal'. But the journal, and other publications such as *The Times*, favoured the 'miasmatic' theory of disease – that disease was invariably conveyed in foul air – which generally prevailed at the time. Its origin can be traced back to the father of medicine, Hippocrates (*c*. 460–370 BC), who held that certain fevers were associated with damp, hot places where the air was foul.

PP. 18–19   1855 **LONDON WATER SAMPLES** — LONDON, UK. THESE SAMPLES FROM DIFFERENT SOURCES AND COMPANIES IN LONDON ENABLED THE COMMITTEE FOR SCIENTIFIC INQUIRIES IN RELATION TO THE EPIDEMIC OF 1854 TO ASSESS THE LEVELS OF IMPURITY IN THE CAPITAL'S DRINKING WATER; YET STILL THEY WERE NOT ENTIRELY CONVINCED THAT WATER, NOT AIR, WAS THE EPIDEMIC'S CAUSE!

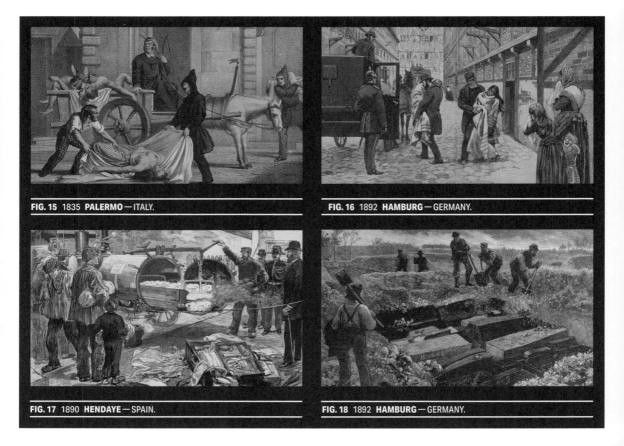

FIG. 15 1835 **PALERMO** — ITALY.

FIG. 16 1892 **HAMBURG** — GERMANY.

FIG. 17 1890 **HENDAYE** — SPAIN.

FIG. 18 1892 **HAMBURG** — GERMANY.

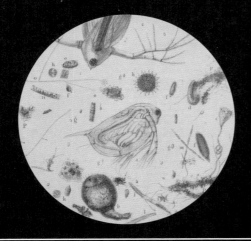

FIG. 19 FROM CISTERN OF **CHELSEA WATER COMPANY**.

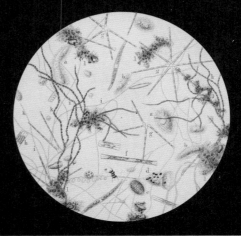

FIG. 20 FROM CISTERN OF **EAST LONDON COMPANY**.

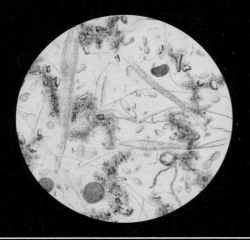

FIG. 21 FROM WELL AT **MILL CORNER, HADLEY**.

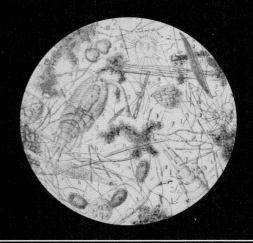

FIG. 22 FROM WELL IN **BAILEY'S YARD, CLERKENWELL**.

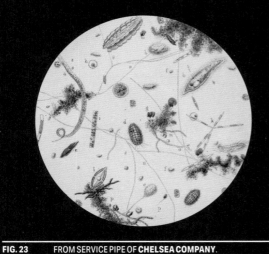

FIG. 23 FROM SERVICE PIPE OF **CHELSEA COMPANY**.

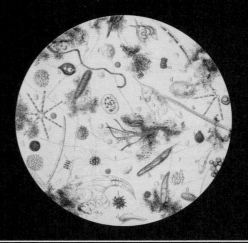

FIG. 24 FROM SERVICE PIPE OF **HAMPSTEAD COMPANY**.

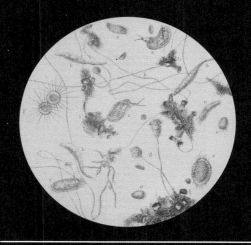

FIG. 25   FROM CISTERN OF **KENT COMPANY**.

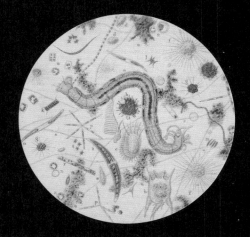

FIG. 26   FROM CISTERN OF **SOUTHWARK + VAUXHALL COMPANY**.

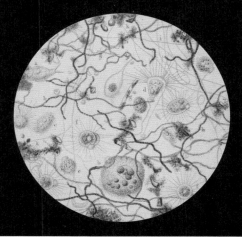

FIG. 27   FROM WELL IN **SANDGATE**.

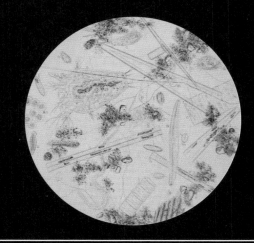

FIG. 28   FROM WELL AT **READING ROOM, ROMSEY**.

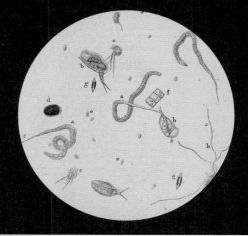

FIG. 29   FROM SERVICE PIPE OF **KENT COMPANY**.

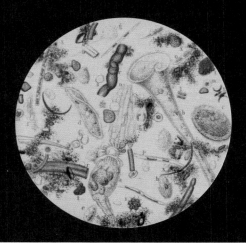

FIG. 30   FROM SERVICE PIPE OF **SOUTHWARK + VAUXHALL COMPANY**.

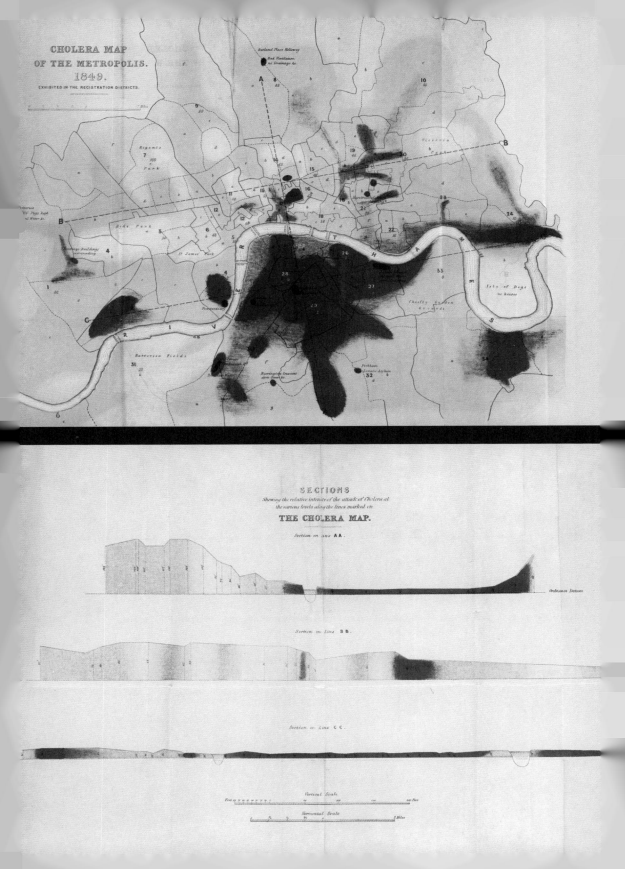

CHOLERA MAP
OF THE METROPOLIS.
1849.
EXHIBITED IN THE REGISTRATION DISTRICTS.

SECTIONS

Shewing the relative intensity of the attack of Cholera at
the various levels along the lines marked on

THE CHOLERA MAP.

Section on line AA.

Section on Line BB.

Section on Line CC.

Vertical Scale

Horizontal Scale

Among the most fervent advocates of the theory was Florence Nightingale (1820–1910), who in her classic *Notes on Nursing* (1859) inveighed against the practice of laying drains beneath houses as odours escaping from them might carry scarlet fever, measles and smallpox into homes. An even more prominent advocate of the miasmatic theory was the public-health campaigner Sir Edwin Chadwick (1800–90) who argued that 'all smell is disease'. Late in life, he called for the erection of an edifice such as the Eiffel Tower in London – this, by some unspecified means, would draw down clean air from the upper atmosphere and distribute it in the streets, thereby expelling foul air and, with it, harmful germs.

These ideas may now seem foolish, but at the time they seemed reasonable. Cholera flourishes in hot weather, and the dry summertime heat also exacerbated the foul smell emanating from the human sewage that had filled rivers such as the Thames, Seine and Elbe by 1840. This process was worsened by the rapid increase in urban populations. London's populace doubled from less than 1 million in 1801 to almost 2 million in 1841, while in the same period that of Paris grew from just over 500,000 to almost 1 million. Between 1850 and 1890, the population of Hamburg expanded from about 180,000 to more than 500,000, and Berlin grew from 450,000 to closer to 2 million. Because of the stench, people would avoid walking near rivers when the temperatures rose, so when citizens began to die in their thousands of a disease which, though carried in water, was invisible in water to the naked eye, it was reasonable to assume that the smell was killing them. Misconceptions can have their uses, however: it was this false belief that enabled Sir Joseph Bazalgette (1819–91), during the hot, parched summer of 1858 in London with its accompanying 'Great Stink', to gain the authority to build the sewers that still serve the city today.

A neglected hero of medical science, Dr John Snow (1813–58) was the person responsible for overturning the 'miasmatic' orthodoxy. Born in York into a labourer's family, he was apprenticed to a surgeon at the age of fourteen and became a member of the Royal College of Surgeons in 1838. Snow had a practice in Broad Street, Soho (now Broadwick Street, off Carnaby Street) and during the 1848–49 epidemic, which killed 14,137 Londoners, he observed that citizens drawing water from a well near his practice succumbed to cholera whereas workers who drank beer at a nearby brewery did not. The well was close to a sewer; brewing destroys many germs. Since citizens and brewery workers were all breathing the same air, it seemed likely to Snow that the cholera lay in the water rather than the air. His 1849 publication *On the Mode of Communication of Cholera* is now regarded as one of history's greatest contributions to medical science, but was dismissed at the time as contrary to the orthodox 'miasmatic' explanation of disease transmission. During the 1853–54 epidemic, which carried off 10,738 citizens, Snow drew a map of the cholera deaths near his surgery, dramatically illustrating the peak in fatalities around the pump and the low incidence near the brewery (see page 22). He served on the Committee for Scientific Enquiry into the 1854 epidemic, a group whose dominant figure was the Chief Statistician William Farr (1807–83); the committee's report turned undignified somersaults to refute the evidence placed by Snow before their eyes. It concluded that if the Broad Street pump was the cause of deaths, then it was because its water had been infected by noxious odours, and that the

FIGS. 31–32 1849 **CHOLERA MAP OF THE METROPOLIS** — LONDON, UK.
CHOLERA MAPS SUCH AS THESE ENABLED THE AUTHORITIES
TO IDENTIFY THE AREAS MOST AFFECTED BY THE CHOLERA
EPIDEMIC THAT RAVAGED LONDON BETWEEN 1848 AND 1849.

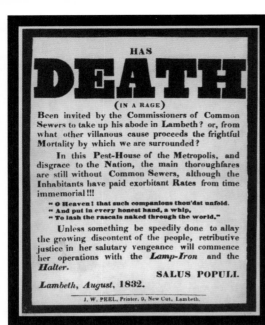

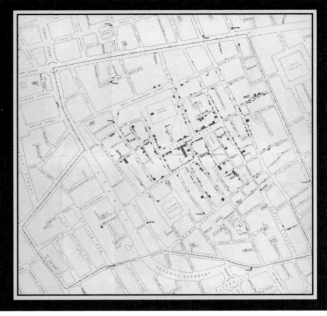

FIG. 33 1832 **CHOLERA PROTEST POSTER** — LONDON, UK. RESIDENTS OF LAMBETH COMPLAINED THAT DESPITE EXORBITANT RATES THEIR STREETS STILL HAD NO PROPER SEWERS, WITH OFTEN FATAL CONSEQUENCES.

FIG. 34 1854 **MAP SHOWING DEATHS FROM CHOLERA IN BROAD STREET** — LONDON, UK. JOHN SNOW'S MAP SHOWS A CONCENTRATION OF DEATHS AROUND THE BROAD STREET PUMP, AND FAR FEWER BY THE BREWERY WHERE WORKERS DRANK BEER RATHER THAN WATER.

brewery workers were protected from the foul air because it didn't blow around corners! John Snow died in 1858, his theories still not accepted, and, as a teetotaller, is ironically commemorated by a pub bearing his name close to the site of his former surgery, with a reproduction of the pump nearby.

In the meantime, the world's most famous scientist had entered the debate. In 1855, Michael Faraday (1791–1857) travelled by steamboat from London Bridge to Hungerford Bridge and on 7 July, he wrote a letter to *The Times* about his journey:

> *The appearance and smell of the water forced themselves at once upon my attention. The whole of the river was an opaque, pale brown fluid...The smell was very bad and the whole river was a real sewer...The condition of the Thames may, perhaps, be considered as exceptional but it ought to be an impossible state instead of which, I fear, it is rapidly becoming the general condition. If we neglect this subject we cannot expect to do so with impunity, nor ought we to be surprised if, ere many years are over, a hot season gives us sad proof of the folly of our carelessness.*

A *Punch* cartoon followed the letter, depicting 'Faraday giving his card to Father Thames and we hope the dirty fellow will consult the learned professor.' And later the same year Charles Dickens (1812–70) wrote the first instalments of the novel that became *Little Dorrit*, in which he lamented the fact that the Thames, the great artery of Britain's commerce and prosperity, had become a 'deadly sewer'.

This event coincided with the Committee for Scientific Enquiry's conclusion that water was, in effect, innocent of transmitting disease. Another eleven years and a final epidemic passed before William Farr was converted. In 1866, there was a severe outbreak of cholera that killed 5,596 people in only 3 sq km (1 sq mile) of Whitechapel. Farr led the resulting enquiry and drew attention to the role of the water closet, which was growing in popularity from the late 18th century: 'The water-closet system had the advantage of carrying nightsoil out of the house but the incidental and not necessary disadvantage of discharging it into the rivers from which the water supply was drawn.' His investigation traced the origin of the Whitechapel epidemic to a labourer called Hedges, who lived in Bromley by Bow. Hedges and his wife had died of cholera and their water closet discharged into the River Lea, close to the East London Water Company's reservoir at Old Ford. Farr had calculated that a high proportion of cholera deaths occurred among customers of the East London Company and, despite denials and obstruction on the part of the firm, he discovered that it had failed to install effective filters between the river and its reservoirs. Farr's anger at being deceived is reflected in his report:

> *For air no scientific witnesses have been retained, no learned counsel has pleaded; so the atmosphere has been freely charged with the propagation and the illicit diffusion of plagues of all kinds; while Father Thames, deservedly reverenced through the ages, and the water gods of London, have been loudly acclaimed immaculate and innocent. In vain did the sewers of London pour their dark streams into the Thames and the Lea...Dr Snow's theory turned the current into the direction of water...the theory of the East wind, with cholera on its wings, assailing the East End of London is not at all borne out.*

So William Farr was converted, and Dr John Snow posthumously justified. As William Farr reached his belated conclusions about the role of infected water, Joseph Bazalgette was building the great civil engineering works that would finally banish cholera from London. Bazalgette neither knew nor much cared whether the problem lay in the water or the air. He just knew that his sewers were an important

---

FIG. 35 1832 **A DEAD CHOLERA VICTIM** — SUNDERLAND, UK. AN EARLY VICTIM OF CHOLERA (TURNED THE DISTINCTIVE BLUE COLOUR ASSOCIATED WITH THE DISEASE) IN SUNDERLAND WHERE THE DISEASE FIRST ENTERED BRITAIN IN 1831.

FIG. 36 1828 **MONSTER SOUP, COMMONLY CALLED THAMES WATER**. A CARTOONIST'S VIEW OF THE HORRORS OF THAMES WATER WHEN SEEN THROUGH A MICROSCOPE IN 1828, THREE YEARS BEFORE CHOLERA ARRIVED IN BRITAIN.

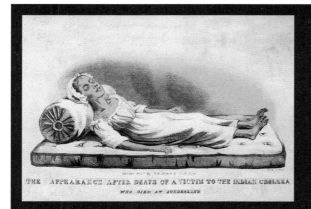

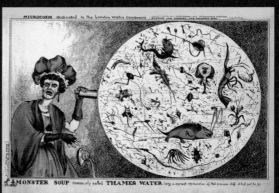

part of the answer. In 1883, the German physician and microbiologist Robert Koch (1843–1910) finally identified the cholera bacillus *Vibrio cholerae* in water in India. The way had been prepared in the 17th century by Antony van Leeuwenhoek (1632–1723), a Dutch cloth merchant and maker of lenses, who built a microscope with a magnification of 200 times, enabling him to observe in his spittle 'many very little living animalcules, very prettily a-moving. The biggest sort had a very strong and swift motion and shot through the spittle as a pike does through the water.' These were germs. In 1885, a zoologist published an article entitled 'The Fauna of the Hamburg Water Main' that identified sixty species of organisms, many of them harmful, with creatures as big as eels and fish being detected in the water mains. In the intervening centuries, the development of fields such as microscopy and other techniques for examining water enabled scientists to understand both the means by which it could transmit diseases such as dysentery, typhoid and cholera and the ways in which it could be purified.

By 1892 the idea of cholera as waterborne had become much more widely accepted by the public and media, as demonstrated by the *Illustrated London News* accompanying a sensational story about the 1892 Hamburg cholera outbreak headed 'Death in the Cup' with an engraving of a small girl drinking water from a vessel held to her lips, claiming that she had died hours later. It was also this knowledge that helped Robert Koch – finally appointed in a rare example of sound judgment by Kaiser Wilhelm II (1859–1941) on behalf of the Prussian government – in bringing the devastating Hamburg outbreak to and end. Koch was given dictatorial powers to bring the epidemic under control, and despite the mockery of the newspaper *Hamburger Fremdenblatt* which observed that 'Herr Koch is the intellectual father of the cholera bacillus' and the complaint of the burgomeister that at the time of the epidemic 'It was the Imperial Health Office and Professor Koch who ran things here', Koch took vital steps to end the epidemic. He first toured the infected areas, and found himself so aghast at the backward state of affairs that he declared 'Gentlemen, I forget that I am in Europe'. He swiftly took action and instructed the police to commandeer the wagons of a local brewery to tour the working-class areas of Hamburg with supplies of fresh, uncontaminated water. Boiling stations were set up on streets and notices issued telling people not to drink unboiled water or milk. Public baths were closed and the sale of raw fruit from barrows was forbidden for fear that it had been washed in infected water. Koch also ensured that filtration beds were installed for the water supplies. In 1905, Koch became one of the earliest winners of the Nobel Prize for Medicine.

As late as 1894, the definitive *History of Epidemics in Britain*, edited by the eminent but controversial physician Charles Creighton (1847–1927), still expressed scepticism that cholera was carried in water. Then again, he also doubted the existence of germs or the effectiveness of vaccination. But cholera had done its work. It had obliged governments, and city authorities, to take seriously their duty to protect citizens from death by epidemic disease. Whether it was the water or the air, cities had to be cleaned up and the only way to do that at the time was by ambitious, expensive and often heroic engineering projects. Many misunderstandings, errors and arguments occurred along the way, but in the pages that follow we will see how systems that were inherited from the ancient world and survived the Middle Ages were adapted to create facilities that keep us safe in the 21st century.

FIG. 37   1912 **DECIMATION AT THE HANDS OF CHOLERA.** AS LATE AS 1912, CHOLERA, BEARING A SCYTHE ASSOCIATED WITH THE ANGEL OF DEATH, IS DEPICTED DECIMATING TROOPS FROM THE FRENCH COLONY OF SENEGAL.

Le Petit Journal

ADMINISTRATION
61, RUE LAFAYETTE, 61

Les manuscrits ne sont pas rendus

*On s'abonne sans frais
dans tous les bureaux de poste*

5 CENT.   SUPPLÉMENT ILLUSTRÉ   **5** CENT.

23me Année ** Numéro 1.150

DIMANCHE 1er DÉCEMBRE 1912

ABONNEMENTS

	SIX MOIS	UN AN
SEINE et SEINE-ET-OISE..	2 fr.	3 fr. 50
DÉPARTEMENTS...........	2 fr.	4 fr. »
ÉTRANGER..............	2 50	5 fr. »

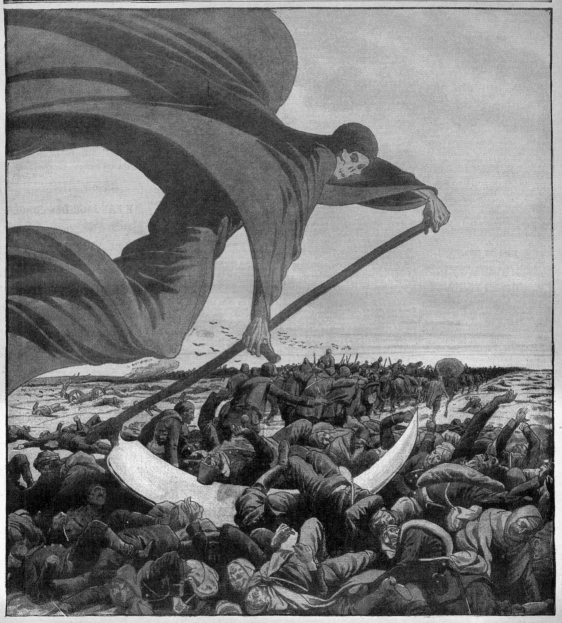

LE CHOLÉRA

PIONEERS OF PLUMBING

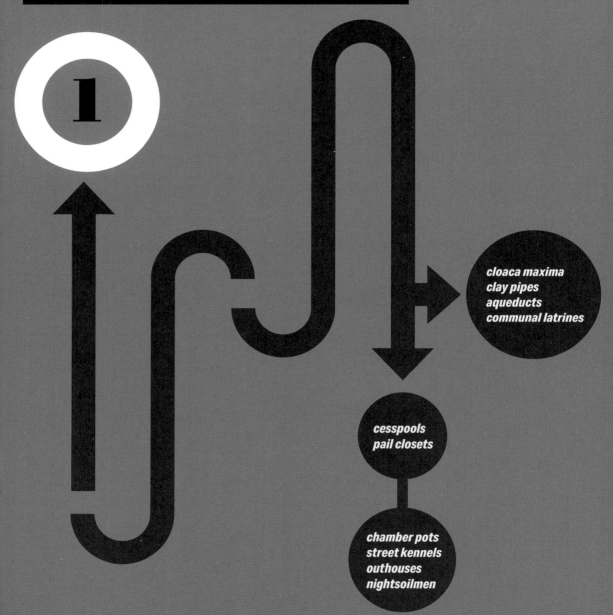

1

cloaca maxima
clay pipes
aqueducts
communal latrines

cesspools
pail closets

chamber pots
street kennels
outhouses
nightsoilmen

[I. SANITATION IN THE ANCIENT WORLD]

[II. SEWAGE IN THE STREETS]

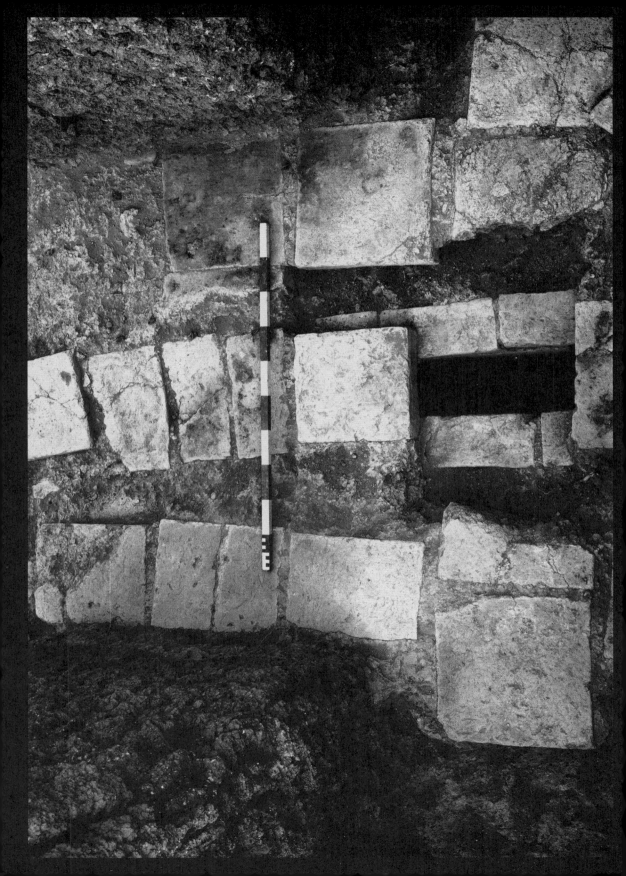

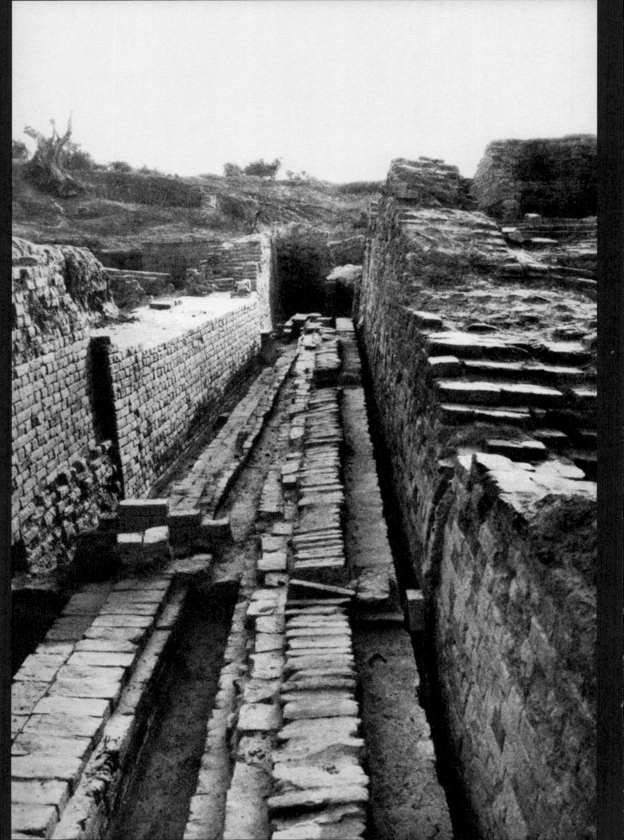

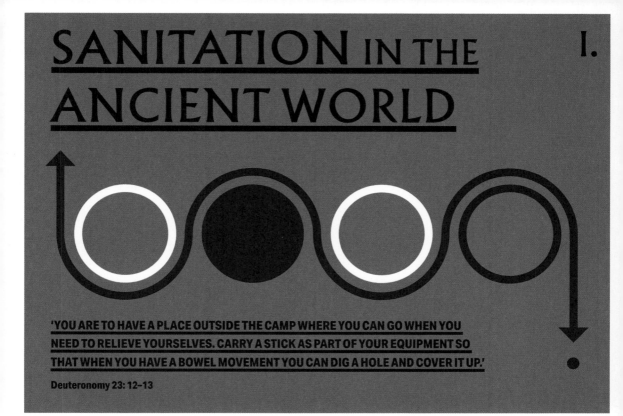

SANITATION IN THE ANCIENT WORLD

'YOU ARE TO HAVE A PLACE OUTSIDE THE CAMP WHERE YOU CAN GO WHEN YOU NEED TO RELIEVE YOURSELVES. CARRY A STICK AS PART OF YOUR EQUIPMENT SO THAT WHEN YOU HAVE A BOWEL MOVEMENT YOU CAN DIG A HOLE AND COVER IT UP.'

Deuteronomy 23: 12–13

M oses' injunction to the children of Israel, as they approached the Promised Land, to 'dig a hole and cover it up' when they found they had a 'bowel movement' was appropriate for a nomadic people crossing the arid plains of Moab on the eastern shore of the Dead Sea. Perhaps they were the first words ever spoken concerning personal hygiene and sewage disposal. Yet by the time they were recorded, in Jerusalem in the 7th century BC, the towns and cities of the eastern Mediterranean and Middle East were already equipping themselves with the beginnings of modern sanitation systems more sophisticated than that advocated by Moses. It is in these early urban communities that we see the origins of the systems of water supply and waste disposal upon which our civilization depends. And from the time of Moses himself, the 1st millennium BC, there are references in texts to a toilet demon, Šulak, who supposedly lurked in the vicinity of the dark holes in the ground with their sinister contents, threatening to bring bad luck upon the house. An essential feature of healthy living, sewers still inspire a certain unease, especially when anything threatens to go wrong with them.

First, they depend upon an efficient water supply. Once water is provided to a community, whether from a river, lake or reservoir, some means must be found to dispose of it after it has been used for washing,

---

P. 27   722–705 BC **DRAIN** — KHORSABAD, IRAQ. THIS DRAIN RAN BENEATH THE THRESHOLD OF A LARGE RESIDENCE OUTSIDE THE CITADEL. THE SITE OF KHORSABAD WAS EXCAVATED BY AMERICAN ARCHAEOLOGISTS BETWEEN 1928 AND 1935.

FIG. 1 ←   *c.* 2000 BC **STREET DRAINS** — MOHENJO-DARO, PAKISTAN. EXCAVATIONS OF MOHENJO–DARO IN THE 1930s REVEALED COVERED DRAINS LINING THE MAIN STREETS. THESE WERE USED TO CARRY WASTEWATER AWAY FROM RESIDENCES.

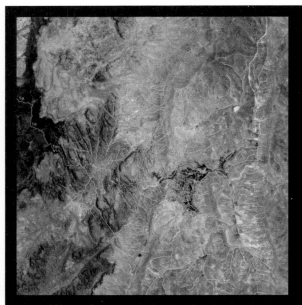

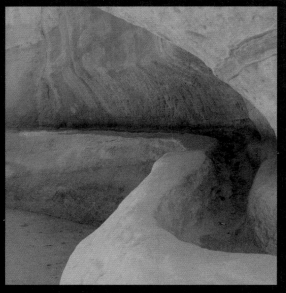

FIG. 2   **SATELLITE IMAGE OF WATERWAYS** — PETRA, JORDAN.
THE NABATAEANS, WHO INHABITED PETRA IN THE 4TH CENTURY BC,
CONTROLLED THEIR WATER SUPPLY THROUGH A SOPHISTICATED
SYSTEM OF DAMS, CISTERNS AND CONDUITS.

FIG. 3   **WATER CONDUIT** — PETRA, JORDAN. COVERED WATER
CHANNELS BROUGHT WATER INTO THE CITY FROM THE SPRING
IN WADI MUSA. THESE CONDUITS RAN ALONG THE SIQ, THE
MAIN PASSAGE THROUGH THE MOUNTAIN INTO THE CITY.

cooking, drinking, hygiene or other purposes. The oldest urban communities are to be found in the
Middle East in the area formerly known as Mesopotamia (covering parts of modern Iraq, Turkey, Iran,
Syria and Jordan), where towns and cities were built to take advantage of the waters of the rivers Tigris,
Euphrates and Jordan. The area was also the site of the first wells, some of which were dug as early as
6,500 BC in the vicinity of Nazareth, north of Israel. By about 3,800 BC, there is evidence of the use of
lavatories in domestic dwellings in cities such as Ur and Uruk in Babylon (modern Iraq). These consisted
of deep cylindrical pits lined with rings of baked clay 40–70 cm (16–28 in.) in diameter, with holes in the
sides through which liquid could escape into the surrounding earth. These were in effect early cesspits.
Sometimes, the cylinders were connected by sloping pipes, moulded from clay, to sewers in the street,
above or below ground; those underground were accessed via manholes with stone covers. The sewage,
along with rainwater, was carried away to rivers, though some sewers incorporated traps that allowed
the liquid to pass while holding the solids, which could then be dug out and used as fertilizer. Later
refinements included the addition of raised steps on which the users could plant their feet (like WCs
still occasionally encountered in parts of rural France) and a closet in a palace in Tell Asmar (Iraq) had
seats. But not all citizens were so sophisticated. In Babylon itself, whose ancient site is about 80 km
(50 miles) south of Baghdad, many citizens simply threw their sewage into the streets, along with their
garbage, where it became mixed with mud and was eventually covered by clay. This raised street levels
and steps had to be built down to reach some of the houses.

In the Nabataean city of Petra (now in Jordan and a World Heritage site), a network of aqueducts,
pipes and conduits harvested water and conducted it to cisterns, using a filtration system of stones,
sand and charcoal to cleanse it of impurities. And in Egypt, in the 1st and 2nd millennia BC, clay and

later copper pipes were used to bring cold and hot water into the homes (and occasionally tombs, owing to the custom of providing the dead with all they would need in the afterlife) of aristocrats. Some incorporated limestone toilets equipped with drainage channels while others made do with clay pots containing sand that could be carried away and emptied, often in the streets, to be washed away by rain – early ancestors of the earth closets still found in some rural areas. According to the Greek historian Herodotus (c. 484–c. 425 BC), most Egyptians in the city of Herakopolis threw their waste into the streets, though in Book II of his *Histories* he acknowledged that 'in the elite and religious quarters there was a deliberate effort made to remove all wastes, organic and inorganic, to locations outside the living and communal areas, which usually means the rivers'.

In the ancient settlement of Lothal in Gujarat, north-west India, which was inhabited from the 4th century BC, groups of homes and sometimes individual properties drew water from wells and shared a system of channels that conducted wastewater from bathrooms to covered drains in the streets. Elsewhere in the Indus valley, where the river that gives India its name flows though the Punjab, there were early schemes of urban sanitation in the period about 2,000 BC. At about the same time, a sophisticated water-management system was constructed in the city of Mohenjo-Daro, close to the river Indus in the Sind province of Pakistan. When the Indus changed its course owing to an earthquake, the city was abandoned, covered in sand by the passage of time and thereby preserved until it was rediscovered in the 1930s. Both private and public buildings were equipped with toilets and water was used for washing and bathing. Waste from buildings passed to a sump which, when about three-quarters full, emptied the liquid on the surface into drainage channels in the streets; these conducted the liquid to the Indus. The channels were covered with paving stones, which could be removed so that the channels could be cleared of debris, including accumulated sewage, and the contents taken to fields beyond the city walls. There was also evidence of tapered terracotta pipes, which fitted into each other, so that lengths of piping could be tailored to the needs of buildings and streets. More remote rural settlements had pierced cylinders like those in Mesopotamia.

FIGS. 4–5   *c.* 300 BC **A DRAIN AND WELL** — LOTHAL, INDIA. DRAINS, MANHOLES AND CESSPOOLS KEPT THE CITY CLEAN AND DEPOSITED THE WASTE IN THE SABARMATI RIVER, WHICH WAS WASHED OUT DURING HIGH TIDE.

FIG. 6   *c.* 2000 BC **STREET DRAINS** — MOHENJO-DARO, PAKISTAN. EXCAVATIONS HAVE SHOWN THAT NEARLY EVERY HOUSE IN THIS ANCIENT CITY CONTAINED BOTH A BATHING AREA AND DRAINAGE SYSTEM.

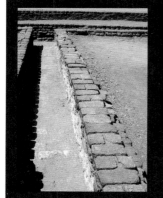
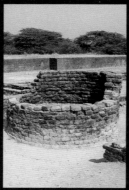
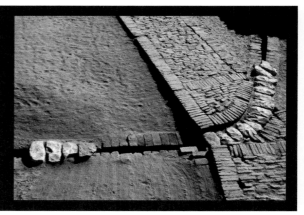

Farther east again, in the ancient Chinese city of Pingliangtai, which arose in about 2,000 BC, there are earthenware sewage pipes beneath the streets, though these may date from the 5th to 8th centuries BC. By the 2nd century BC, the palace of a monarch of the Western Han dynasty – whose name has unfortunately been lost to history – had a latrine with running water, a seat and an armrest. The ancient city of Chang'an had been settled in Neolithic times and was strategically located on the Silk Road, serving as a capital for successive dynasties. Now known as Xi'an, in Shanxi province, it had a population of about 500,000, an unimaginable number for a European city of the time. By 200 AD, it was equipped with a sophisticated system of earthenware pipes to supply water and sewers, some of them built of brick, to remove waste. One of them, excavated in 2008, is 2 m (6 ft 6 in.) wide. These are possibly the earliest sewers built from brick, the material favoured many centuries later by the engineers designing sewers for the great cities of the Industrial Revolution.

Evidence has been found in Minoan Crete of underground pipes, made of clay, bringing water into buildings, including public lavatories and some private homes and dating from the 2nd and 3rd millennia BC. The royal palace at Knossos had a latrine on the ground floor above which, on the roof, was a reservoir to collect rainwater, fulfilling the function of a water tank in the loft of a modern dwelling. The latrine had a wooden seat and an earthenware pan and was probably flushed by the rooftop reservoir. The archaeologist Sir Arthur Evans (1851–1941) suggested that during prolonged spells of dry weather the latrines In the Palace of Minos at Knossos were flushed by water poured into them by servants. Some of these drains are still in use after 4,000 years and some are large enough to stand in. Such is the complexity of the drainage network that it may have given rise to the legend of the Minotaur's labyrinth. Further evidence of a flushing toilet was found on the island of Santorini, north of Crete, which was buried in a volcanic eruption in about 1,627 BC and is consequently well preserved.

These early communities made use of sewage in a way that was to become commonplace in later centuries. Raw human (and animal) sewage contains harmful pathogens, but when composted for about six months it made excellent fertilizer at a time when chemical fertilizers were unknown.

FIG. 7 100–200 AD **CHINESE MODEL OF LATRINE AND PIGSTY.**
THIS TERRACOTTA MODEL ILLUSTRATES AN INNOVATIVE METHOD
OF REUSING SEWAGE. MODELS SUCH AS THESE WERE DESIGNED
TO BE BURIED WITH THEIR OWNERS.

FIGS. 8-10 **CERMAMIC PIPE DRAINS** — YONGCHUAN, CHINA.
THESE CERAMIC PIPES FEATURED AS PART OF THE STORM
AND SEWERAGE SYSTEM CREATED BY FIRST EMPEROR QIN
(259 –210 BC), THE FIRST EMPEROR OF A UNIFIED CHINA.

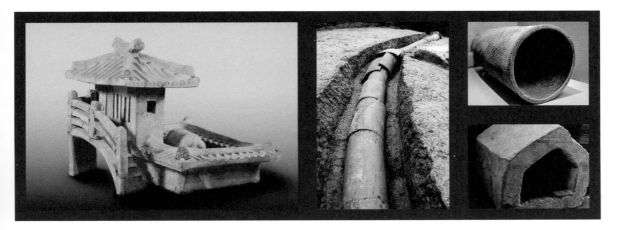

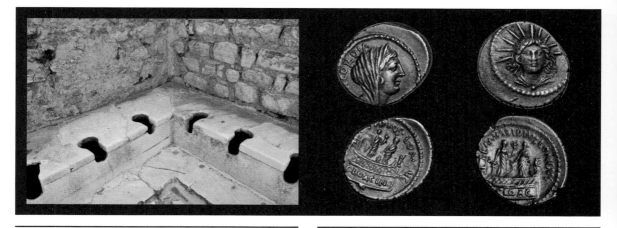

FIG. 11 1–100 AD **LATRINES IN THE SCHOLASTICA BATHS** — TURKEY.
THIS LUXURIOUS PUBLIC TOILET FACILITY WAS KEPT COOL IN THE
SUMMER BY A CENTRAL POOL OF CLEAN WATER.

FIG. 12 42 BC **COINS FEATURING THE ROMAN GODDESS CLOACINA.**
COINS MINTED BY ROMAN MONEYER LUCIUS MUSSIDIUS LONGUS
SHOW BOTH THE SEWER GODDESS AND HER SHRINE.

> ## 'THANKS TO HUMAN FERTILIZER, THE EARTH IN CHINA IS STILL AS YOUNG AS IN THE DAYS OF ABRAHAM. CHINESE WHEAT YIELDS A HUNDRED AND TWENTY FOLD.'
>
> *Les Misérables,* Victor Hugo (1862)

In Mesopotamia, the Indus Valley, China and Crete, sewage was being used for this purpose in prehistoric times. In Puglia, in southern Italy, the settlement of Murgia Timone has a network of cisterns for filtering and storing water dating from the 4th millennium BC. Between 2,500 and 3,000 BC, in the Stone Age village of Skara Brae in the Orkney Islands to the north of Scotland, pipes made of stone were lined with the bark of trees to bring water into homes and to conduct the waste out, along with small rooms that may have been used as indoor toilets.

According to its own mythology, the city of Rome was founded in 753 BC. In fact, its marshy and mosquito-ridden site alongside the river Tiber was settled between 1,000 and 900 BC by a variety of tribes. It was Rome's fifth king, Tarquin the Elder (reigned 616–578 BC) who – following some severe floods – employed Etruscan engineers to build the celebrated Cloaca Maxima ('Greatest Sewer'), partly to remove sewage but principally as a means of draining the city's swamps. Built of stone, the Cloaca later drew on streams from the hills of Rome to flush away surface water and debris from the Forum and elsewhere and bear it to the Tiber. It was thought to be governed by its own goddess, Cloacina. As Rome expanded and was eventually served by eleven aqueducts, the Cloaca was regularly flushed by the output of public baths and fountains including the Baths of Diocletian and Trajan. The Cloaca was originally an open channel, though according to the historian Titus Livy (64 or 59 BC–12 or 17 AD), writing many centuries later, an underground section was created during the reign of Tarquinius Superbus, Rome's seventh and last king, who reigned from 535 to 509 BC. o———————→ 36

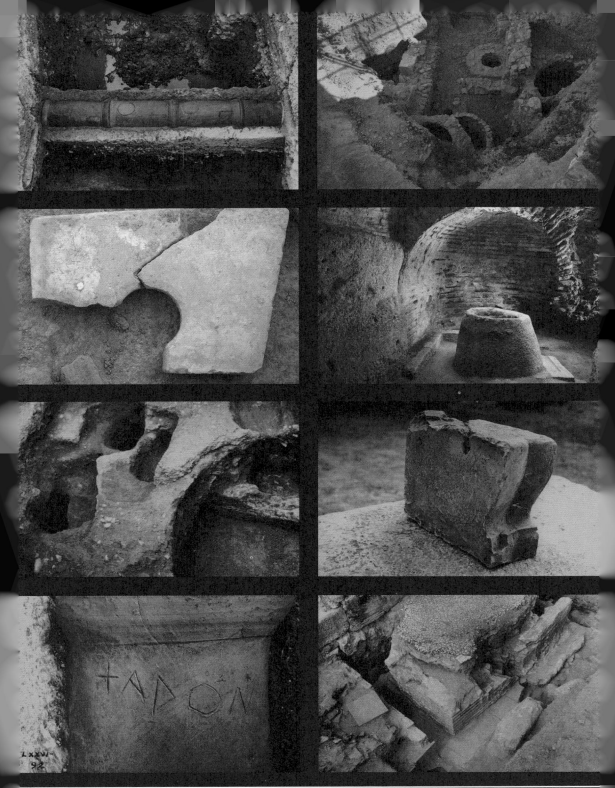

FIGS. 13-21 WELLS AND PIPES IN THE ATHENIAN AGORA — ATHENS, GREECE. LOCATED IN THE HEART OF ANCIENT ATHENS, THE AGORA WAS A SOCIAL AND POLITICAL HUB. 20TH-CENTURY EXCAVATIONS HAVE REVEALED OVER 400 WELLS, ALONG WITH PIPES FOR THE SUPPLYING FOUNTAINS WITH CLEAN WATER AND REMOVING WASTEWATER. **FIG. 19** SHOWS A PIPE INSCRIBED WITH 'ΧΑΠΟΝ', PERHAPS THE NAME OF THE SLAVE WHO LAID IT.

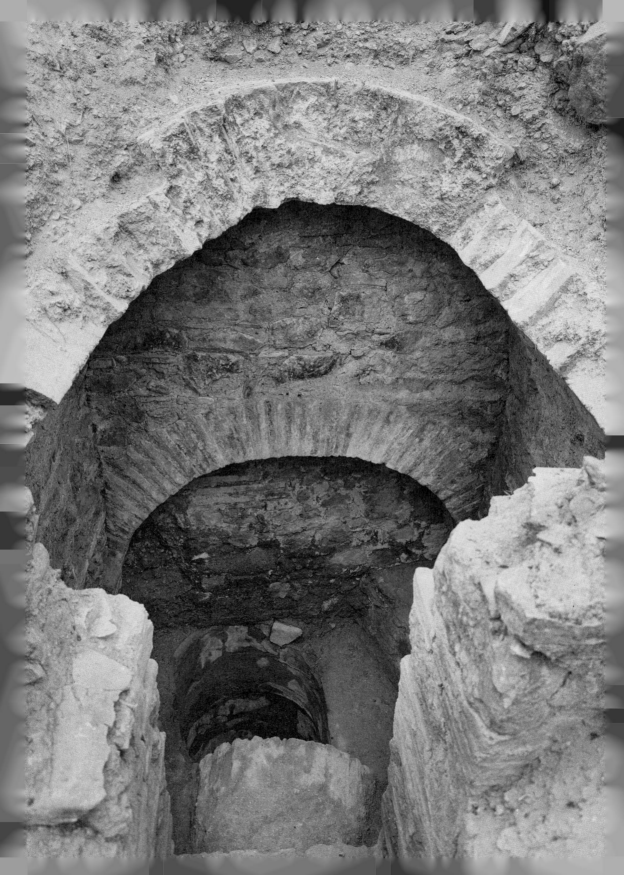

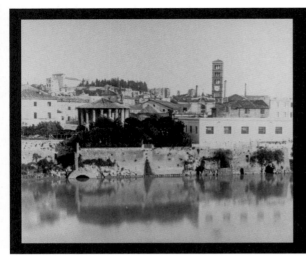
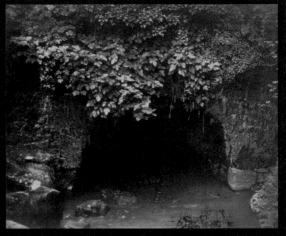

FIG. 22 6TH CENTURY BC **OUTLET OF THE CLOACA MAXIMA** — ROME, ITALY. TO THE LEFT OF THE PHOTOGRAPH THE CLOACA MAXIMA SEWER IS HALF SUBMERGED IN THE TIBER, WHERE IT DISCHARGED EFFLUENT.

FIG. 23 6TH CENTURY BC **OPENING OF THE CLOACA MAXIMA** — ROME, ITALY. IN THE 1860s THE CLOACA MAXIMA WAS A 'MUST SEE' OBJECT ON THE GRAND TOUR CIRCUIT THE WEALTHY TOOK THROUGH EUROPE.

At about the same time, Hippocrates was writing his treatise *Airs, Waters and Places*, which argued for the health benefits of clean, uncontaminated water, and Athens was using lead and bronze pipes to bring water to the city. Brick-lined conduits, including one between the Acropolis and the hill of the Pnyx, delivered rainwater and human waste to a basin beyond the city limits. One of the conduits, the 'Great Drain', was 2.4 m (7 ft 10 in.) deep. From there the excrement was diverted to the river Cephissus to irrigate and enrich the soil of orchards and fields beyond the city. In the 2nd century BC in the city of Pergamon (in what is now the province of Izmir in north-western Turkey), a water supply was brought from the Madradag mountains, a drop of 900 m (2,953 ft) along a pipe 42 km (26 miles) in length. The pipes, which operated under considerable pressure, were made of fired clay with a diameter of 16–20 cm (6–8 in.) and the wastewater was taken away through stone collectors sunk in the streets and covered by stone plates.

The historian Dionysius of Halicarnassus (60 BC–*c*. 7 AD) claimed that 'The extraordinary greatness of the Roman Empire manifests itself above all in three things: the aqueducts, the paved roads and the construction of the drains.' This claim was made at the time of the first emperor of Rome, Augustus, as the city was being rebuilt. The whole length of the Cloaca Maxima was gradually covered over during the time of the Roman republic and empire, by which time it was connected to other smaller sewers. These served public latrines and bathhouses, which were often found together as the water from the baths could flush the latrines. The 'Sewer of Judith' collected water from the baths of Agrippa and the Pantheon and drove a mill called the Mulino di Bella Judith until 1889. In places, the Cloaca Maxima is 3.2 m (10 ft 6 in.) wide and 4.2 m (13 ft 9 in.) high. In the 18th century, the artist Giovanni Piranesi (1720–78) created images of the mouth of the Cloaca Maxima, making it a 'must-see' feature of the Grand Tour for young English gentlemen completing their education. Some of the sewers were buried beneath the streets, while others remained open and were used for the disposal of garbage. Some reports suggest that the body of the emperor Heliogabalus (ruled 218–222 AD) was dumped into a public sewer after he was assassinated by the Praetorian Guard. The latter were supposed to

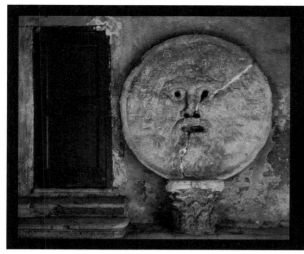

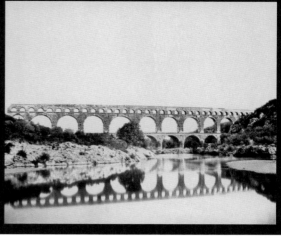

FIG. 24   *c.* 1ST CENTURY AD **THE MOUTH OF TRUTH** — ROME, ITALY. ONCE A HUGE DRAIN COVER, THE MOUTH OF TRUTH NOW ADORNS THE PORTICO OF SANTA MARIA IN COSMEDIN, ROME.

FIG. 25   *c.* 50 AD **PONT DU GARD** — GARDON RIVER, FRANCE. ARCHITECT AGRIPPA'S MAGNIFICENT PONT DU GARD AQUEDUCT BRIDGE WAS CONSTRUCTED TO CONVEY WATER TO THE CITY OF NÎMES.

form the personal protection of the emperor but were notoriously fickle and unsentimental about the means by which they disposed of those who offended them, so he may have met his fate in this way, though more sensitive commentators suggest that his corpse found its way straight into the Tiber and bypassed the sewers. It is more likely that the body of Saint Sebastian, martyred during the persecutions overseen by the emperor Diocletian in about 304 AD, was thrown into the sewer, an act depicted in a painting by Ludovico Carracci (1555–1619) in 1612. The body was supposedly rescued from that ignominious fate by a pious lady called Lucina and reburied in a church now called San Sebastiano Fuori le Mura ('Saint Sebastian outside the walls').

In classical times, the sewers were rarely connected to private residences, which depended upon cesspools until such connections were made in about 100 AD, using terracotta pipes. Cities including Pompeii and Herculaneum were similarly equipped. In Pompeii, there were cesspits within buildings and beneath pavements ranging in size from less than 1 m to 10 m (3 to 33 ft) in depth and the forum was equipped with a public latrine with wooden, bench-like seats supported by stones protruding from the wall. It also appears that the paved streets were used to convey rainwater, wastewater and sewage, including animal waste, from the city, with stepping stones being provided at intervals to enable people to cross them unsullied. During the time of Augustus (reigned 27 BC–14 AD), his son-in-law and minister Marcus Agrippa (62/64 BC–12 BC) was responsible for managing Rome's water supply. The Romans recognized that spring water brought at a distance from beyond city boundaries was suitable for drinking while rain and wastewater from public baths was more adequate for flushing sewers and cleaning streets, a method adopted by Georges-Eugène Haussmann (1809–91) in Paris in the 19th century. Agrippa is credited with supervising the construction of the magnificent Pont du Gard to convey water to the French city of Nîmes and is also recorded as having travelled along the Cloaca Maxima on a voyage of inspection. Its outlet may still be seen draining rainwater into the Tiber close to the Ponte Rotto, although the sewers that were once connected to it are now linked to a modern sewerage system. A circular stone called 'The Mouth of Truth', which can still be seen on display in the portico of Rome's Santa Maria in Cosmedin, was probably a drain cover to give access to the sewers beneath the Temple of Hercules.

By the 4th century AD, Rome had more than a hundred public latrines, many of them featuring several adjacent seats and requiring payment for use. An excellent example of one such facility (known as a 'forica') survives at Ostia, the port of Rome, about 16 km (10 miles) west of the city, where lead was used for the supply of water before it was used in Rome itself. Public latrines were not always connected to the Cloaca. Some were equipped with cesspits that were also used to dispose of garbage and, occasionally, human remains (including casualties from the games in the Colosseum). Urine was collected in amphorae, which were placed outside the premises of fullers, who used the liquid, together with fullers' earth, to remove oil from sheepskins and to fix dyes. It was also used for tanning leather. Other Roman communities also benefited from sewerage, notably the Slovenian city of, Celje, which in 45 AD, during the reign of the emperor Claudius, became the city of Claudia Celeia. Many of its Roman streets have survived, with a pronounced camber on the road surface channelling rainwater to the edges of the streets, where it entered the drains.

Constantinople, capital of the Eastern or Byzantine Roman Empire, also had sewers, which are used today to feed modern treatment works. Known as Istanbul since the early 20th century, the city retains its huge colonnaded cistern, dating from the time of the emperor Justinian in the 6th century AD, which covers almost 10,000 sq m (2.5 acres) and holds 833 litres (220 gallons) of water. It can be visited (and featured in the 1963 James Bond film *From Russia with Love*). By the 2nd century AD British cities, including London and York, were also equipped with public latrines. London had at least three. One was on London Bridge, from which the waste was deposited straight into the river; of the others, both equipped with cesspools, one was south of Fleet Street's present site and the other was at Queenhithe, to the south of the present site of St Paul's Cathedral. Roman cities also had sewers for the disposal of water, some of these being made of hollowed-out elm logs. Some, for rain and garbage, often ran along the middle of streets and were known as 'kennels'. There were also 'laystalls' which were specifically for dumping rubbish, especially cattle dung. Kennels, cesspools and and laystalls were cleared by 'raykers' who collected the contents and dumped it on the shore of the Thames, where it was either washed into the river or collected by dung-boats for sale to farmers.

So by the time of the Roman Empire, a model had been established for the handling of human waste. Some cities already had latrines, including public facilities, whose waste was either sent into rivers or collected and used as fertilizer on farms that surrounded the communities or for industrial processes such as tanning leather or fulling wool. This model was to serve the human population until well into the 18th and 19th centuries, when the growth of the population, especially that proportion living in towns, demanded more radical measures.

FIG. 26   *c.* 500 AD **THE MEDUSA FRIEZE IN THE BASILICA CISTERN** — ISTANBUL, TURKEY. TWO OF THE 336 MARBLE COLUMNS THAT SUPPORT THIS CAVERNOUS CISTERN FEATURE HUGE CARVED HEADS OF MEDUSA AT THEIR BASE.

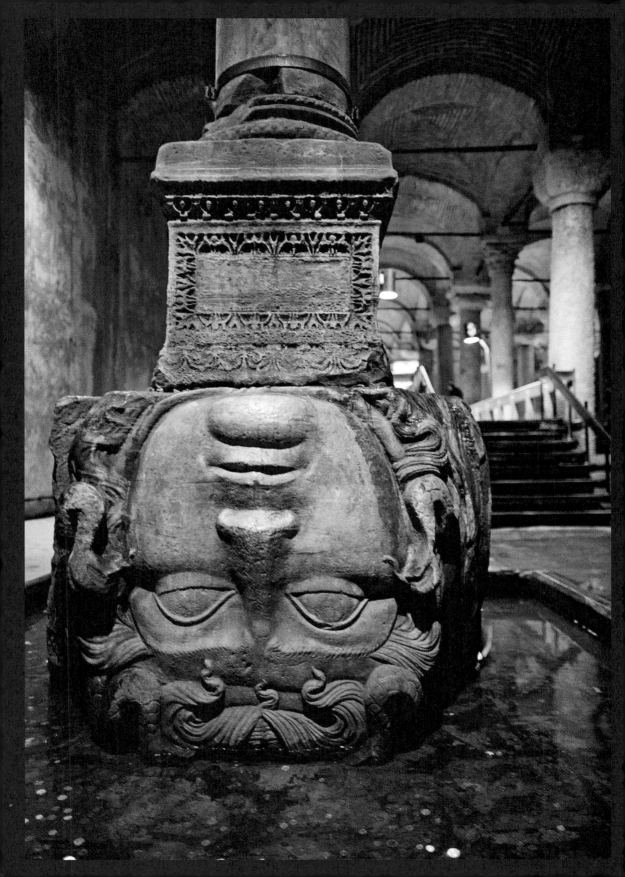

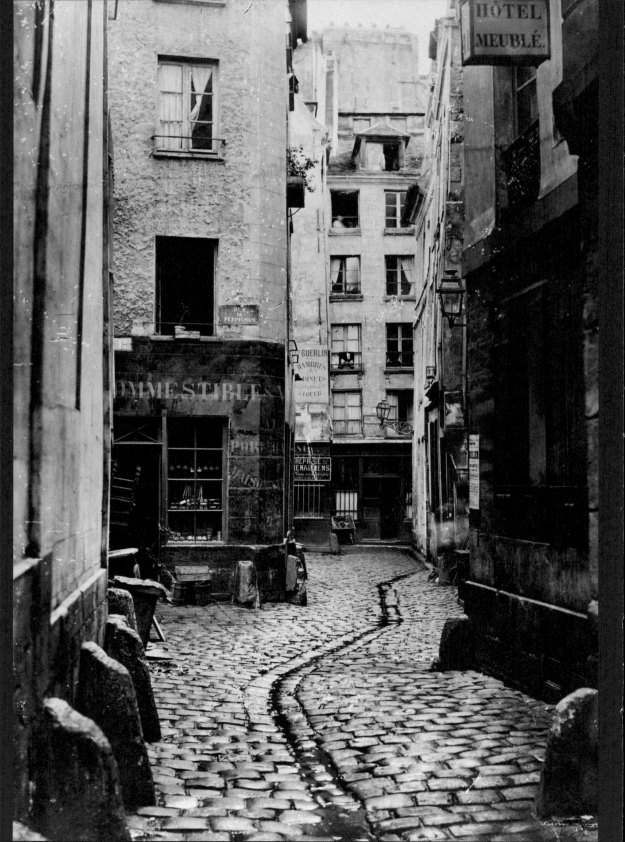

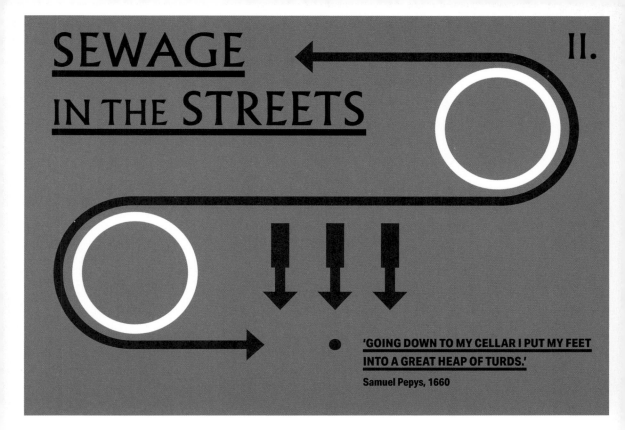

SEWAGE
IN THE STREETS

'GOING DOWN TO MY CELLAR I PUT MY FEET INTO A GREAT HEAP OF TURDS.'

Samuel Pepys, 1660

Many historians consider that the Dark Ages in history extend from the decline of the Roman Empire in the 5th century AD to the early medieval period in the 10th century. This was a turbulent period in European history characterized by invasions by Germanic tribes from the east and Viking raids from Scandinavia in the north. Written records from the time are much rarer than those of the classical period. But this is an embarrassingly eurocentric view. In the 8th century AD, in the Mayan city of Palenque in southern Mexico, a sophisticated system of aqueducts supplied the city with water, using limestone filters to purify it and channels to take away the waste. The civilization of Palenque is overlooked because it mysteriously disappeared from history in about 800 AD and was engulfed by the surrounding forests until it was rediscovered by Spanish invaders in the 16th century and excavated by American and Mexican archaeologists in the 20th century. Elsewhere in South America, the Spaniards inherited waste disposal systems similar to those of Chavín de Huántar in Peru where, in the 1st millennium BC, the residents had exploited the Andean terrain to draw water from the river Mosna as it entered from the mountain slopes and channelled waste to the river where it left the inhabited area. In the 1560s and 1570s, the Spaniards built a water supply and sewerage system for the capital, Lima, using clay pipes and created a corps of *aguadoros* (water carriers, many of them freed African slaves) to collect water from fountains for private

FIG. 1   19TH CENTURY **RUE DES TROIS CANETTES** — PARIS, FRANCE. A 'KENNEL' RUNS DOWN THE CENTRE OF THIS MEDIEVAL STREET. IT IS DESIGNED TO CARRY WASTE THROWN INTO THE STREET TO THE RIVER.

homes, water public squares and kill stray dogs for fear of rabies. In some provincial towns, *aguadoros* persisted until the middle of the 20th century. To this day it is estimated that 1.5 million of Lima's more than 10 million inhabitants are not connected to sewers and in Peru's city of Tumbes, with over 100,000 residents, the water intake is located close to a garbage dump.

At the time of Palenque's decline, the Arab world was flourishing and in the cities within the Islamic territory of Al-Andalus in southern Spain, such as Córdoba and Granada, most houses had latrines that drained to public sewers, while smaller communities used cesspools. The ancient sewers of Córdoba remained in use until the early 20th century. The Moslem city of Murcia had an elaborate system of subterranean sewers that took the waste to beyond the city walls. History records the story of a Christian escaping from Moslem captivity in Algeciras who fled through the sewers and eventually found himself on the seashore, the waste being discharged into the Mediterranean.

Elsewhere in Europe, the means by which human waste was collected and rendered harmless was much the same in 1800 as it was at the height of the Roman Empire. Indeed, in the late 19th century Italy itself, the heart of the former empire, was very poorly served, with half of Italian communes lacking piped water and three-quarters having no sewers. This lack of progress owed something to the decline of towns, many of which lost much of their population when the empire deteriorated. Bologna in Italy and Trier in Germany lost two-thirds of their population. In some Italian cities, an attempt was made to maintain a modest degree of hygiene. In 1346, Milan passed the 'Statutes of the Streets and Waters of the Country of Milan', which forbade householders to transport the contents of cesspits through the streets in the heat of summer. The job was reserved for *cistenari* (cistern men) using carts called *navazze* – despite which a small river passing through the city earned the name 'Nirone' (black) from its foul contents. In Florence, the job was done by *votapozzi*, who sold sludge to farmers as fertilizer and emptied liquid into the Arno. In at least one respect, sanitation actually took a step backwards.

FIG. 2 1830s **SOUTH AMERICAN MAN DRIVING A DONKEY CARRYING WATER CASKS.** THESE MEN WERE KNOWN AS *AGUADOROS* AND CARRIED WATER FROM THE RIVER INTO TOWNS.

FIGS. 3–4 17TH CENTURY **ITALIAN SCAVENGERS.** SCAVENGERS EARNED THEIR LIVING COLLECTING WASTE FROM TOWNS AND SELLING IT TO FARMERS.

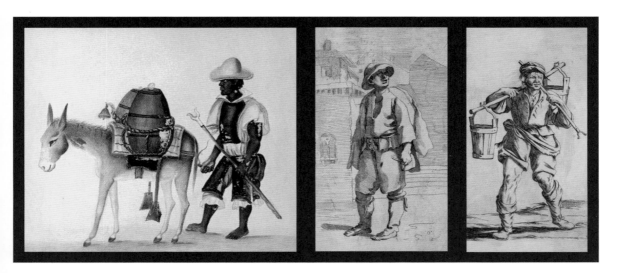

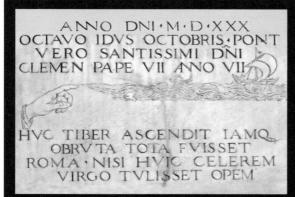

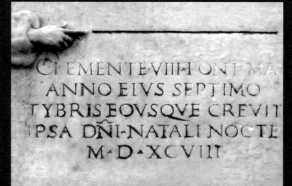

The Romans brought to northern Europe and England the art of brickmaking, examples being still visible in such structures as Hadrian's Wall and the city of Verulamium near St Albans. But when the Romans left in 410 AD, they took this skill with them. Since bricks were essential for the construction of large sewers, the reintroduction of brickmaking to northern Europe from the late Middle Ages was an essential prerequisite for the urban sewers that followed.

Conditions in Rome itself deteriorated during this period. In 537 AD, Vitiges – the king of the Ostrogoths – severed eleven aqueducts supplying the city with water in furtherance of a siege. The siege failed but the damage remained and it was not until 1587 that fresh supplies were brought to the diminished population of the city by new aqueducts. It was only in the 1870s that significant improvements were made to the sewerage system and between 1180 and 1870 it is estimated that catastrophic floods affected the city on average every thirty-one years as the Tiber overflowed, its polluted waters backing up into the underground sewers and water supplies and bringing cholera, typhoid and other waterborne diseases to the citizens. At last, in the 20th century, brick embankments put a stop to these disastrous floods.

Yet sophisticated systems for processing sewage did exist in this period. Monasteries were among the pioneers. At the great Benedictine monastery of Cluny in Burgundy, founded in 910 AD, a building was constructed with forty individual latrines, but the pioneers were the monasteries of the Cistercian Order. The order was founded in 1098 in Cîteaux, near Nuits-St-Georges a small town in Burgundy renowned for its wine. A monastery still flourishes at Cîteaux, but the order swiftly expanded throughout Europe. The Cistercians wished to lead a simple life, far from cities, and sought remote locations, close to rivers, where land was plentiful and often very fertile. These were communities of several hundred people led by an abbot and including monks, novices and lay brothers who did much of the manual work and lived as part of a self-contained community. Their English sites, despite having been ransacked by local people for building materials after they were plundered by Henry VIII, show signs of the sophisticated use of water for drinking, washing, waste disposal and industry. Channels were dug to deliver water from a river to basins or ponds where sediment would settle before the water was taken through pipes made of hollowed-out tree trunks, clay or lead, to be used for a variety of purposes. Some would go to

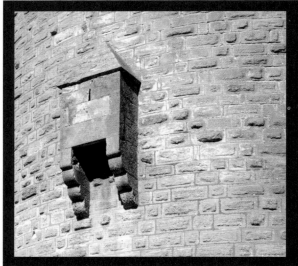
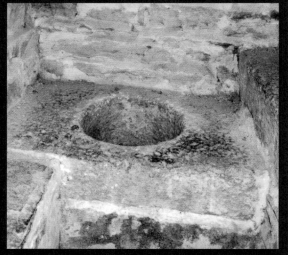

FIG. 7 **EXTERIOR OF LATRINE IN AIGUES-MORTES** — FRANCE.
THE TOILET PROTRUDES FROM THE WALL OF THE BATTLEMENTS
OF THE CITY. ANY WASTE FELL DIRECTLY TO THE GROUND BELOW.

FIG. 8 **INTERIOR OF LATRINE IN FOUGERES CASTLE** — FRANCE.
NO MORE THAN A CUPBOARD SPACE, THE MEDIEVAL LATRINE
WAS A SIMPLE SHAFT HOLE CUT INTO A MASONARY SEAT.

basins for drinking water or for brewing beer; some to ponds where fish were bred; some would provide power for water mills to grind corn; some would be used for cleaning wool (the Cistercians were big sheep farmers, especially in England) and the wastewater from these would pass beneath the communal latrine house, known as the *reredorter*, before returning to the river downstream from the monastery. A Cistercian monastery in Amsburg, Germany, shows evidence of all these uses and in England one of the finest examples is Fountains Abbey near Ripon in Yorkshire, where traces of many of these workings may still be glimpsed in the ruins. In medieval castles of the period, similar, if more primitive methods were employed. Visitors to Aigues-Mortes, a very well-preserved fortified town in the Camargue in southern France, cannot fail to notice holes in the battlements through which occupants were able to empty their bladders and bowels – this cannot have made the prospect of besieging the town any more enticing for attacking forces!

Within cities, different arrangements were required and systems as sophisticated as those of the Cistercians were rare. One such example was in the small walled city of Dubrovnik in Croatia, which acquired a system of sewers in the late 13th century while it was under the sovereignty of Venice; Venice itself depended upon tides to wash out to sea the waste that it tossed into its canals. Parts of the Dubrovnik system are still in use. Also in Croatia is the Palace of Diocletian in Split, built early in the 4th century AD, for which water was brought 7 km (4.3 miles) by aqueducts, and wastewater, faeces and rainwater was conveyed to the Adriatic by underground sewers 2.2 m (7 ft 2 in.) high by 1.15 m (3 ft 9 in.) wide. The palace remained occupied by residents and merchants of the city, who benefited from Diocletian's water supply and waste systems. Elsewhere, as in Roman cities, cesspools in the basements of some buildings were used as latrines while 'kennels' (open channels or 'canals') in streets received household and industrial waste. This would often be thrown from windows overhanging the streets, accompanied by a warning shout such as '*Tout à la Rue*' (Paris) or '*Gardy loo*' (Glasgow). This combination of waste products, mixed with mud on unpaved roads, produced a foul-smelling mixture;

rain would wash some of the waste into the kennels and rivers and some of it into buildings. Attempts to bring order to this situation were sporadic and generally ineffective. In 1539, King Francis I issued a decree requiring every new house in Paris to have its own cesspool, but this did nothing for the tenements that already existed without them. Notoriously contaminated wells on the Left Bank of the Seine served a community of bakers, the popularity and high esteem of their bread being evidently unaffected by this misfortune. A century later, in 1630, a survey of Paris's twenty-four covered sewers revealed that every one of them was broken or clogged with waste and the following century the mayor set a fine of 100 livres for anyone found dumping garbage in them, accompanied by corporal punishment for their servants! In the 17th century, the town council of Berlin was attempting to keep the sewers clear by organising the sweeping of solid wastes into heaps and specifying the times and places that chamber pots could be emptied into the river Spree.

Cesspools had to be regularly emptied by 'raykers' or 'gong-fermors', later known as 'nightsoilmen', who were well paid by occupants of buildings for removing the contents and made a further profit by selling it to farmers whose fields, in medieval times, were close to cities. Early attitudes to human waste acknowledged that it had to be removed from living quarters but also recognized that it could be a useful source of fertilizer. Some was buried, as enjoined by Moses in Deuteronomy, some was dumped in rivers by 'raykers', but much was diverted to fields as a source of nutrition for crops. In 1281, thirteen men took five nights to clear the cesspools of Newgate prison, each man being paid sixpence a night, which was three times the normal wage for a labourer. The trade continued for centuries. In the 1840s, the going rate for a load of animal waste delivered to a farmer by a nightsoilman was two shillings and sixpence, about a day's wage for a labourer, and as late as 1904 the Grand Junction Canal Company was conveying 45,669 tonnes of such manure from Paddington Basin to the farms of Hertfordshire. The systematic use of sewage farming was practised at Craigentinny Meadows in Edinburgh where, from 1750, the land was successfully worked in this way. As late as 1885, a gazetteer of Scotland boasted that the 2.6-sq km (652-acre) estate was valued at £5,739 per annum because the land had 'been under regular sewage irrigation for upwards of 85 years and yielded 50 to 70 tonnes of grass 49

FIG. 9   **1348 FRENCH ILLUMINATION OF BOCCACCIO'S**
DECAMERON. IN THIS SCENE A YOUNG MAN FALLS INTO
A SEWER FROM A LATRINE PERCHED BETWEEN TWO HOUSES.

FIG. 10   **1559 SECTION OF *DUTCH PROVERBS* BY PETER BRUEGHEL**
THE ELDER. A LATRINE OVER A RIVER ILLUSTRATES THE PROVERB
'IT HANGS LIKE A PRIVY OVER A DITCH', MEANING 'IT'S OBVIOUS'.

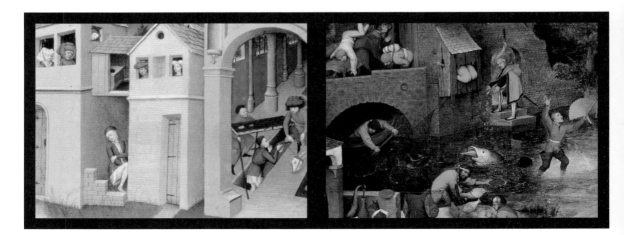

The description of Romney Marsh

The Sea

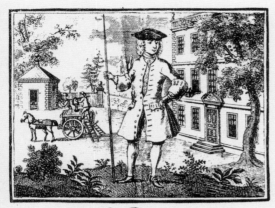

John Wigly
Nightman.

At the Black Bull opposite
Poland Street in Oxford Road,
L O N D O N.
Performs the above Business to the
Satisfaction of all Persons that employ
Him at Reasonable Rates.

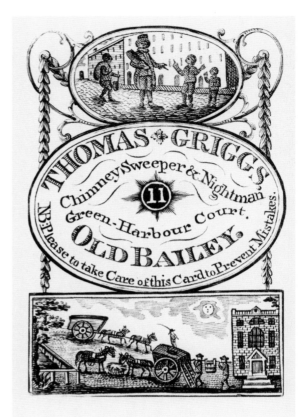

THOMAS GRIGGS
ChimneySweeper & Nightman,
11
Green-Harbour Court.
OLD BAILEY.
N.B. Please to take Care of this Card to Prevent Mistakes.

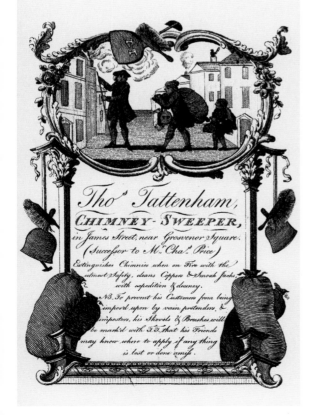

Tho. Tattenham,
CHIMNEY-SWEEPER,
in James Street, near Grosvenor Square,
(Successor to Mr. Chas. Price)
Extinguishes Chimnies when on Fire with the
utmost Safety, cleans Coppers & Smoak Jacks
with expedition & decency.
N.B. To prevent his Customers from being
imposed upon by vain pretenders &
impostors, his Shovels & Brushes will
be mark'd with T.T. that his Friends
may know where to apply if any thing
is lost or done amiss.

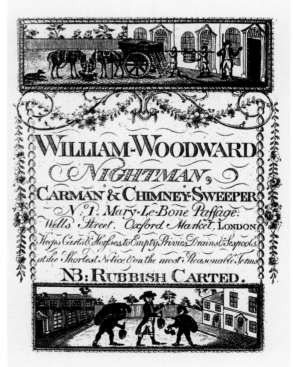

WILLIAM-WOODWARD
NIGHTMAN,
CARMAN & CHIMNEY-SWEEPER
No. 1. Mary-Le-Bone Passage.
Wells' Street, Oxford Market, London,
Keeps Carts & Horses to Empty Privies, Drains & Sesspools
at the Shortest Notice Upon the most Reasonable Terms
NB: RUBBISH CARTED.

per acre sold at prices as high as £44 an acre to "cow-keepers"'. The practice continued well into the 20th century in rural areas of the USA, central Europe, China, and Japan. Indeed today's sewage treatment works – examples of very sophisticated chemical and biological engineering – are still often referred to as 'sewage farms', a term that reflects their origins but no longer their technology. During Queen Elizabeth I's reign (1558–1603), other uses were found for the nightsoilmen's merchandise. At the time of the Armada in the late 16th century, saltpetre was extracted from the waste and used as an ingredient in gunpowder for the queen's ships. Thus did recycled excrement play its part in helping Sir Francis Drake to protect the realm.

Unemptied cesspools were a threat to life as well as health and comfort. In 1184, the Holy Roman Emperor Frederick I (reigned 1155–90), commonly known as 'Frederick Barbarossa' on account of his red beard, summoned his nobles to a diet (a kind of parliament) in the German city of Erfurt. According to a later account: 'The emperor…had occasion to go to the privy, whither he was followed by some of the nobles, when suddenly the floor that was under them began to sink; the emperor immediately took hold of the iron grates of a window, whereat he hung by the hands till some came and succoured him. Some gentlemen fell to the bottom, where they perished.' The nightsoilman's task was not without its perils either. It is recorded that in 1328, in London, one 'Richard the Rayker' fell through the rotten boards of his own privy and, in the words of a contemporary 'drowned monstrously in his own excrement'.

The perils associated with poorly constructed and maintained cesspools were well understood in medieval times. In 1189, the first mayor of London, Henry Fitzalwyn (c. 1135–1212), in an early form of building regulations, decreed that the 'necessary chamber [cesspool] should be at least two and a half feet from the adjacent building if it was made of stone and three and a half feet if made of other materials', such as wood. This was to prevent leakage from cesspits affecting neighbouring properties. It was not altogether successful. In 1290, some Carmelite friars of London petitioned Parliament to 'abate a nuisance [viz. a great stench] which prevents them from performing their religious duties' and by 1300, according to John Stowe's *Survey of London*, Sherbourne Lane's Sweetwater Bourne had become so foul that it had become known as 'Shiteburne Lane'. At about the time of Fitzalwyn's decree, the king of France, Philip II (reigned 1180–1223) was overseeing the creation of open sewers known in England as 'kennels' in the middle of paved streets in Paris and in 1348 King Philip VI formed Paris's first corps of sanitation workers to clean the streets. In 1370, the provost (mayor) of Paris, Hugues Aubriot (d. 1382 or 1391), began to cover over these kennels to create subterranean sewers. In Antwerp, the authorities encouraged the open sewers to be covered over by allowing citizens to extend their houses over them.

If cesspools were not regularly emptied, then problems arose – often for neighbours. In 1328, William Sprot, a Londoner, complained that his neighbours William and Adam Mere had allowed their cesspool to overflow into his property. In 1711, Jonathan Swift complained about the disgusting 'sweepings from butchers' stalls, dung, guts and blood, drowned puppies, stinking sprats all drenched in mud, dead cats and turnip tops' which that passed through the streets as sewers overflowed in heavy rain.

○——————→ 52

FIGS. 12–15 ADVERTISEMENT CARDS FOR NIGHTSOILMEN — LONDON, UK.
18TH- AND 19TH- CENTURY ADVERTISEMENTS FOR NIGHTSOILMEN, WHO OFTEN DOUBLED AS CHIMNEY SWEEPS.

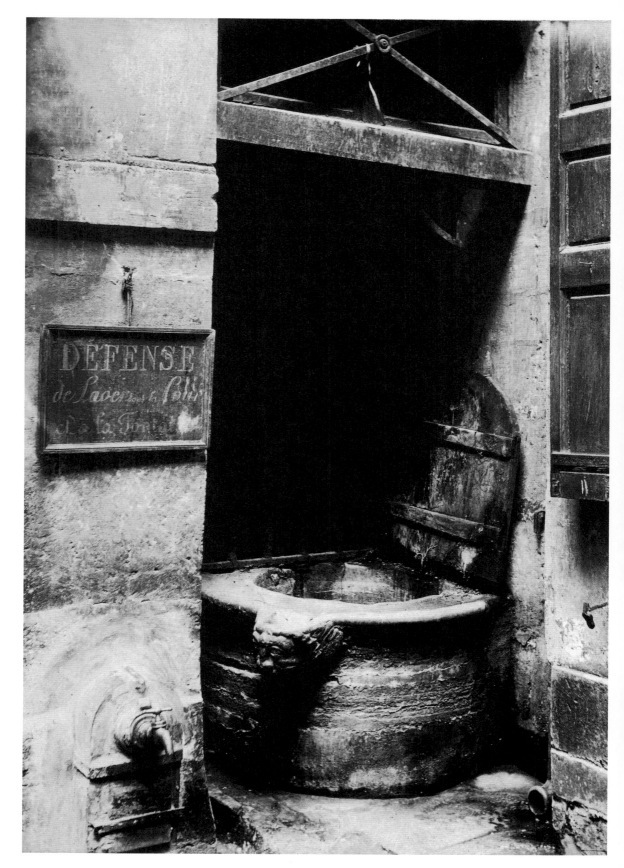

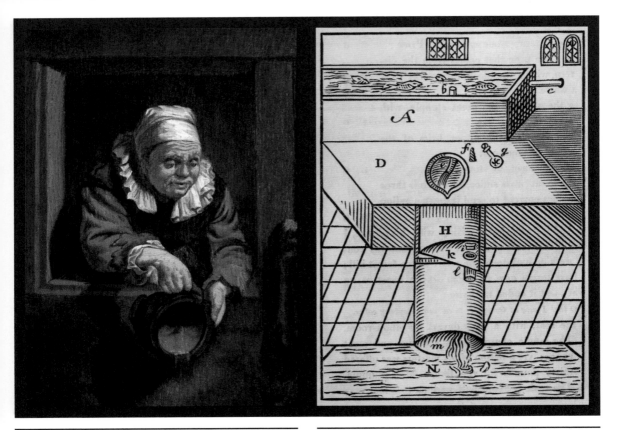

FIG. 18 *c.* 1670 **WOMAN EMPTYING A CHAMBER POT**. MIND YOUR HEADS! A WOMAN EMPTIES A CHAMBER POT INTO THE STREET IN LEYDEN, NETHERLANDS. THIS METHOD OF SEWAGE DISPOSAL WAS USED ACROSS EUROPE.

FIG. 19 1596 **SIR JOHN HARINGTON'S DESIGN FOR A FLUSHING WATER CLOSET**. TWO MODELS BASED ON THE AJAX DESIGN WERE BUILT. HOWEVER, TWO CENTURIES PASSED BEFORE THE USE OF WCS BECAME WIDESPREAD.

Apart from human faeces, horse droppings and urine there was also the problem of garbage, notably waste not only from homes but also from grocers, butchers, fishmongers and slaughter-houses. In 1307, the pollution of London's Fleet River was attributed to waste from butchers and tanners at Smithfield cattle market. The waste in the streets would often be consumed by pigs and chickens, who added their own excrement to that of those households, which, lacking cesspools, emptied chamber pots into the street. As in classical times, these were deposited in kennels or laystalls (dumps), from which they would be removed by raykers at intervals unless the contents were first washed into the river. By the reign of Edward III (reigned 1327–77), the city had grown to a point where the accumulation of rubbish had outrun the ability of the raykers and their employers to dispose of it, so in 1357 the king addressed the mayor and sheriffs of the City of London in the following terms:

> *Whereas now, when passing along the water of Thames, we have beheld dung and filth accumulated in diverse places in the said City upon the bank of the river aforesaid and also perceived the fumes and other abominable stenches arising there from we do command you that you cause as well the banks of the said river, as the streets and lanes of the same City, and the suburbs thereof, to be cleared of dung and other filth without delay and the same when cleaned to be so kept.*

There is still a Laystall Street in Clerkenwell.

Over the centuries that followed, many attempts were made to bring some order to the sewerage of towns. Commissioners were appointed, decrees issued and penalties exacted for failing to observe them, all with little effect. Experiments were carried out adding lime and other chemicals to sewage in order to suppress or mask the odour. The readier availability of drinking water added to the problems of wastewater disposal, an example being the construction by Sir Hugh Myddleton (1560–1631) of the New River, which brought fresh water from Ware in Hertfordshire to London in the early 17th century. It still supplies London with water, though the elm pipes that connected the supply to the homes of its first customers, such as the father of the poet John Milton, have been replaced by more modern materials. In the meantime, however, some technical advances were made that would oblige the authorities reluctantly to acknowledge the need for substantial public expenditure to make cities safe places to live.

In 1596, an otherwise unknown courtier at the court of Queen Elizabeth I, Sir John Harington (1560–1612), published a book entitled *The Metamorphosis of Ajax: A Cloacinean Satire*, which described an invention of his own design: a water closet with a flushing mechanism to wash away faeces and urine and mask the smell. He installed one at his own home, Kelston, near Bath in Somerset; and another at Richmond Palace, one of the homes of his godmother, the Queen. Perhaps his invention reflected the appalling conditions in which even the wealthy lived at the time. Ahead of visits from Queen Elizabeth I, Bess of Hardwick (1527–1608) had to ask her servants to clean her two great houses, Chatsworth and Hardwick Hall, seeking out excrement from corners, cupboards and other spaces where residents had relieved themselves. Neither of Harington's devices (or the houses they served) survives. For two centuries, his great gift to the world was forgotten. It was only in the 19th century that it was rediscovered – with disastrous consequences for public health.

FIG. 20   **THE WATERHOUSE BY ISLINGTON** — LONDON, UK.
FROM 1613 ONWARDS THE NEW RIVER BROUGHT WATER
FROM WARE IN HERTFORDSHIRE TO ISLINGTON IN LONDON.

FIG. 21   **THE NEW RIVER, ISLINGTON** — LONDON, UK.
THE NEW RIVER HEAD NEAR SADLER'S WELLS. IT STILL
SUPPLIES WATER TO THE LONDON RING MAIN.

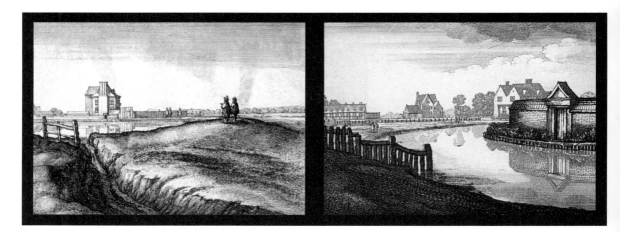

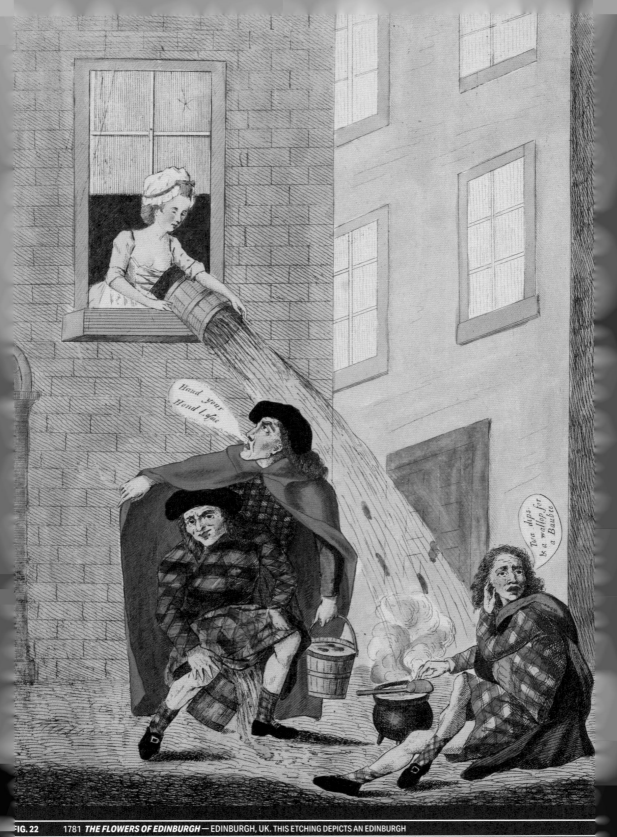

FIG. 22 1781 *THE FLOWERS OF EDINBURGH* — EDINBURGH, UK. THIS ETCHING DEPICTS AN EDINBURGH

HOUSEWIFE EMPTYING A BUCKET OF WASTE FROM A FIRST-FLOOR WINDOW ONTO A MAN BELOW.

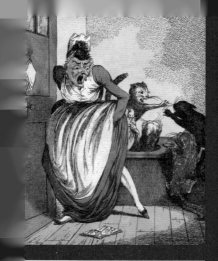

FIG. 23 1801 *DISSENTIONS IN THE CABINET*. CHARLES WILLIAMS.

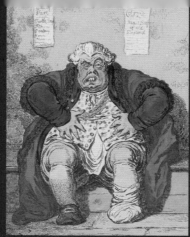

FIG. 24 1796 *NATIONAL CONVENIENCES*. JAMES GILLRAY.

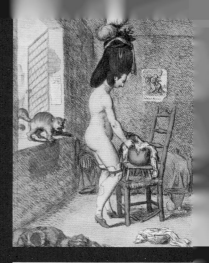

FIG. 25 1779 *THE WHORE'S LAST SHIFT*. JAMES GILLRAY.

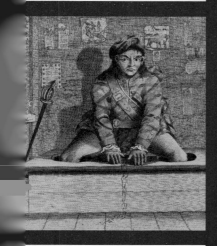

FIG. 26 1745 *SAWNEY IN THE BOG HOUSE*. CHARLES MOSLEY.

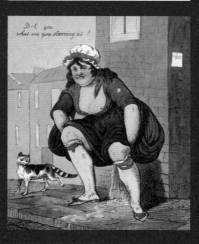

FIG. 27 1799 *INDECENCY*. ISAAC CRUICKSHANK.

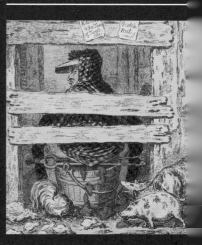

FIG. 28 1796 *NATIONAL CONVENIENCES*. JAMES GILLRAY.

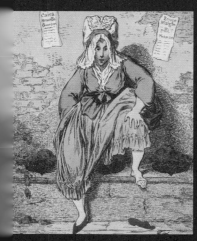

FIG. 29 1796 *NATIONAL CONVENIENCES*. JAMES GILLRAY.

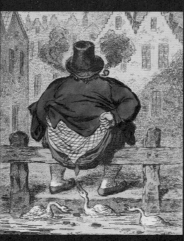

FIG. 30 1796 *NATIONAL CONVENIENCES*. JAMES GILLRAY.

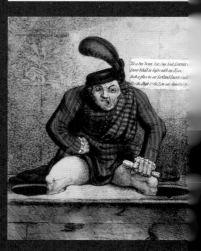

FIG. 31 1779 *SAWNEY IN THE BOG HOUSE*. JAMES GILLRAY.

SUBTERRANEAN INFRASTRUCTURES

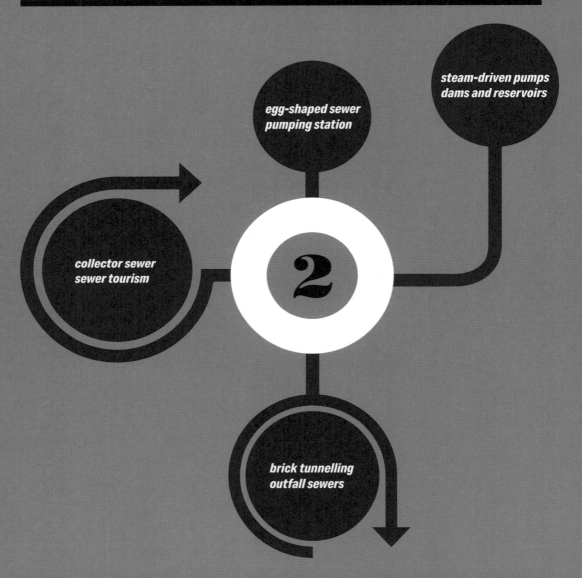

steam-driven pumps
dams and reservoirs

egg-shaped sewer
pumping station

collector sewer
sewer tourism

2

brick tunnelling
outfall sewers

[I. THE CLEANSING OF PARIS]

[II. LONDON & THE GREAT STINK]

[III. WORLDWIDE ADAPTATIONS]

[IV. RAISING STREETS]

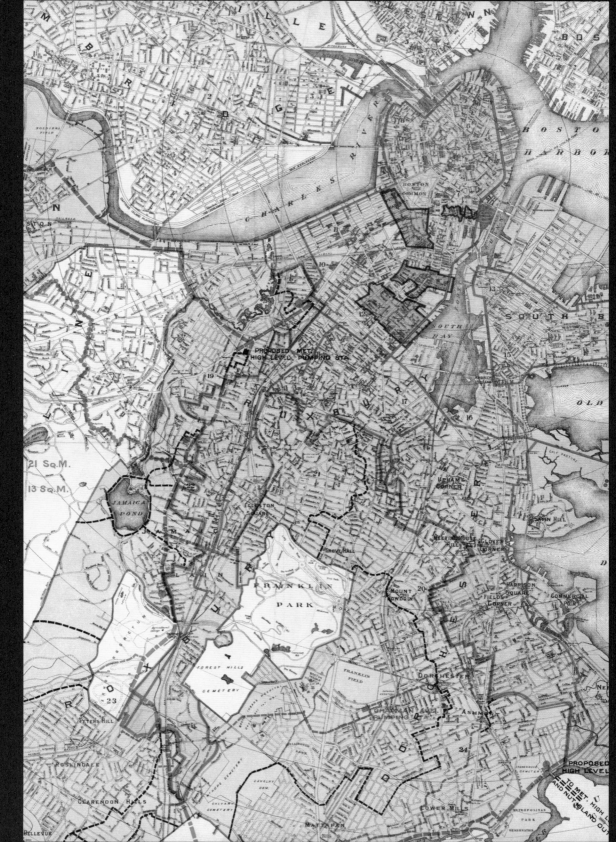

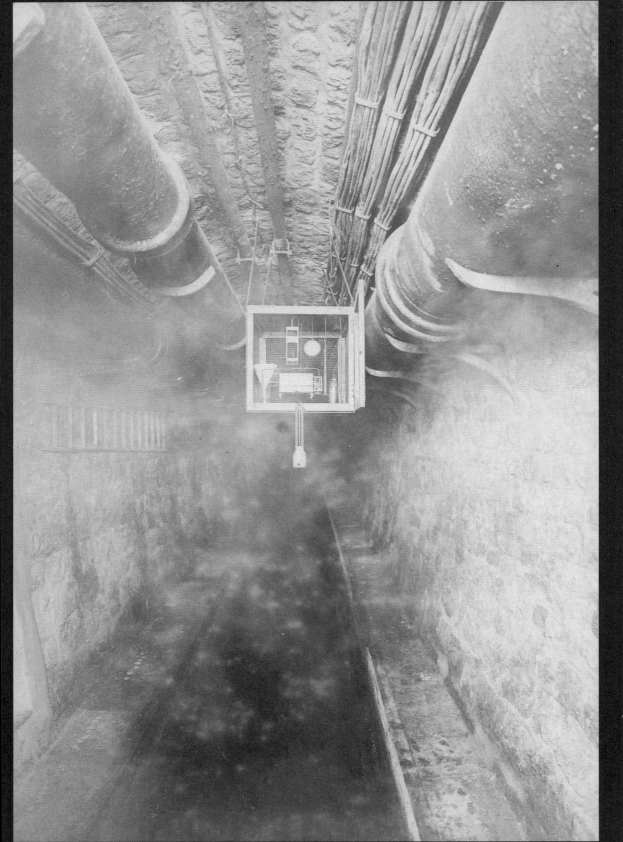

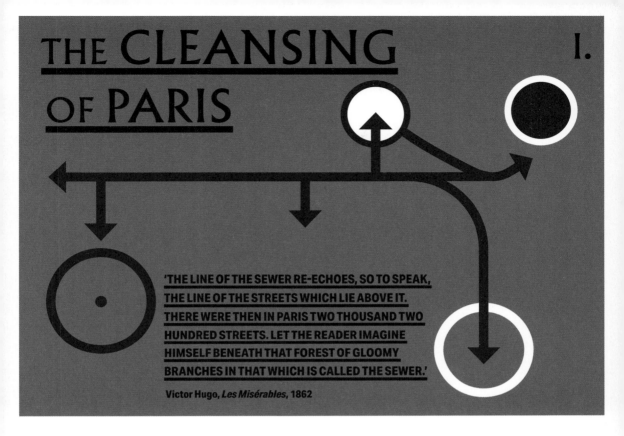

THE CLEANSING OF PARIS

'THE LINE OF THE SEWER RE-ECHOES, SO TO SPEAK, THE LINE OF THE STREETS WHICH LIE ABOVE IT. THERE WERE THEN IN PARIS TWO THOUSAND TWO HUNDRED STREETS. LET THE READER IMAGINE HIMSELF BENEATH THAT FOREST OF GLOOMY BRANCHES IN THAT WHICH IS CALLED THE SEWER.'

Victor Hugo, *Les Misérables*, 1862

The sewers of Paris have occupied an infamous place in the nation's history and literature. In 1791, the Jacobin revolutionary Jean-Paul Marat sheltered in the sewers while fleeing from his enemies and it was probably in those fetid depths that he contracted or exacerbated the skin disease that required him to be immersed for much of his time in a medicinal bath (he would eventually be murdered in it by Charlotte Corday – the subject later of a famous painting by Jacques-Louis David). And in Victor Hugo's *Les Misérables* (1862), set in the period 1815–32, the principal protagonist, Jean Valjean, makes his escape from the villainous police inspector Javert through them, along with his wounded friend Marius. The cleaning of the sewers was sporadic and mostly dependent upon rainfall and sewermen equipped with *rabots* – poles 2 m (7 ft) long, with paddles at right angles, which were used to free accumulated sewage. The notoriety of the sewers was such that Emperor Napoleon III (1808–73) – nephew of the former emperor Napoleon Bonaparte – incorporated them in a plan to recreate the French capital and rid it of the wretched conditions of the poorer classes described in Hugo's novel, conditions that caused nine riots between 1825 and the one that made Louis Emperor Napoleon III in 1852. ○——————➤ 62

P. 57 1902 **BOSTON DRAINAGE SYSTEM** — BOSTON, USA. THE RED LINES SHOW THE INTERCONNECTING SEWERS OF THE SOUTH METROPOLTIAN SYSTEM AND THE MAIN DRAINAGE SYSTEM.

FIG. 1 ← 1893 *L'ÉGOUT RIVOLI* — PARIS, FRANCE. THE GREAT SEWER BENEATH RUE DE RIVOLI, WITH THE DISTINCTIVE RAISED SIDES FOR WORKERS TO WALK ALONG.

FIG. 2   1789 *LES ÉGOUTS DE PARIS.*

FIGS. 2–3 MAPS OF THE SEWERS **(FIG. 2)** AND WATER SUPPLIES **(FIG. 3)** OF PARIS IN 1789, PRIOR TO HAUSSMANN'S RENOVATIONS.

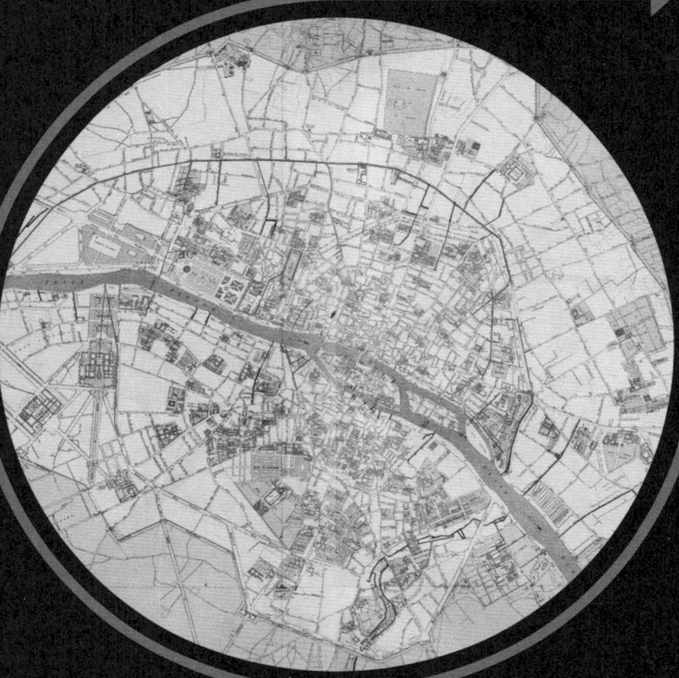

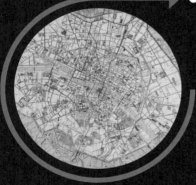

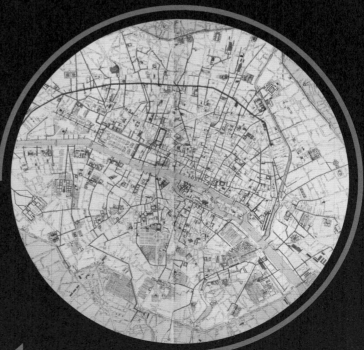

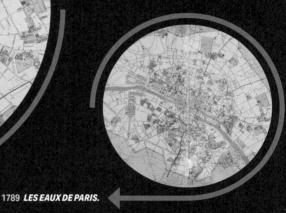

FIG. 3   1789 *LES EAUX DE PARIS.*

FIG. 4   1854 *LES EAUX DE PARIS.*

FIGS. 4–5 THESE MAPS OF WATER **(FIG. 4)** AND SEWERS **(FIG. 5)** SHOW HAUSSMANN'S PLANS BEGINNING TO TAKE SHAPE.

FIG. 5   1854 *LES ÉGOUTS DE PARIS.*

FIG. 6   1878 *LES ÉGOUTS DE PARIS.*

FIGS. 6–7 BY 1878 THE NETWORK OF SEWERS (**FIG. 6**) AND WATER SUPPLIES (**FIG. 7**) IS MUCH DENSER, AS HAUSSMANN'S SYSTEM EXPANDS.

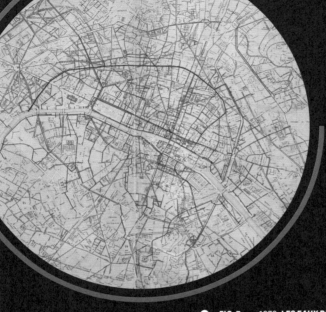

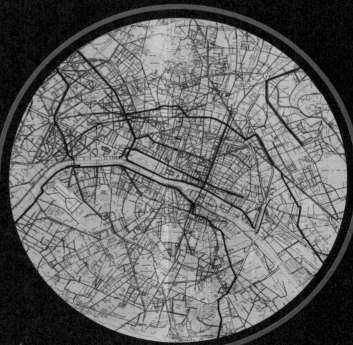

FIG. 7   1878 *LES EAUX DE PARIS.*

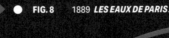

FIG. 8   1889 *LES EAUX DE PARIS.*

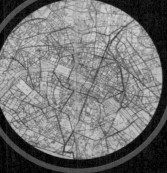

FIGS. 8–9 BY 1889 SOME FURTHER ADDITIONS HAVE BEEN MADE AS THE POPULATION OF PARIS CONTINUES TO GROW.

FIG. 9   1889 *LES ÉGOUTS DE PARIS.*

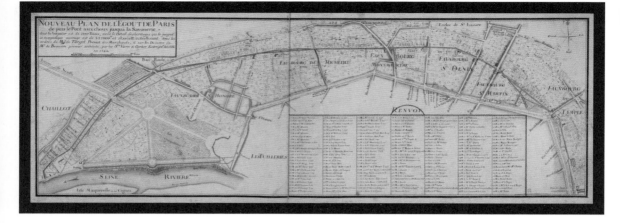

FIG. 10   1738 **NEW PLAN OF THE SEWER OF PARIS** — PARIS, FRANCE.
THIS SYSTEM OF SEWERS WAS DESIGNED BY JEAN BEAUSIRE, CHIEF
OF PUBLIC WORKS IN PARIS BETWEEN 1684 AND 1740. HE IS ALSO
REMEMBERED FOR HIS FOUNTAINS, SEVERAL OF WHICH ARE STILL
IN OPERATION TODAY.

In December 1848, after the eighth such demonstration, Louis Napoleon was chosen as president of
the French Republic promising stability, justice and prosperity for all. The disruptive tendencies of his
fellow citizens did not pass unnoticed by the new president. They were to inform his ambitious plans
for the reconstruction of the French capital, whose narrow streets and foul slums lent themselves to the
construction of barricades and the breeding of discontent. Napoleon persuaded his fellow Frenchmen
to grant him something approaching dictatorial powers which, alone, would guarantee the peace
and which he deployed to reconstruct the French capital.

Louis had spent his early years in exile, some of it in England, where he came to admire London's parks
and the works of John Nash (1752–1835) in the creation of thoroughfares such as Regent Street. Louis
envisaged the reconstruction of the French capital as part of his plan to perpetuate his rule. Narrow
passages and alleyways would be replaced by broad boulevards suitable for the deployment of artillery
and cavalry. Pure water would be brought from distant springs to replace the waters of the Seine into
which the city's waste was emptied. And finally, magnificent sewers beneath the streets would take
the waste to a point downstream where it would no longer threaten the health of the populace.
Moreover, the unemployed masses who were the principal source of discontent would be usefully
occupied in the reconstruction of the city. And the achievement was colossal. The English sanitary
reformer Edwin Chadwick informed the Emperor, his host on a visit to the French capital, that his
city was 'fair above, foul below' and added: 'It was said of Augustus that he found Rome brick and
left it marble. May it be said of you that you found Paris stinking and left it sweet.'

To achieve his vision, the Emperor needed a public servant with the qualities to carry it out and he
found him in the person of Georges-Eugène Haussmann (1809–91), prefect of Bordeaux, who had
attracted the attention of Louis Napoleon during a visit to Bordeaux in his campaign to become ruler.
He instructed Victor de Persigny (1808–72), his interior minister, to interview Haussmann. De Persigny
recorded his impressions:

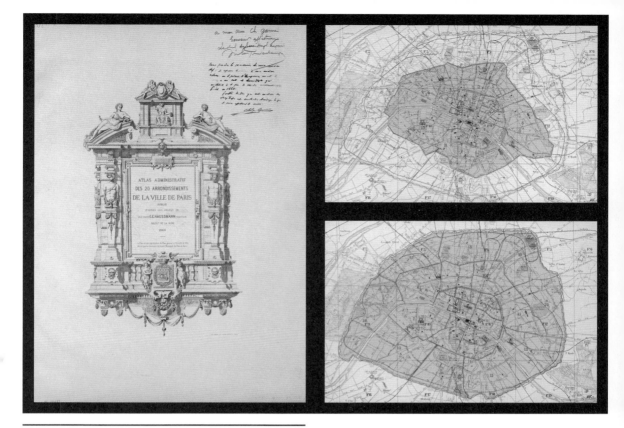

FIGS. 11–13 1868 **TITLE PAGE AND MAPS FROM AN ADMINISTRATIVE ATLAS OF PARIS, COMMISSIONED BY HAUSSMANN** — PARIS, FRANCE. THESE MAPS SHOW THE EFFECTS OF NAPOLEON'S DECISION TO ENLARGE PARIS BY ANNEXING ELEVEN COMMUNES AND PLACING THEM UNDER HAUSSMANN'S AUTHORITY.

It was Monsieur Haussmann who impressed me the most. I had in front of me one of the most extraordinary men of our time; big, strong, vigorous, energetic, and at the same time clever and devious, with a spirit full of resources. I told him about the Paris works and offered to put him in charge.

It was an inspired choice. Haussmann, who was over 2 m (6 ft) tall, had the qualities that the job, and the Emperor, demanded and between 1853 and 1870 he executed Louis Napoleon's vision. The boulevards were 20–40 m (66–132 ft) wide compared to the 1–2 m (3–7 ft) of the alleys they replaced, many of the thoroughfares radiating from grand squares such as the Place de l'Arc de Triomphe and the Place de la Bastille. Moreover, they were connected to the railway stations, so they would also enable troops to be brought swiftly into the city to subdue rioters. In all, 418 km (260 miles) of new, broad streets replaced narrow warrens and passages. Some critics complained that the city of Honoré de Balzac and Victor Hugo had disappeared and in 1867, as Haussmann's projects proceeded relentlessly, the historian Léon Halévy begged: 'There will be a twentieth century. Let us leave something for them to do!' But as long as he had the support of Napoleon III, Haussmann's own determination was more than enough to face down his critics.

○————————➤ 67

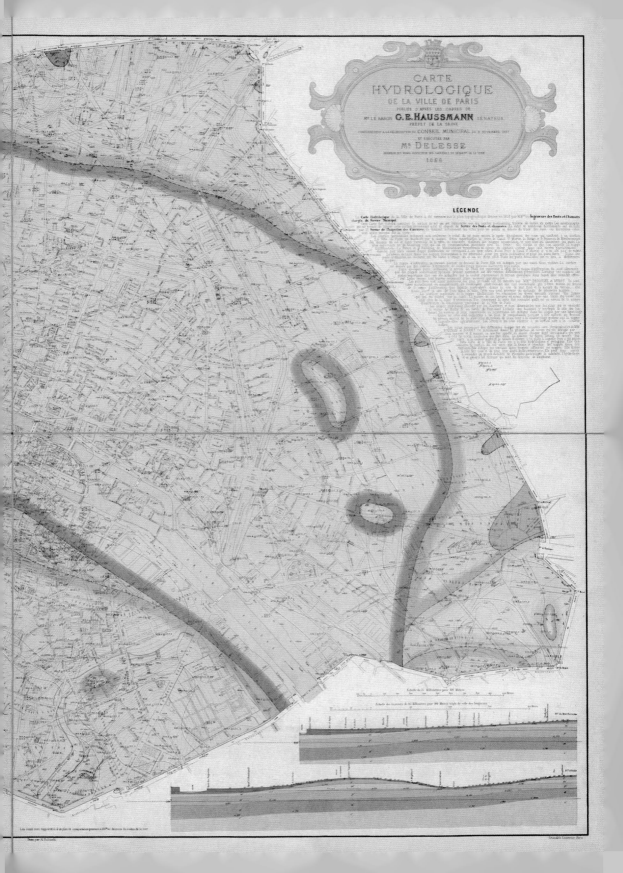

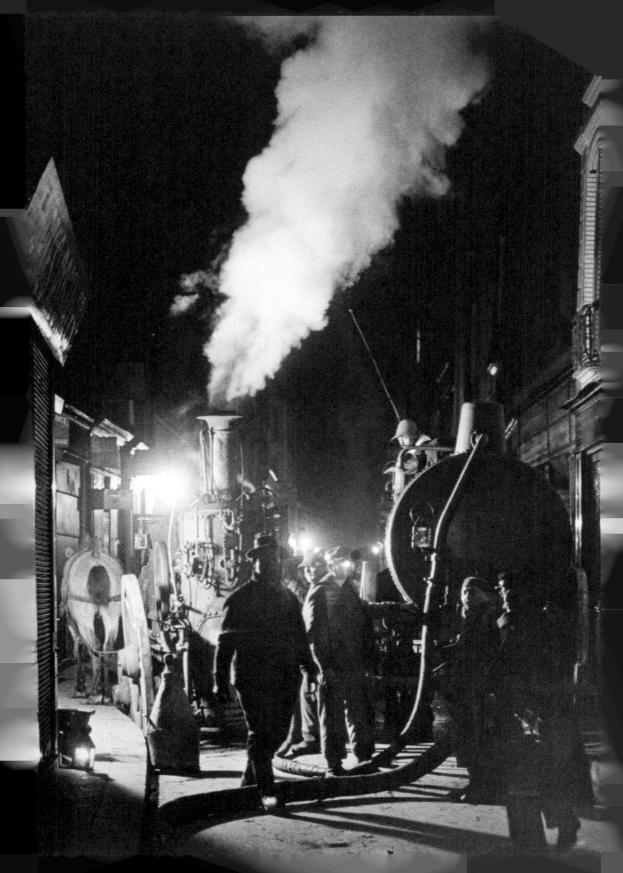

Before he could execute the Emperor's ambitious plans, however, he needed an engineer with the necessary technical expertise. Having created a new *Service des égouts et eaux* ('service of sewers and water') in 1855 Haussmann's choice fell upon Eugène Belgrand (1810–78), a graduate of the prestigious École Polytechnique and later of the École Nationale des Ponts et Chaussées, whose knowledge of geology and water management had impressed Haussmann in supplying water to the Burgundian town of Avallon. Haussmann interviewed Belgrand and recorded: 'I was astonished to find in this large, bald man, whose peasant exterior gave no hint of superior intelligence, a highly accomplished geologist and hydrologist.' Belgrand's skills in water management were important because in the early stages of his work Haussmann's main concern was the improvement of the water supply to Paris, whose rapidly expanding population was served mainly by supplies drawn from the Seine, into which the 142 km (88 miles) of existing sewers emptied much of their contents. This mostly consisted of street garbage, horse droppings and urine, since solid human excrement was collected at night by teams of nightsoilmen (known as *vidangeurs*) and delivered to farmers or to foul-smelling dumps.

In the late 18th century, an idea had arisen that waste, including sewage, could be a source of wealth. The basic idea lay in the potential for sewage to be used as an exceptionally good fertilizer, which could be used to successfully increase the productivity of land. Various early proponents suggested ways in which this alchemy of gold from sewage could be achieved. French novelist Nicolas-Edme Restif (1734–1806) suggested that instead of Parisians dumping their waste in the Seine they could sell it to farmers to fund a public street-cleansing service. Philosopher Pierre Leroux's (1797–1871) 'Circulus' theory proposed that the recycling of human waste would improve soil fertility so much as to allow the yield from the fields to easily keep pace with population growth. Moreover he suggested that 'each would religiously gather his dung to give it to the state, that is to say the tax collector, in place of a tax.' Fellow Channel Islands exile, Victor Hugo, visited Leroux and joined him as an advocate of the 'Circulus'. His strong views on the matter even made it into *Les Misérables* where he wrote, in reference to Paris's waste disposal via the Seine, that 'Paris throws 25 million francs a year into the water. And this is no metaphor. We believe we are purging the city. We are weakening the population.' The wealth thus discarded 'if used for welfare and for pleasures, would double the splendour of Paris. Its marvellous fete, its gold flowing from full hands, its splendour, its luxury, its magnificence, is its sewer.' German chemist Justus von Liebig (1803–73) developed the idea further by identifying the importance of minerals such as potassium in plant nutrition, and on these grounds criticised the practice of dumping sewage into rivers and seas as a shocking waste of valuable fertilizer. In England the Revd Henry Moule (1801–80) devised a practical application of this concept with his 1850s invention of a 'dry earth closet'. This consisted of a receptacle (such as a bucket) full of earth into which faeces and urine were received and then buried under another layer of earth. This could be repeated until the receptacle was full at which point the contents could be emptied onto the owner's garden as an effective fertilizer.

Meanwhile, cholera epidemics were believed to be caused by a 'miasma' of foul air arising from pollution and although this was not correct (water itself being the culprit) it was beginning to be appreciated that water drawn from a river as polluted as the Seine had become was, at the very least, unpalatable.

FIG. 15 1931 ***CESSPOOL CLEANERS WITH THEIR PUMP, RUE RAMBUTEAU*, BRASSAÏ** — PARIS, FRANCE. CESSPOOL CLEANERS PUMPING OUT THE CONTENTS OF A CESSPOOL IN THE CENTRE OF PARIS.

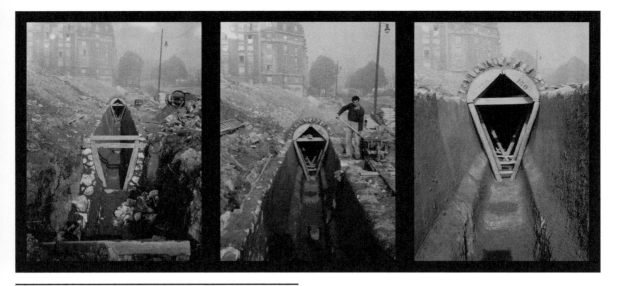

FIGS. 16–18 1920s **DEVELOPMENT OF THE PARIS SEWERS** — PARIS, FRANCE. AS PARIS GREW ITS SEWER SYSTEM WAS ALSO REQUIRED TO EXPAND. HERE FURTHER EGG-SHAPED SEWERS ARE ADDED.

> 'HE DREW A PICTURE OF THE WHOLE OF PARIS OPENING THE FLOODGATES OF ITS SEWERS AND RELEASING THEIR FERTILIZING FLOOD OF HUMAN MANURE...THE GREAT CITY WOULD BE RESTORING TO THE LAND THE LIFE WHICH IT HAD RECEIVED FROM IT.'
>
> **Émile Zola**, *La Terre* **(1887)**

Belgrand built a series of aqueducts and conduits to bring drinking water from the river Dhuis, a sub-tributary of the Marne to the east of Paris, and the river Vanne to the south-east; to conserve this *eau potable*, the sullied waters of the Seine were used for street cleaning. To this day, the expressions *eau potable* and *eau non potable* are commonly seen in Paris and elsewhere in France. Having improved the water supply, Belgrand turned his attention to the infamous sewers of Paris. Belgrand increased their mileage fourfold, to almost 800 km (497 miles), to deal with the extra flow emanating from the improved water supply. And Belgrand's sewers were not like the narrow passages in which Marat had hidden. The smaller street sewers were egg-shaped, in accordance with the latest designs to concentrate and hence speed the movement of liquid at times of low flow, but at 2.3 m (7 ft 6 in.) high and 1.3 m (4 ft 3 in.) wide they were large enough for a man to stand comfortably to clear obstructions and execute repairs. However, Belgrand is mostly remembered for his colossal

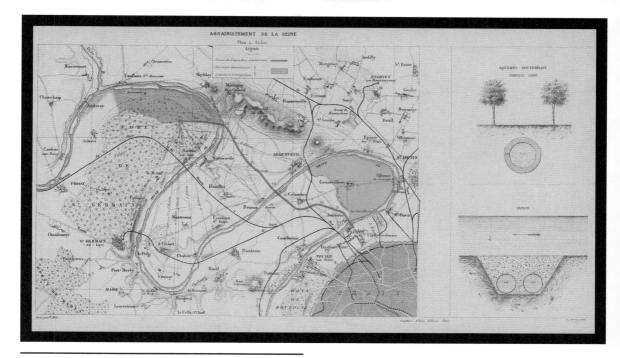

FIG. 19 **SANITATION OF THE SEINE** — PARIS, FRANCE. SEWAGE WAS
TAKEN TO ASNIÈRES, 24 KM (15 MILES) FROM THE CENTRE OF PARIS.
IT IS NOW THE SITE OF A WASTEWATER TREATMENT PLANT.

'collector' sewers, which gathered the waste from street sewers and conveyed it to the Seine at
Asnières – then just beyond the City boundary. In doing so, he took advantage of a bend in the
Seine, so the outfall at Asnières was almost 8 km (5 miles) downstream from the centre of Paris.
Moreover, since the Seine through Paris is not tidal the flow of the river immediately conveyed
the sewage downstream.

The scale and nature of these sewers was expressed by Haussmann in heroic language:
'Subterranean galleries are the internal organs of the great city and they function like those of
the human body…secretions are mysteriously performed and public health maintained without
disturbing the running of the city or spoiling its beauty.' There were eleven of these main sewers,
amounting to 64.3 km (40 miles) in length. The largest, the outfall to Asnières, is over 5 km (3 miles)
long and measures 4.3 m (14 ft) high and 5.5 m (18 ft) wide – more than four times the capacity of
the sewers that were being constructed at the same time by Joseph Bazalgette in London, a much
larger city. A narrow channel in the bottom of the sewer is itself 3.5 m (11 ft 5 in.) wide by 1.35 m
(4 ft 5 in.) deep. The sewer was completed in 1859. A siphon conveyed the sewage from the collectors
on the Left Bank and added it to that of the Right Bank so that it could all be taken to the Asnières
outfall. The siphon, near the Pont d'Alma, consisted of two sealed iron tubes, 150 m (492 ft) long,
which were lowered into the Seine attached to iron weights. The river was closed to traffic for a week
while this was done. This was not a popular move, but the authority of the Emperor made it possible.
It is hard to imagine it being done in London, where Joseph Bazalgette had to contend with the
demands of quarrelsome MPs and councillors.

o——————▷ 82

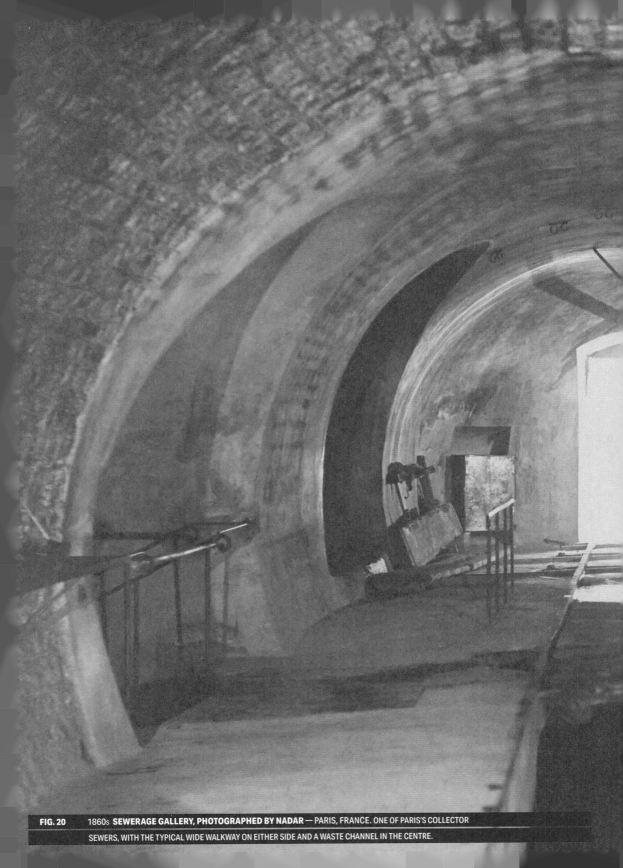

FIG. 20   1860s **SEWERAGE GALLERY, PHOTOGRAPHED BY NADAR** — PARIS, FRANCE. ONE OF PARIS'S COLLECTOR
SEWERS, WITH THE TYPICAL WIDE WALKWAY ON EITHER SIDE AND A WASTE CHANNEL IN THE CENTRE.

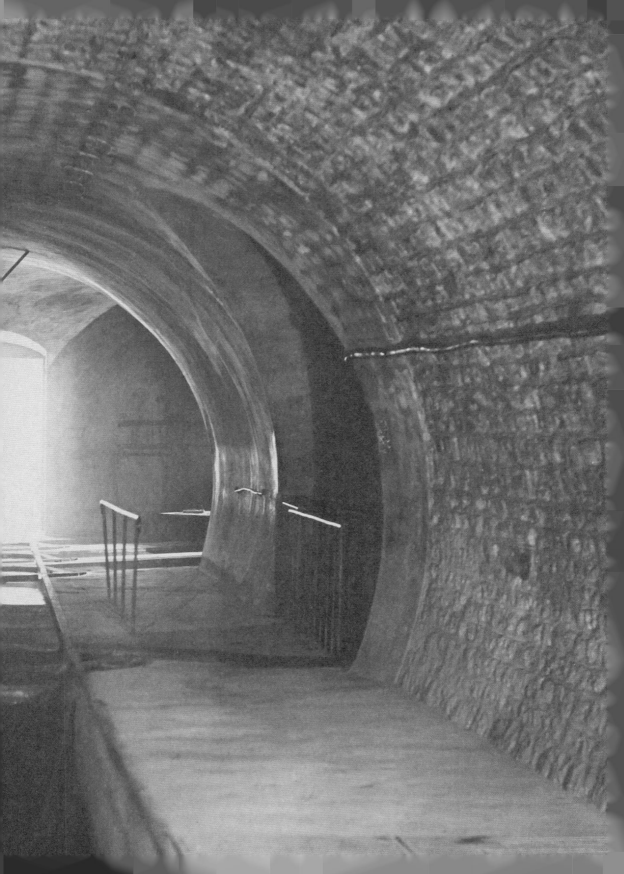

TYPES DE GA

TYPE N.º 2

GALERIE DU BOULEVARD SÉBASTOPOL

Renfermant deux conduites d'eau une de 1ᵐ10 pour l'eau de Source
et une autre de 0ᵐ60 d'eau d'Ourcq.. Décharge du collecteur des coteaux

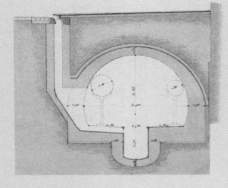

COLLECTEUR GÉNÉRAL, conduisant le

PARTIE CONSTRUITE EN TRANCHÉE

Agencement d'un regard pour descendre dans la galerie

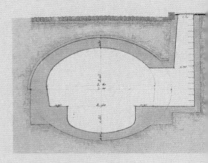

TYPE N.º 7

GALERIE de la rue de Rivoli

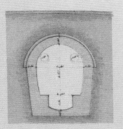

TYPE N.º 5

COLLECTEURS du quai de Gèvres, des coteaux entre
les Bᵈˢ de Strasbourg et Malesherbes, Avenues Bosquet
et Duquesne, de la Villette et de la Plaine St Denis, etc

GALERIE

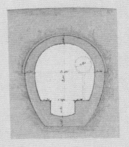

TYPE N.º 9

GALERIE des Bᵈˢ du Temple et Beaumarchais,
de la Rue Rambuteau et d'une partie des Bᵈˢ extérieurs

TYPE N.º 10

GALERIE destinée à recevoir deux conduites
d'eau de 0ᵐ90 et de 0ᵐ30 de diam'

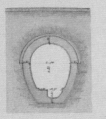
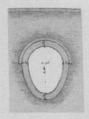

TYPE N.º 13

EGOUT des voies de moyenne importance

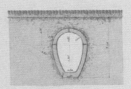

BRANCHEMENT DE REGARD D'ÉGOUT

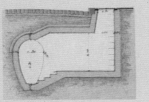

COLLECTEURS dont le curage s'effectue au moyen de bateaux vannes
EGOUTS a rails dont le curage se fait au moyen de wagons vannes
Autres EGOUTS dont la force et l'espacement des traits varient suivant l'importance de
Dimensions des EGOUTS anciens indiqués au moyen d'une fraction dont le numéra
Regards d'Egout placés sur l'axe de la galerie
Regards d'Egout avec branchement sur le côté de la galerie
Bouches d'Egout ou Entrées d'eau
Les Côtes bleues indiquent les altitudes du sol des rues, des trappes de regards, et
Les Côtes rouges donnent les altitudes des radiers des Egouts
Les maçonneries des types de I à II sont diminuées d'un tiers dans leur épaisseur q
lorsque le mortier de ciment est employé

Gravé chez Avril fͬᵉˢ et Wuhrer, 52, r Gay-Lussac.

ERIES D'ÉGOUTS.

PE Nº 1

Égouts de Paris de la Place de la Concorde au Pont d'Asnières

COLLECTEURS de la Bièvre, des quais de la rive droite entre la
place du Châtelet et celle de la Concorde

PARTIE CONSTRUITE EN SOUTERRAIN
Agencement d'une chambre de sauvetage et du puits de service

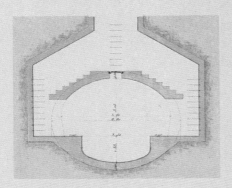

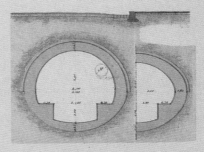

E Nº 4
rd St Michel au dessous
ard St Germain

TYPE Nº 6
1. COLLECTEURS des coteaux jusqu'au Bᵈ de Strasbourg, des Ternes
des Quais, jusqu'au Bᵈ de Sébastopol, de la rue Nᵈ des pᵗˢ Champs
2. GALERIES du Bᵈ St Michel au dessus du Bᵈ St Germain

TYPE Nº 8
GALERIE de la rue de Puébla, d'une partie
du Bᵈ Haussmann, du Bᵈ des Capucines, etc.

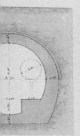

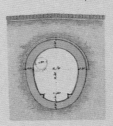

TYPE Nº 11
GALERIE destinée à recevoir deux conduites d'eau
construite rue Pigalle.

TYPE Nº 12
ÉCOUT ordinaire des voies importantes

PE Nº 14
des petites rues

TYPE Nº 15
BRANCHEMENT PARTICULIER

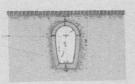

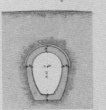

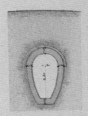

BRANCHEMENT DE BOUCHE D'ÉGOUT
ou entrée d'eau

CENDE

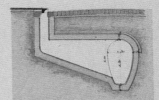

ente la hauteur sous clef et le dénominateur la largeur de l'Égout à la naissance de la voûte.

d'eau

ont faites avec mortier de ciment ; pour les types Nº 12, 13, 14, et 15, on a indiqué les épaisseurs admises

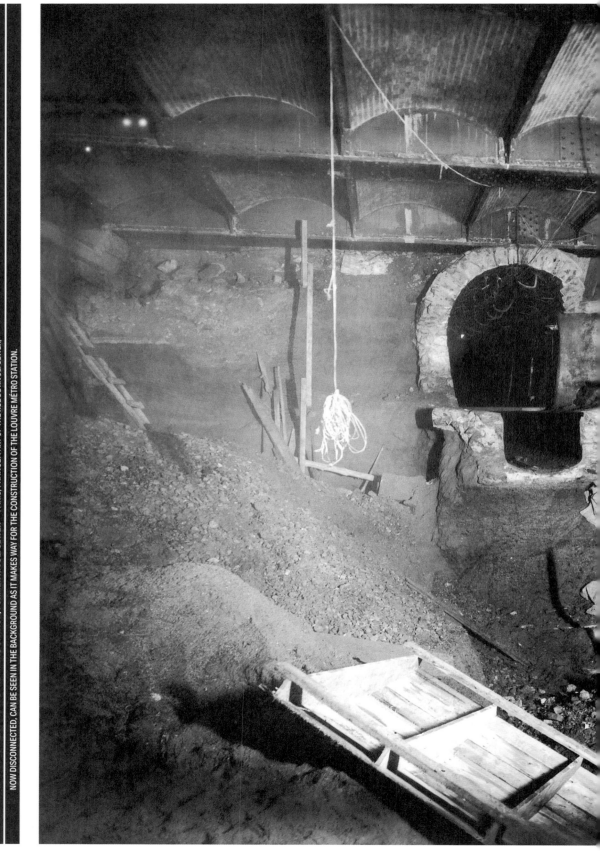

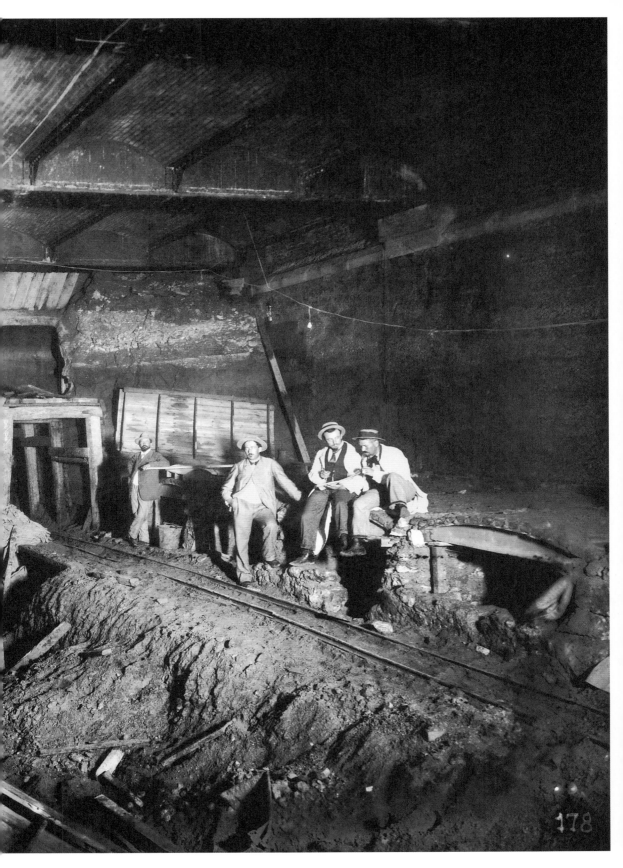

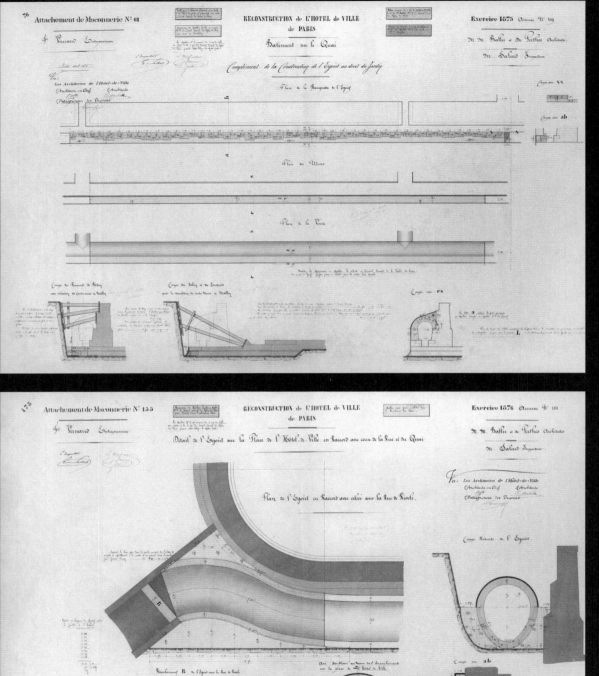

FIG. 23 ↑ 1875 **CONSTRUCTION OF THE SEWERS BENEATH**
THE NEW HÔTEL DE VILLE — PARIS, FRANCE. PLANS
FOR THE SEWER BENEATH THE RIVERFRONT AND GARDEN.

FIG. 24 ↓ 1876 **CONSTRUCTION OF THE SEWERS BENEATH**
THE NEW HÔTEL DE VILLE — PARIS, FRANCE.
PLANS FOR THE SEWER BENEATH THE RUE DE RIVOLI.

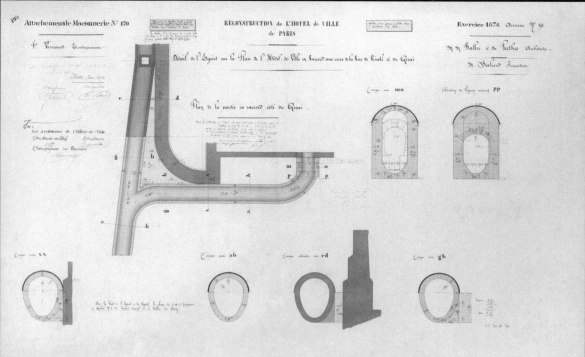

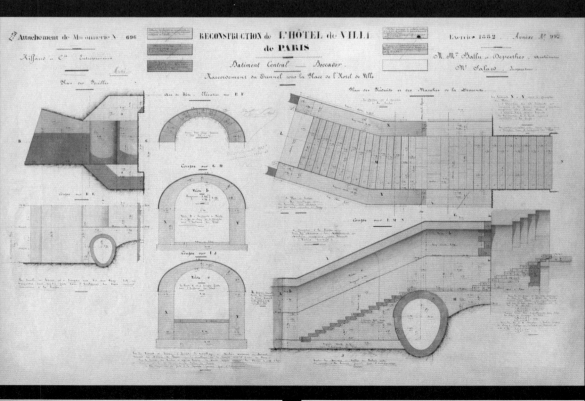

FIG. 25 ↑ 1876 **CONSTRUCTION OF THE SEWERS BENEATH THE NEW HÔTEL DE VILLE** — PARIS, FRANCE. PLANS FOR THE SEWER CONNECTING RUE DE RIVOLI AND THE QUAYSIDE.

FIG. 26 ↓ 1882 **CONSTRUCTION OF SEWERS BENEATH THE NEW HÔTEL DE VILLE** — PARIS, FRANCE. PLANS FOR THE SEWER BENEATH THE HÔTEL DE VILLE.

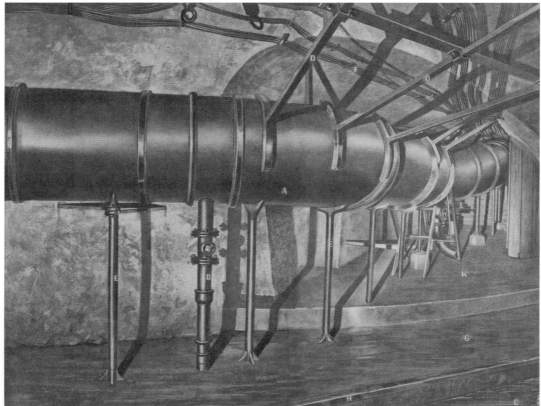

FIGS. 27–30 1872–87 COLLECTOR SEWERS OF PARIS — PARIS, FRANCE. FOUR VIEWS OF ONE OF THE MAIN COLLECTOR SEWERS. THE WASTE CHANNEL IS CLEARLY VISIBLE,

AS ARE THE SEPARATE PIPES RUNNING ALONG THE SIDES CARRYING BOTH DRINKING WATER AND WATER FROM THE SEINE USED TO FLUSH THE STREETS.

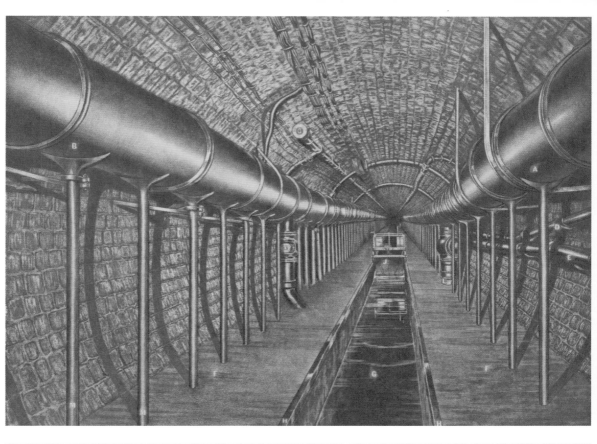

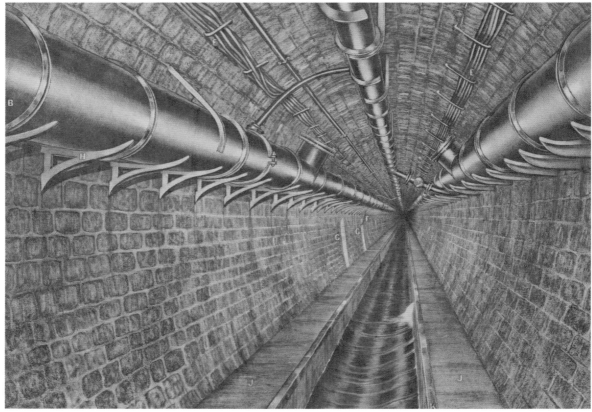

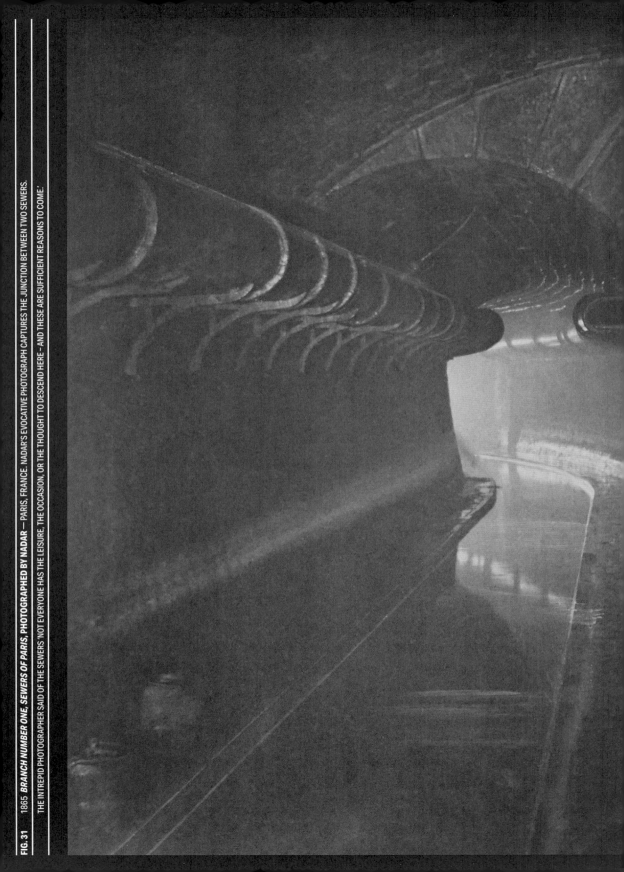

FIG. 31 1865 *BRANCH NUMBER ONE, SEWERS OF PARIS*, PHOTOGRAPHED BY NADAR — PARIS, FRANCE. NADAR'S EVOCATIVE PHOTOGRAPH CAPTURES THE JUNCTION BETWEEN TWO SEWERS.

THE INTREPID PHOTOGRAPHER SAID OF THE SEWERS 'NOT EVERYONE HAS THE LEISURE, THE OCCASION, OR THE THOUGHT TO DESCEND HERE – AND THESE ARE SUFFICIENT REASONS TO COME.'

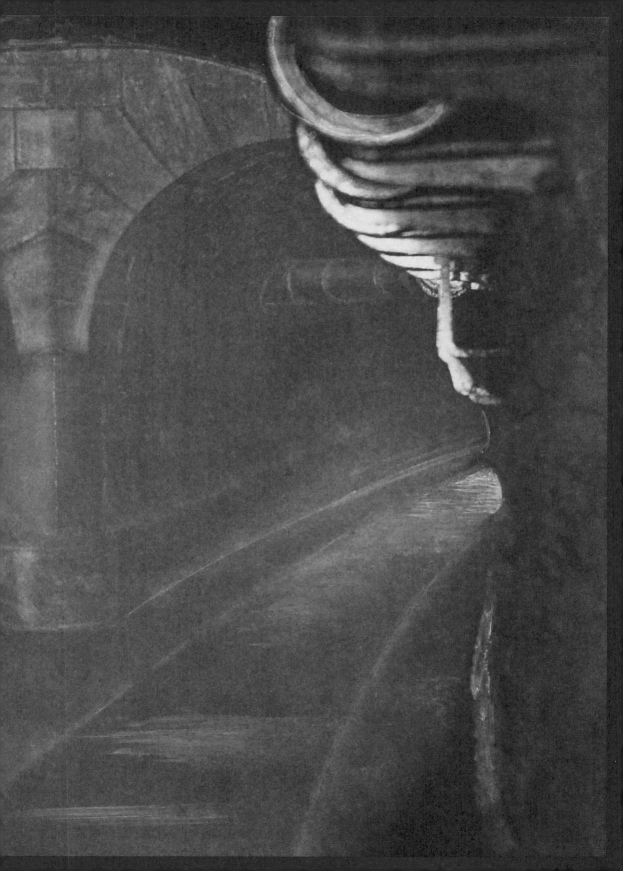

Belgrand's collector sewers were designed to be cleaned by specially designed *bateaux-vannes* (sewer boat) that measured about 2 m (6 ft 6 in.) by 1.5 m (4 ft 11 in.) and travelled along the central channel of each sewer, pushing before them any waste that had accumulated in the water. Smaller sewers were cleared by *wagons-vannes* (sewer cart), which operated in a similar manner. Having propelled their loads of grit, garbage, sewage and other rubbish to the point at which it was collected or expelled to the Seine, the vehicles were then hauled back to the start point on ropes by teams of sewermen, against the current. The process was described by an observer in 1902:

> *Flushing is accomplished by boats or carts at the front of which is fixed a shield...The shields or flood-gates are pierced with holes large enough to permit water to force itself through, but small enough to check more solid matter. The flood gates are lowered into the current and the body of water which forms before them makes an energetic wash.*

FIG. 32   1878 **WELL DRESSED VISITORS** — PARIS, FRANCE. BELGRAND'S SEWERS WERE DESIGNED TO BE ADMIRED, AND QUICKLY BECAME A FASHIONABLE ENTERTAINMENT IN THE CITY, WITH VISITORS GUIDED THROUGH IN RELATIVE LUXURY.

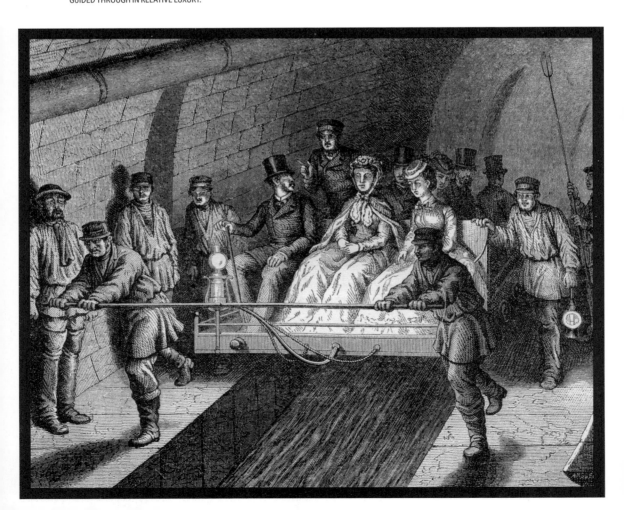

The siphons were cleared by a large ball that was propelled along them by the flow of water, pushing debris ahead of it. And the collector sewers also incorporated galleries along the sides together with separate iron pipes for drinking water and water from the Seine to flush the streets above the sewers. This was a clever arrangement for which later generations of engineers would be grateful, since it made it possible to repair and replace these pipes without digging up the roads beneath which they were buried.

The sewers of Belgrand and Haussmann were designed to be seen. They contained signs indicating the names of the streets above and during the 1867 Paris Exposition, Haussmann arranged for 400 visitors a day to be conducted though the sewers in *bateaux* and *wagons* while others could walk along the walkways that ran along the sewers 'so neat and clean that a lady might walk along them from the Louvre to the Place de la Concorde without bespattering her dainty skirts'. Lit by gas lamps (Haussmann saw no future for electricity), both King Louis I of Portugal and Tsar Alexander II of Russia made the trip, the latter personally conducted by Haussmann and Belgrand. These trips became a regular feature of the city's entertainment. In 1894, one visitor described the *bateau-vanne* as 'a veritable gondola with carpeted floor and cushioned seats; lit up by large lamps, less picturesque perhaps than a Venetian but much more luminous.' Guidebooks assured the nervous visitor that the visit, lasting forty-five minutes, was one 'in which ladies need have no hesitation in taking part'. An article in *Harper's Weekly* described 'ladies in stylish costumes, light bonnets and high heels', while one American visitor commented that 'the presence of lovely women can add charm to a sewer'! The journalist Louis Veuillot (1813–83) commented, with a touch of irony, 'People who have seen everything say that our sewers are possibly the most beautiful thing in the world!' Belgrand's sewers were certainly spectacular but their size and accessibility meant that, as late as the 1960s, Paris's prefect of police was concerned that they might be used as hiding places for terrorists from the OAS (Secret Army Organization) intent on assassinating General Charles de Gaulle because of what they regarded as his betrayal of French interests in Algeria. Several unsuccessful attempts were made to assassinate de Gaulle, but none from Haussmann's sewers. o——————▶ 90

FIG. 33 1903 **VISITORS TO THE SEWERS IN A CART** — PARIS, FRANCE. THE PARISIAN SEWERS REMAINED A POPULAR TOURIST ATTRACTION INTO THE 20TH CENTURY, WITH VISITORS ENJOYING TOURS IN ESPECIALLY DESIGNED SEWER CARTS.

FIG. 34 1920 **VISITORS TO THE SEWERS IN A BOAT** — PARIS, FRANCE. TOURISTS COULD ALSO EXPLORE THE SEWERS BY BOAT. THE VESSELS WERE LED THROUGH THE SEWERS BY SEWERMEN FROM THE WALKWAYS.

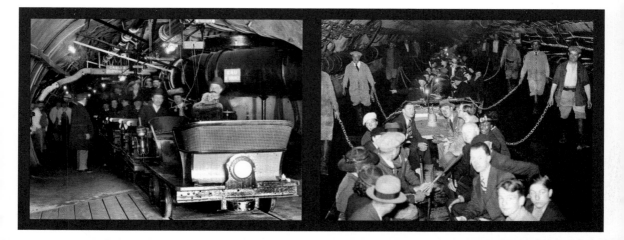

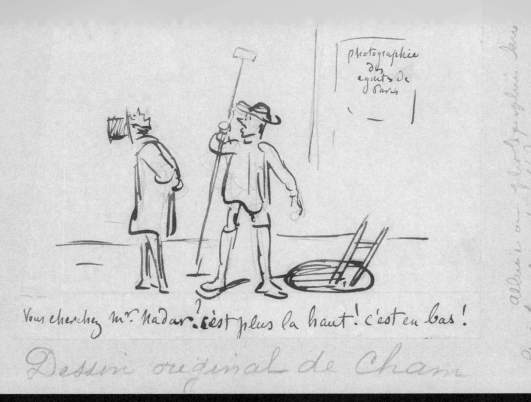

Vous cherchez mr Nadar? c'est plus la haut! c'est en bas!

Dessin original de Cham

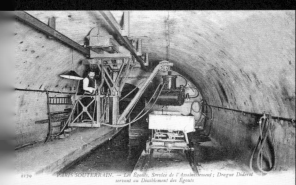

PARIS SOUTERRAIN. — Les Égouts, Service de l'Assainissement; Drague Diderot servant au Désablement des Égouts

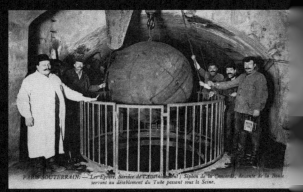

PARIS SOUTERRAIN. — Les Égouts, Service de l'Assainissement; Siphon de la Concorde, descente de la Boule servant au désablement du Tube passant sous la Seine.

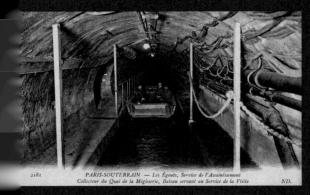

PARIS-SOUTERRAIN — Les Égouts, Service de l'Assainissement Collecteur du Quai de la Mégisserie, Bateau servant au Service de la Visite

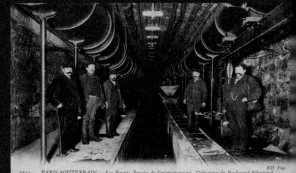

PARIS-SOUTERRAIN. — Les Égouts, Service de l'assainissement, Collecteur du Boulevard Sébastopol.

FIG. 35 ↑ **1864 LOOKING FOR MR NADAR? HE'S DOWNSTAIRS!** — PARIS, FRANCE. THIS CONTEMPORARY CARTOON SUGGESTS THE LIKELIHOOD OF FINDING PHOTOGRAPHER NADAR IN PARIS'S SEWERS.

FIGS. 36–39 ↓ **CLEANING THE PARIS SEWERS** — PARIS, FRANCE. MECHANICA AND MANUAL METHODS WERE USED TO REMOVE OBSTRUCTIONS; NOTE THE LARGE BALL FOR CLEARING THE SIPHON.

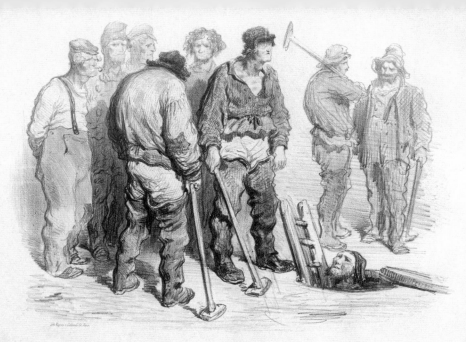

Rats (d'igout)

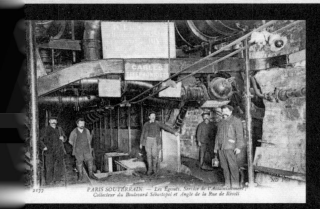

2177   PARIS SOUTERRAIN. — Les Égouts. Service de l'Assainissement ;
Collecteur du Boulevard Sébastopol et Angle de la Rue de Rivoli   ND Phot.

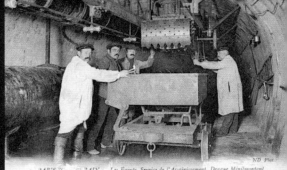

PARIS SOUTERRAIN. — Les Égouts. Service de l'Assainissement, Drague Ménilmontant
servant au désablement des Égouts   ND Phot.

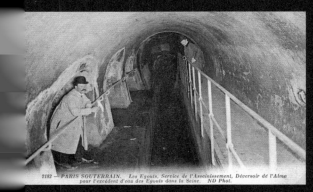

2182 — PARIS SOUTERRAIN. Les Égouts. Service de l'Assainissement, Déversoir de l'Alma
pour l'excédent d'eau des Égouts dans la Seine.   ND Phot.

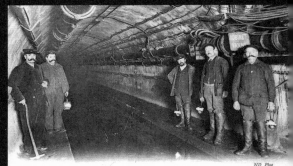

2176   PARIS SOUTERRAIN. — Les Égouts. Service de l'Assainissement ; Collecteur du Boulevard Sébastopol   ND Phot.

FIG. 40 ↑   1854 **SEWER RATS** — PARIS, FRANCE. SEWER RATS,
OR 'FLUSHERS', WERE SENT DOWN THE SEWERS EQUIPPED
WITH PADDLES TO REMOVE OBSTRUCTIONS.

FIGS.   **PARIS UNDERGROUND** — PARIS, FRANCE.
41–44 ↓   POSTCARDS CREATED TO FULFIL PUBLIC INTEREST
IN THE SUBTERRANEAN WORLD.

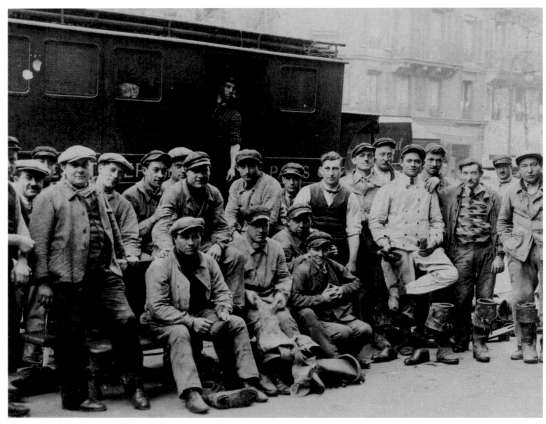

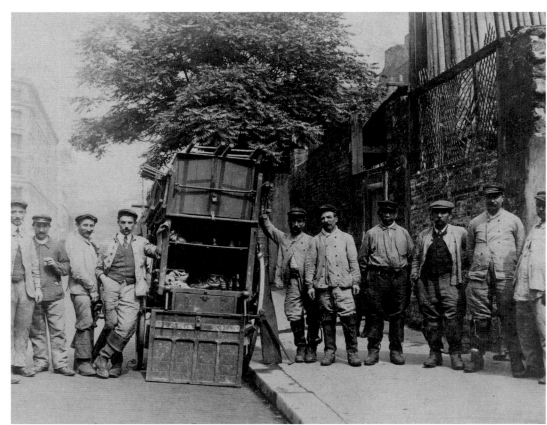

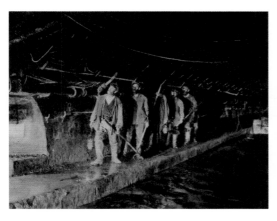
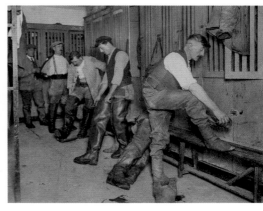
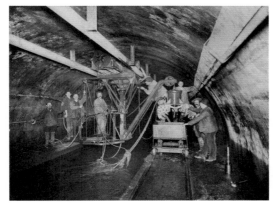
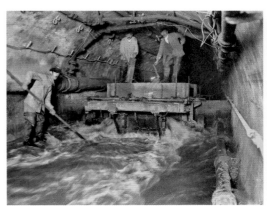
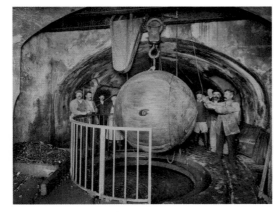
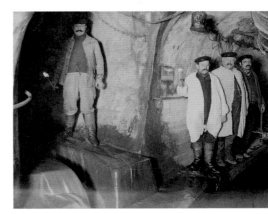
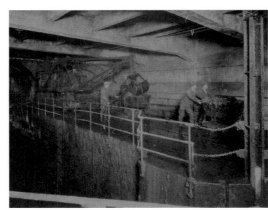
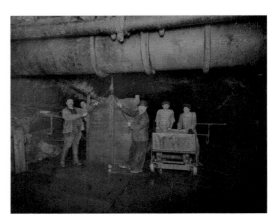

FIGS. 47–54   CLEANING THE SEWERS OF PARIS — PARIS, FRANCE. TEAMS OF SEWERMEN USING VARIOUS METHODS AND APPARATUS FOR CLEARING THE SEWERS OF OBSTRUCTIONS. THE LARGE BALL WORKED BY BEING PROPELLED ALONG THE TUNNELS BY THE FLOW OF WATER, PUSHING ANY DEBRIS AHEAD OF IT.

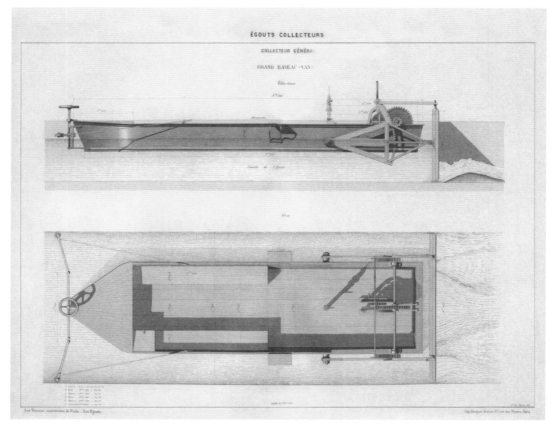

COLLECTEUR GÉNÉRAL

VANNE DE BARRAGE ET SA CHAMBRE.

COLLECTEUR GÉNÉRAL
Coupe en Long

COLLECTEUR GÉNÉRAL
Coupe en Travers.

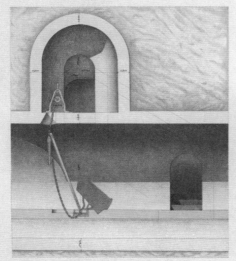
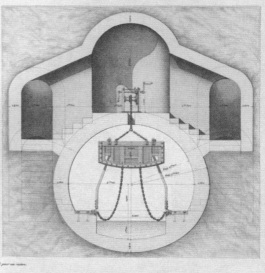

Échelle de 0^m025 pour un mètre.

Pl. 8.

DRAGUE POUR ÉGOUTS
ÉLÉVATION
Échelle de 0^m025.

WAGONNET A BASCULE
pour les petits égouts à rails
VUE DE FACE

COUPE

VUE LATÉRALE

Échelle de 0^m025.

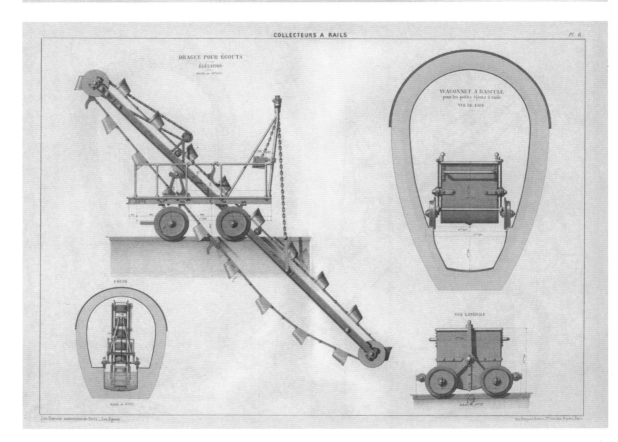

And yet Belgrand's magnificent sewers had one great weakness. They collected the rain that fell on Paris and the debris of the streets washed down by water drawn from the Seine – mud, garbage, horse droppings, sand, dust and gravel – but they did not remove human excrement. Haussmann did contemplate a separate pipe within the sewers to dispose of excrement, but only a very short section was built near Asnières. He favoured 'separators' in buildings (in effect, filters) through which liquid could pass, including urine, but faeces would continue to be collected throughout the Second Empire and beyond by fifty teams of nightsoilmen. Haussmann wasn't really interested in human faeces and certainly didn't want it fouling his showpiece sewers. He really contributed little to the solution of the problem that was Bazalgette's chief concern in London, and in 1883 it was estimated that at least 25,000 wells were still being polluted by cesspools during heavy rain.

Some experiments were conducted by Adolphe Mille (1812–94), chief engineer to the city of Paris, at La Villette and Gennevilliers, spreading the waste collected by the nightsoilmen over formerly barren fields and Haussmann himself acknowledged that the increase in fertility (and hence rents) was encouraging. Eventually, 5,000 hectares (19 sq miles) were used for this purpose and in the 1980s, long after the city had adopted modern sewage-treatment practices, La Villette was transformed into a public park. Eventually it was left to Adolphe Mille himself to introduce the process of including faeces in the system by which the city's waste was collected and processed through the sewers. Haussmann would not have approved.

It was the colossal cost of Haussmann's works that led to his downfall. In the face of mounting criticism of the cost, Napoleon III dismissed him. Within a year, Napoleon III himself had been deposed following the routing of his armies in the Franco-Prussian War and he fled into exile in Chislehurst, Kent. It has been estimated that Haussmann's works in Paris cost about £100 million, compared with Bazalgette's total expenditure of about £21 million (including the construction of streets, bridges and parks) to serve a population one-and-a-half times that of Paris with a more comprehensive system. The defeat of the French army in that war was attributed to the fact that the soldiers were ill-trained and equipped with antiquated guns. If some of the money spent on Paris had been devoted to re-equipping the army, a different outcome might have been expected.

Belgrand was rewarded for his work by being elected to France's Académie des Sciences, (founded in 1666 and similar to Britain's Royal Society) and by his being one of seventy-two names of scientists, engineers and mathematicians whose names are engraved on the Eiffel Tower beneath the first balcony. Haussmann's name was not among them, but the Paris we see and admire today is his legacy and that of Napoleon III as well as Belgrand. The magnificent Boulevard Haussmann is itself a worthy monument to its creator. But not the sewers, which – though magnificent – fulfilled only a part of their task.

FIG. 59   1865 *TRAVELLING THE SEWER BY BOAT*, BY NADAR —
PARIS, FRANCE. SEWERMEN IN ONE OF THE LARGER
BATEAUX-VANNES, CLEARING ONE OF THE COLLECTOR SEWERS.

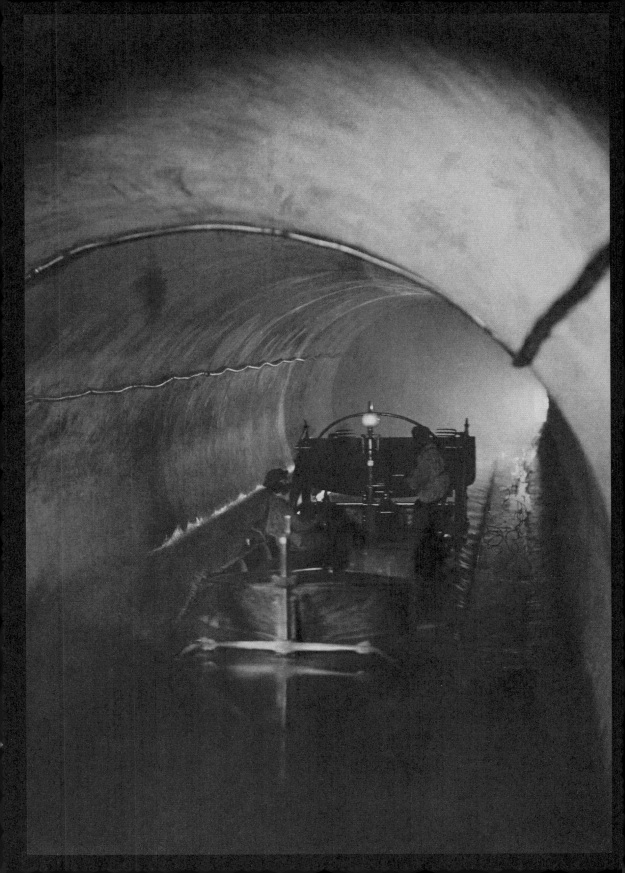

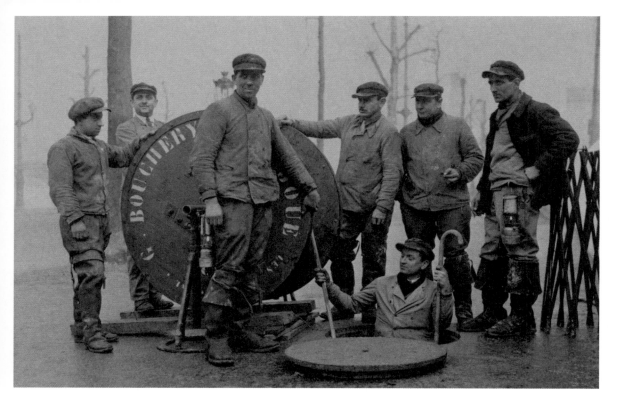

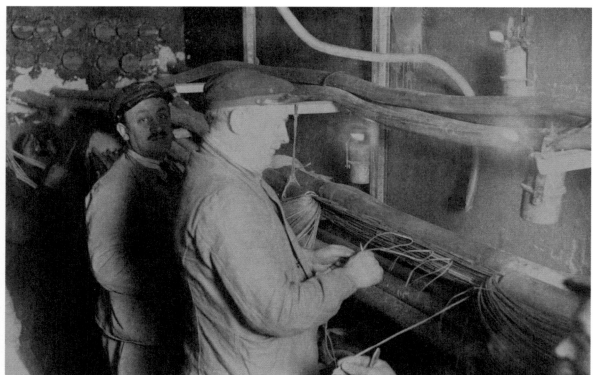

FIGS. 60–61 1928 **LAYING CABLES IN THE SEWERS** — PARIS, FRANCE.

TELEPHONE ENGINEERS USE THE SEWER TUNNELS TO LAY TELEPHONE

CABLES ALONGSIDE PREVIOUSLY INSTALLED WATER PIPES.

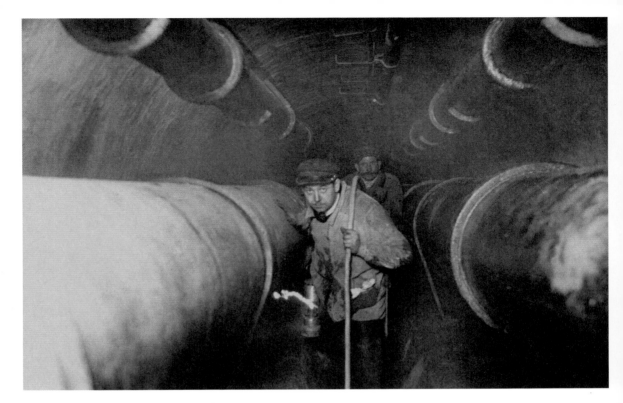

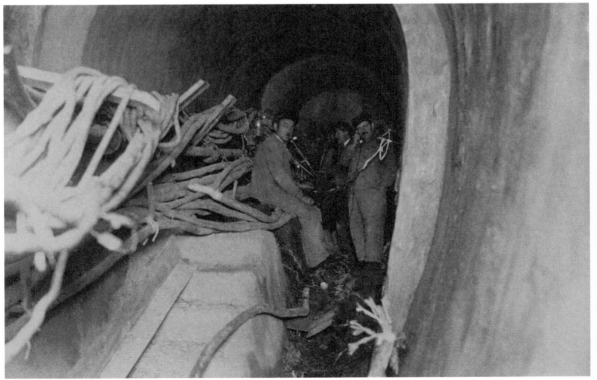

FIGS. 62–63 1928 **LAYING CABLES IN THE SEWERS** — PARIS, FRANCE.

WATER PIPES AND TELEPHONE CABLES COMPETE FOR SPACE

IN PARIS SEWERS.

THIS SEWER BENEATH THE AVENUE DE SAINT-MONDE IS BEING DEMOLISHED TO MAKE WAY FOR A NEW LINE FOR THE MÉTRO.

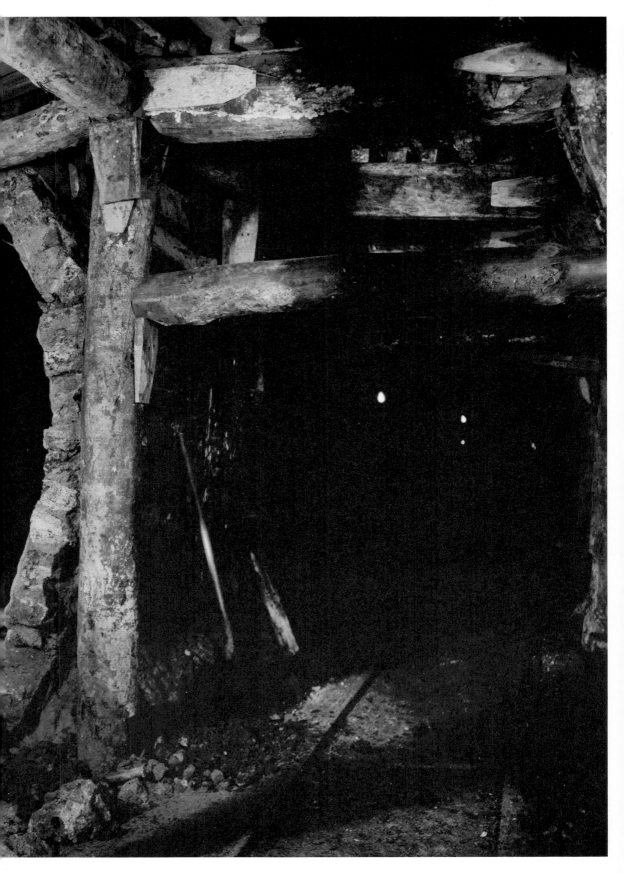

FIGS. 65–73 1897–98 **EXTENDING THE SEWER NETWORK** — PARIS, FRANCE. THESE PHOTOGRAPHS CAPTURE THE PROGRESS OF THE WORK TO EXTEND THE AQUEDUCT OF ACHÈRES

TO MÉRY-SUR-OISE AND TRIEL-SUR-SEINE. CONCRETE PIPES DEVELOPED BY MUNICIPAL ENGINEER AIMÉ BONNA (1855–1903) WERE USED FOR THESE EXTENSION WORKS.

Prolongement de l'émissaire général des eaux d'égout vers Triel.
2ᵉ lot de l'aqueduc

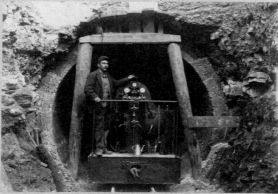

Entrée du souterrain de l'Hautie (côté de Triel)

19 Octobre 1897

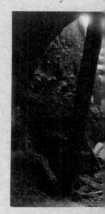

Prolongement de l'é

Tranchée

Prolongement de l'émissaire général des eaux d'égout vers Triel
2ᵉ lot de l'aqueduc

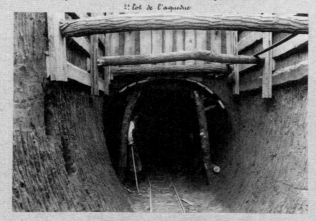

Tête amont du souterrain de Maurecourt

2 novembre 1897

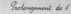

Prolongement de l

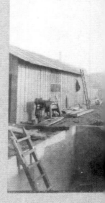

Agrandissement de l'usine de Colombes.

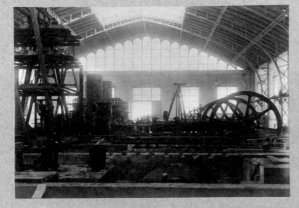

Vue prise dans l'intérieur de la salle des machines

7 février 1898

Raccordement du bassin

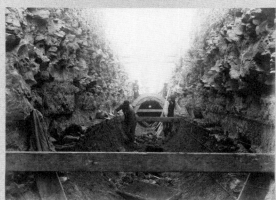

Branche de Méry

Chantier de construction

29 octobre 1897

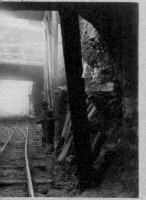

...éral des eaux d'égout vers Triel.
...e l'aqueduc

...terrain de l'Hautie (Côté de Triel).
...l'intérieur du souterrain.

29 octobre 1897

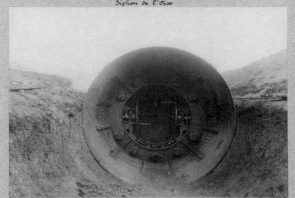

Prolongement de l'émissaire général des eaux d'égout vers Triel.
Siphon de l'Oise

Vue intérieure du bouclier

11 novembre 1897

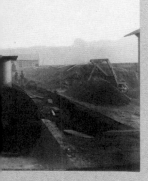

...néral des eaux d'égout vers Triel
...de l'Oise

...sas

11 novembre 1897

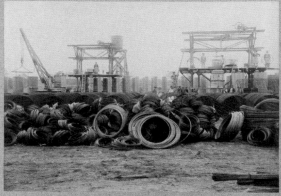

Canalisations (2ᵉ lot). — Chantier des Courlins.

Chantier de fabrication (Vue de face)

27 mai 1898

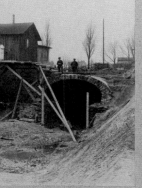

...de Clichy

...eaux d'égout avec la galerie du quai.

25 février 1898

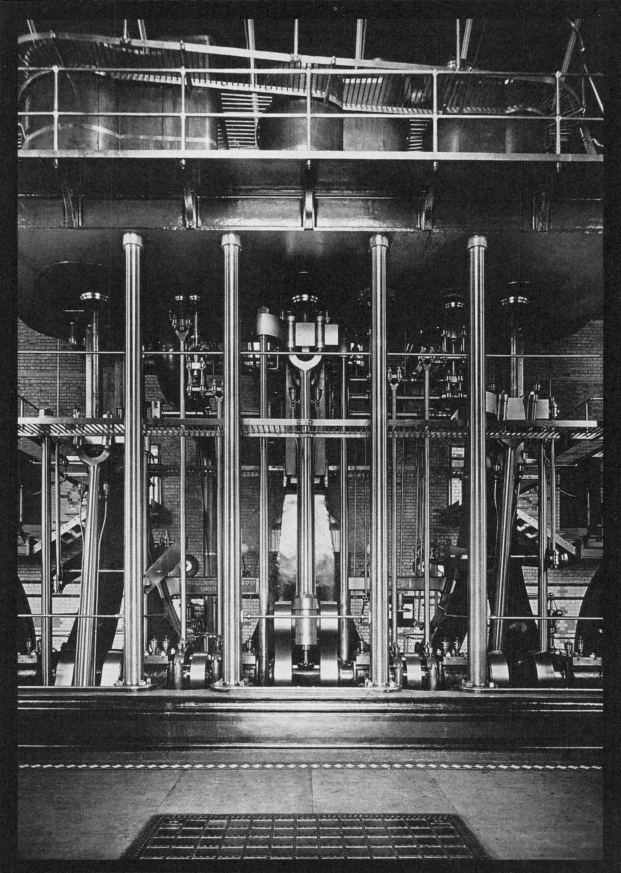

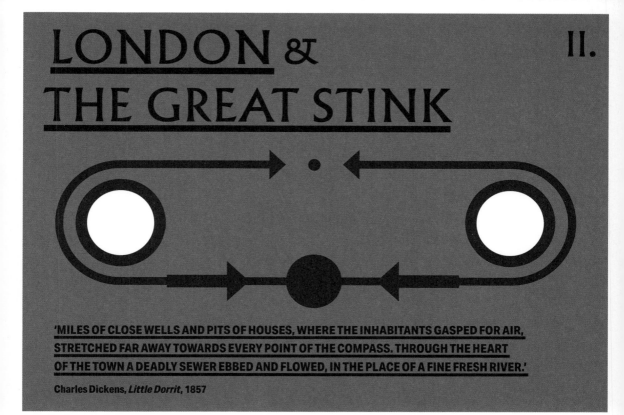

LONDON & THE GREAT STINK

'MILES OF CLOSE WELLS AND PITS OF HOUSES, WHERE THE INHABITANTS GASPED FOR AIR, STRETCHED FAR AWAY TOWARDS EVERY POINT OF THE COMPASS. THROUGH THE HEART OF THE TOWN A DEADLY SEWER EBBED AND FLOWED, IN THE PLACE OF A FINE FRESH RIVER.'

Charles Dickens, *Little Dorrit*, 1857

F or many years, London, which in 1801 had a population approaching 1 million, had struggled with the system of sewage disposal inherited from medieval times. Cesspools were emptied by nightsoilmen, who sold the contents to farmers just outside the city. Public sewers in and beneath the streets were intended for the disposal of rainwater, although garbage, including butchers' offal, was surreptitiously dumped in them and the kennels, as had been observed during the reign of Edward III. Nevertheless, the Thames was a reasonably clean river and salmon – the litmus test of water quality – were still being caught in the first decades of the 19th century. But three factors now combined to interrupt these arrangements. First, London grew and the countryside moved farther away. Moorfields and Spitalfields ceased to be fields by the end of the 18th century, so the nightsoilmen had to carry their sewage a greater distance. Secondly, from 1847, a more effective fertilizer became available in the form of guano (solidified bird droppings), imported from islands off the coast of Chile. The Gibbs family used the enormous fortune they earned from the trade to build Tyntesfield, now a National Trust property in Somerset. The nightsoilmen struggled to compete.

FIG. 1   **THE RIVERDALE ENGINE AT MORELANDS PUMPING STATION** — LONDON, UK. THE PUMPING STATION WAS BUILT BY THE SOUTHWARK & VAUXHALL WATER CO. TO PUMP WATER FROM THE THAMES AT MOLESEY LOCK TO DISTANT RESERVOIRS.

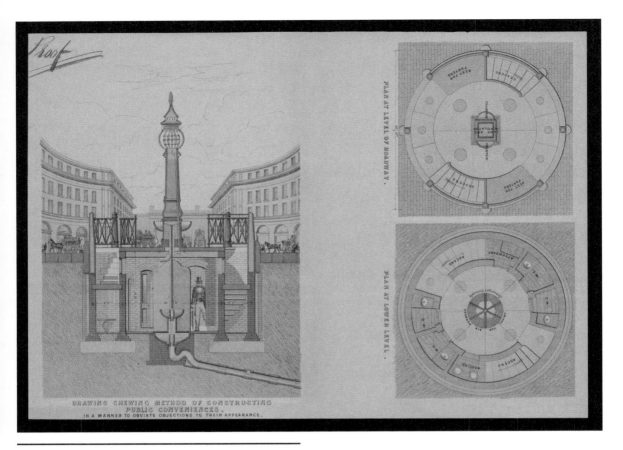

FIG. 2   1858 **JENNINGS' PUBLIC TOILET DESIGN** — LONDON, UK.
GEORGE JENNINGS PROPOSED THIS DESIGN TO THE CITY OF LONDON.
ALTHOUGH IT WAS NOT IMPLEMENTED, LONDON'S FIRST PUBLIC
TOILETS EVENTUALLY ESTABLISHED IN 1885 DID USE MANY OF THESE
FEATURES – SUCH AS THE INNER RING OF URINALS AND THE GAS
LAMP ABOVE GROUND TO PROVIDE A DRAUGHT FOR VENTILATION.

But the most decisive factor was the introduction of the water closet, whose invention, by Sir John Harington, is described on page 53. In 1775, a patent was registered by a Bond Street watchmaker named Alexander Cummings (1733–1814) for an improved version of Harington's device. In 1778, a Yorkshire-born carpenter and inventor called Joseph Bramah (1748–1814) was asked to install one of the closets in a private home and realized that he could improve the design further and simplify the process by which its components were manufactured. He patented his version of the WC and started to make them in large quantities. He had made and sold over 6,000 closets by 1797 and his company continued to flourish until 1890. A Victorian businessman called Thomas Crapper (1836–1910) started a competitive business in Chelsea in 1861 and nine years later opened a showroom to display his wares, which were advertised under the slogan 'A certain flush with every pull'. The business continued to operate from 120 King's Road, Chelsea until 1966 and still trades, dealing in sanitary fittings online. The products were of high quality, with many still in use – for example at a public house called The Parcel Yard adjacent to the Harry Potter Platform 9¾ at London's King's Cross station. In 1849,

Thomas Twyford (1849–1921) opened a factory for the production of sanitary ware in Stoke-on-Trent and in 1883 began to manufacture the 'Unitas' ceramic closet for export to the world. To this day the word 'unitas' in Russian means 'toilet'. The WC was one of Britain's great gifts to civilization.

But the greatest ingenuity of all was shown by George Jennings (1810–82), who was born in Hampshire and joined the plumbing business of his uncle in Southampton. He is remembered for his enterprise in installing WCs in the Crystal Palace, which housed the Great Exhibition of 1851.

○———————➤ 106

'NO ONE CAN DENY THE GREAT BENEFIT THAT HAS ARISEN FROM THE MAIN DRAINAGE WORKS. THE DISCHARGE OF THE SEWAGE INTO THE RIVER WITHIN THE HEART OF LONDON HAD BECOME INTOLERABLE, AND ITS INTERCEPTION HAS EXERCISED A POWERFUL INFLUENCE IN IMPROVING THE GENERAL HEALTH OF THE METROPOLIS. FOR THE SYSTEM HAS NOT ONLY REMOVED AN OFFENSIVE AND DELETERIOUS ELEMENT FROM THE MOST POPULOUS PART OF LONDON, BUT HAS ALSO PROMOTED GENERAL SALUBRITY.'

Joseph Bazalgette's obituary from the Institution of Civil Engineers (1891)

FIG. 3 **THOMAS CRAPPER'S MARLBOROUGH STREET WORKS IN CHELSEA** — LONDON, UK. THOMAS CRAPPER HIMSELF IS ALLEGEDLY AMONG THE GROUP STANDING OUTSIDE THE WORKS.

FIG. 4 1900 **TWYFORD WORKS** — STOKE-ON-TRENT, UK. THE COMPANY'S CLIFF VALE WORKS, BUILT IN 1887, WERE IDEALLY SITUATED BETWEEN THE TRENT AND MERSEY CANAL, THE RAILWAY AND A MAIN ROAD.

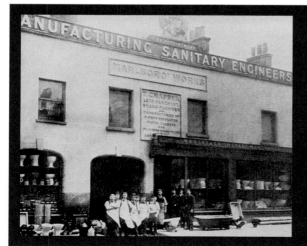

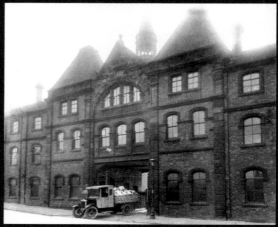

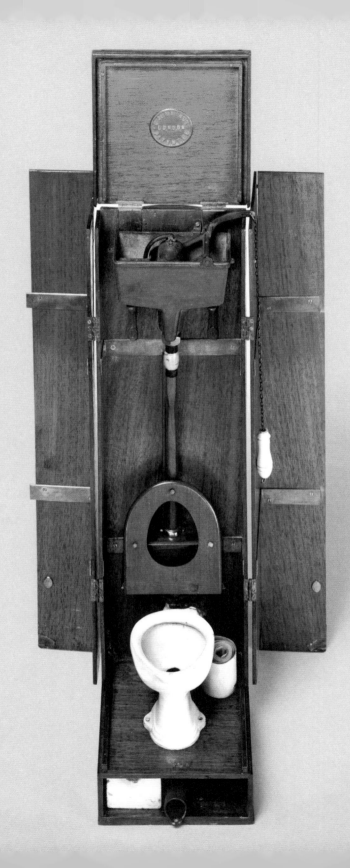

FIG. 5 ↓   1895–1905 **SALES MODEL OF JENNINGS' TOILET** — THIS DESIGN WAS USED IN THE PUBLIC CONVENIENCES AT THE GREAT EXHIBITION OF 1851.

FIGS. 6–11 ↓↓   1894 **TWYFORD'S CATALOGUE** — TWYFORD'S OFFER A SELECTION OF FLUSHING TOILETS IN EARTHENWARE AND PORCELAIN, AND AVAILABLE IN A VARIETY OF DECORATIVE DESIGNS.

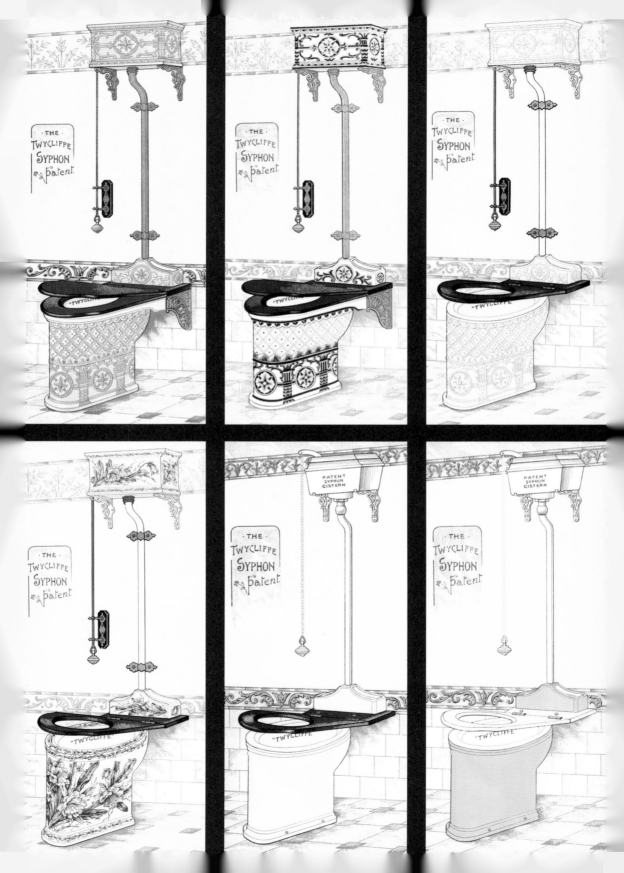

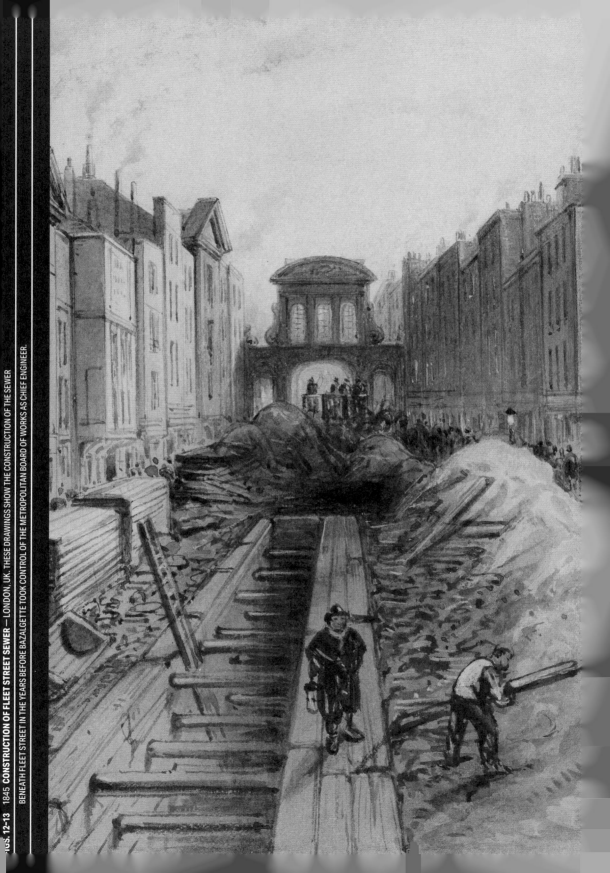

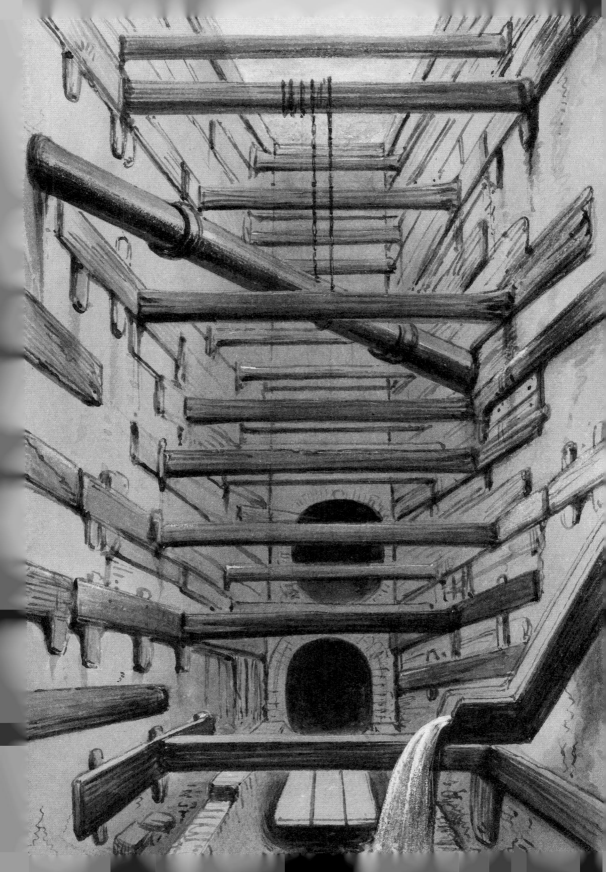

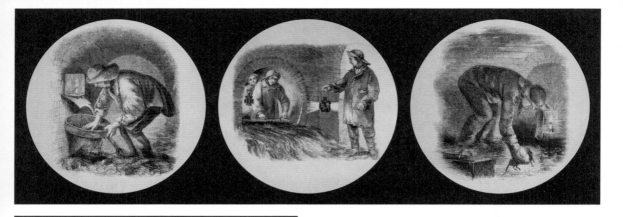

FIGS. 14–16 1851 **MAYHEW'S LONDON** — LONDON, UK. PRIOR TO BAZALGETTE'S WORKS IT WAS MUCH EASIER TO ENTER THE SEWERS. IN *LONDON LABOUR AND THE LONDON POOR*, MAYHEW IDENTIFIES A HOST OF CHARACTERS THAT COULD BE DISCOVERED THERE. HERE ARE ILLUSTRATED THE SEWER HUNTER, WHO SEARCHED FOR COINS AND JEWELLERY, THE RAT CATCHER AND THE SEWER WORKERS EMPLOYED IN FLUSHING THE SEWERS.

Some 827,000 people used these conveniences, many experiencing them for the first time, and each paying one penny for the privilege. This gave us the expression 'spend a penny' and effectively drew attention to the advantages of the devices. But water closets have one major disadvantage when used in conjunction with cesspools. When flushed, they discharged a small amount of faeces and urine, potential fertilizer, and 8 litres (2 gallons) or more of water, rapidly filling the cesspools with liquid that farmers did not wish to buy and which leaked.

It was these conditions, to which Michael Faraday drew attention in 1855, that led to the creation of the Metropolitan Board of Works who began work the following year. The board replaced a multitude of parish vestries, liberties, commissions and similar bodies that had come into existence over centuries. Their aims had been twofold: to spend as little ratepayers' money as they could and to despatch their sewage to the adjacent parish as quickly as possible. Sizes and shapes of sewers were not coordinated and the arrangement was particularly unfortunate for those parishes that were situated in the low-lying parts of London, close to the Thames, where everyone's waste accumulated before entering the river. The Metropolitan Board of Works was the first body established for London as a whole, with authority to construct roads, bridges and parks but above all street drains and intercepting sewers or 'collectors'.

In 1856 Joseph Bazalgette was appointed Chief Engineer to the Metropolitan Board of Works. He was born in England, but was descended from a French grandfather who had arrived in England in the 1770s. He learned engineering, as most did at those times, by being an articled pupil, in his case to Sir John MacNeill (1793–1880) who gave him his first experience of drainage by employing him on land drainage schemes in Northern Ireland. He also worked on railway proposals, which gave him experience in dealing with politicians and he became a member of the Institution of Civil Engineers in 1838. When applying for the post of the Metropolitan Board of Works' chief engineer, his referees were Robert Stephenson (1803–59), designer of *The Rocket*, and Isambard Kingdom Brunel (1806–59).

Bazalgette's was not the first such appointment. In May 1847, James Newlands (1813–71) had been appointed as the first borough engineer in Britain to prepare a comprehensive sewerage plan for the troubled, disease-ridden city of Liverpool, whose population had been swelled by impoverished Irish fleeing the potato famine and who were living in conditions of inconceivable squalor, in flooded cellars without sanitation. Liverpool was at that time the most populous city in Britain beyond London, with a population approaching 400,000. The appointment of Newlands had been preceded, in January of the same year, by the appointment of Dr William Henry Duncan (1805–63) as Britain's first Medical Officer of Health. Together, the two men campaigned, with eventual success, for the construction of sewers and clearance of cellars, which meant that when cholera returned to Britain in 1854 its effects were far less virulent than previous epidemics. Newlands has a claim to have been the first engineer to introduce egg-shaped sewers (sometimes referred to as 'English sewers'), designed to concentrate the liquid in a narrow channel during times of low flow levels. This speeds the movement of the water and the solids it carries, though even the Cloaca Maxima, the ancestor of all large sewers, was higher than it was wide. During the Crimean War, James Newlands was sent to the Crimea as Sanitary Commissioner, earning from Florence Nightingale the accolade: 'Truly I may say that to us 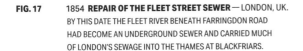 110

110

FIG. 17   1854 **REPAIR OF THE FLEET STREET SEWER** — LONDON, UK.
BY THIS DATE THE FLEET RIVER BENEATH FARRINGDON ROAD
HAD BECOME AN UNDERGROUND SEWER AND CARRIED MUCH
OF LONDON'S SEWAGE INTO THE THAMES AT BLACKFRIARS.

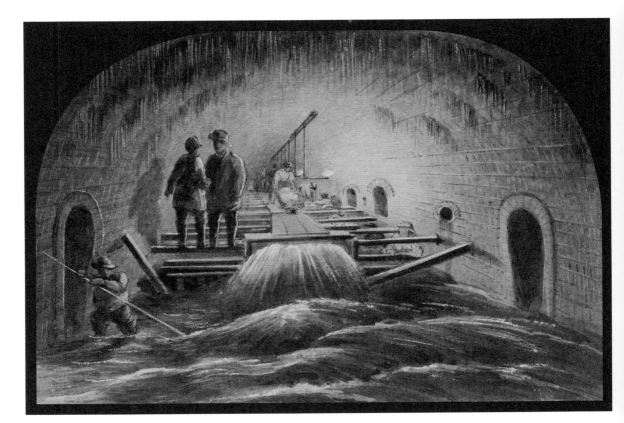

LONDON

LIMEKILN DOCK SEWER

SAVOY STREET SEWER

REGENT STREET SEWER

RANELACH SEWER MAIN

SECTIONS ADOPTED BY THE METROPOLITAN SEWERAGE COMMISSIONERS

Nº 6 Nº 5 Nº 4 Nº 3 Nº 2 Nº 1

SEWER SECTIONS

KING'S SCHOLARS' POND SEWER

LONSDALE SQUARE BRANCH

CITY ROAD BRANCH

DIFFERENT SECTIONS

EXAMPLES OF THE DIFFERENT SHAPES AND DESIGNS OF SEWERS THAT BAZALGETTE INHERITED AND WHICH HE HAD TO INCORPORATE INTO HIS DESIGN FOR A COMPREHENSIVE SYSTEM. TO COLLECT ALL OF LONDON'S SEWAGE AND CONVEY IT TO TREATMENT WORKS AT BECKTON AND CROSSNESS. IT IS INTERESTING TO NOTE THAT ONE SEWER COULD INCORPORATE MULTIPLE DIFFERENT SHAPES THROUGHOUT ITS COURSE, AS DIFFERENT DESIGNS WERE FAVOURABLE TO DIFFERENT LEVELS OF FLOW.

FROM SECTIONS PUBLISHED BY **THE METROPOLITAN BOARD OF WORKS**
J. W. BAZALGATTE, CHIEF ENGINEER, 1857

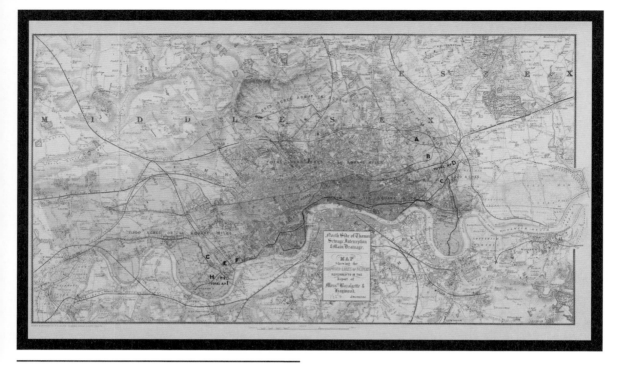

FIG. 18 1854 **PROPOSED LONDON SEWERS** — LONDON, UK.
A PROPOSAL BY JOSEPH BAZALGETTE AND WILLIAM HAYWOOD
FOR THE ESTABLISHMENT OF A NETWORK OF SEWERS ON
THE NORTH SIDE OF THE THAMES.

sanitary salvation came from Liverpool.' Dr Duncan is remembered in Liverpool by a pub named
'Dr Duncan' in his honour in the city centre and a special brew called 'Dr Duncan's IPA'.

Bazalgette set to work without delay. He knew the task ahead of him, as he had previously been
employed by one of the commissions that had done some preparatory work and built some new
street sewers. By June 1856, he was able to submit his plans, a system of intercepting sewers running
parallel to the river. On the north side of the river, he proposed that the sewage was taken mostly
by gravity to Abbey Mills, near West Ham, before being lifted by huge pumping engines into outfall
sewers that took it on to Beckton in Essex for discharge at high tide. On the south side it would be
taken to Crossness, in Kent, where the largest beam engines ever built could lift it into reservoirs
where it was discharged into the river before beginning its voyage to the North Sea.

The legislation setting up the Metropolitan Board of Works required that Bazalgette submit his
designs to the Chief Commissioner of Works, a government minister who had to approve the plans
before work could start. This was Sir Benjamin Hall (1802–67). Hall was himself a civil engineer
who was preoccupied with the rebuilding of the Houses of Parliament on the banks of the Thames
following the disastrous fire of 1834 that had destroyed most of the buildings while preserving
Westminster Hall itself. He was a tall man and is a strong contender for the honour of having given
his name to the bell that sounds the hours in the Parliamentary clock, 'Big Ben'. Hall needed to
be reassured that Bazalgette's system offered enough capacity to deal with the waste of London;

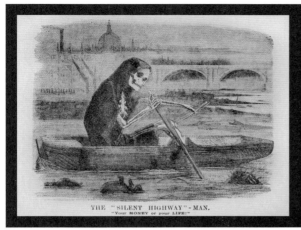

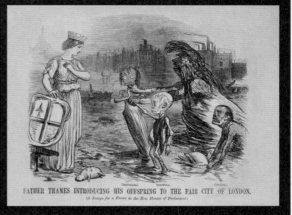

FIG. 19   1858 **'THE "SILENT HIGHWAY" MAN'** — LONDON, UK.
PUBLISHED IN *PUNCH* MAGAZINE ON 10 JULY 1858 DURING
'THE GREAT STINK', THIS CARTOON BY JOHN LEECH SHOWS
THE ALLEGORICAL FIGURE OF DEATH ROWING A BOAT ON
THE POLLUTED RIVER THAMES AS DEAD ANIMALS FLOAT BY.

FIG. 20   1858 **'FATHER THAMES INTRODUCING HIS OFFSPRING
TO THE FAIR CITY OF LONDON'** — LONDON, UK. PUBLISHED IN
PUNCH ON 3 JULY 1858, THIS CARTOON DEPICTS THE DISEASES
OF DIPTHERIA, SCROFULA AND CHOLERA EMERGING FROM THE
THAMES. IN FACT, ONLY CHOLERA IS A WATERBORNE DISEASE.

most importantly, he needed to be persuaded that it would be discharged into the river so far downstream that it would not return to the city on a very high tide. To that end, he engaged two eminent water engineers, James Simpson (1799–1869) and Douglas Galton (1822–99), to examine Bazalgette's calculations. Their opinion was equivocal. Experiments that they undertook with floats suggested that in certain exceptional conditions the sewage could make its way back to Westminster. Hall did not wish to go down in history as the man who, having supervised the reconstruction of the Palace of Westminster, had also authorised sewage works that would poison its atmosphere. Select committees deliberated, engineers pondered and cesspools continued to leak into the soil and river. Bazalgette estimated the additional cost of moving the outfalls beyond his proposed sites at Beckton in Essex on the north bank and Crossness in Kent on the south bank. There followed a suggestion that since the capital's sewage was 'an imperial matter' the cost should be paid by the British Empire, not just by the citizens of the metropolis. This did not long survive the objections of communities beyond London and was unceremoniously abandoned.

There the matter stood until the log-jam was broken by a force of nature. The summer of 1858, three years after the publication of Michael Faraday's letter to *The Times* on the state of the Thames, delivered the hot, dry summer that he had foreseen. Debates in Parliament now took over and on 7 June 1858, *Hansard* reported that 'It was a notorious fact that Hon. Gentlemen sitting in the Committee Rooms and the Library were utterly unable to remain there in consequence of the stench which arose from the river.' Even soaking the curtains of the Palace of Westminster in chloride of lime did little to mask the smell. It is essential to remember that most well-informed people, including MPs, were adherents of the 'miasmatic' theory of disease propagation, which held that germs were spread by foul air, not polluted water. We now know this to be a mistaken view, but it worked for Bazalgette. Fearful that Members of Parliament would be poisoned by the foul stench, a Bill was introduced by Prime Minister Disraeli (who referred to the river as 'That Stygian pool'), which removed Hall's veto, and authorised Bazalgette to start work immediately. The Bill also enabled HM Treasury to underwrite any sums raised by the Metropolitan Board to build the sewers which enabled money to be borrowed at low interest rates.

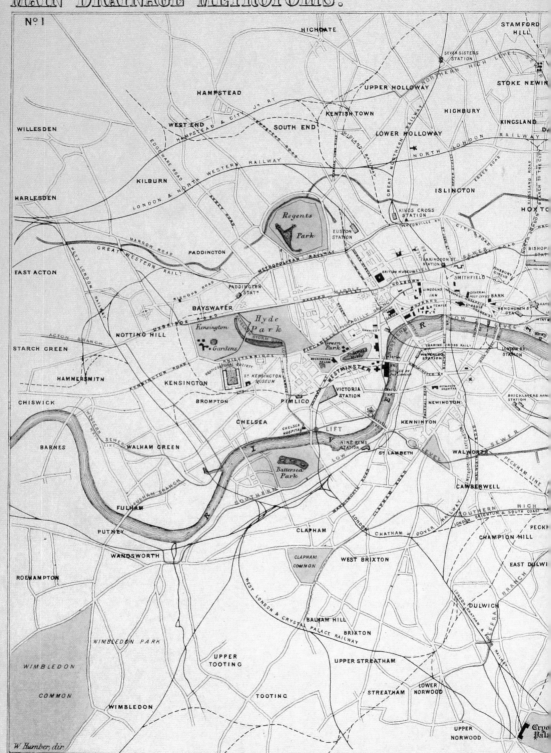

MAIN DRAINAGE METROPOLIS.

Nº 1

W. Humber, dir.

London: Lockwo

WANSTEAD

LEYTON-STONE

LOW LEYTON

...TON

APTON

GREAT EASTERN RAILWAY (CAMBRIDGE LINE)

HOMERTON

HACKNEY WICK

HACKNEY

Victoria Park

OLD FORD

STRATFORD

ILFORD

(COLCHESTER LINE)

LITTLE ILFORD

GREAT EASTERN RAILWAY

ESSEX ROAD

TILBURY FORT & SOUTEND Ry

River Roding

BARKING

TILBURY & SOUTHEND Ry

LIFT ABBEY MILLS

BOW

GREAT EASTERN RAILY

STEPNEY

LIMEHOUSE

...CIAL ROAD

...L RAILWAY

BROMLEY

WEST HAM

ISLE OF DOGS BRANCH

PLAISTOW

EAST HAM

ABBEY MARSH

NORTHERN OUTFALL SEWER

EAST HAM LEVEL

Barking Level

BARKING CREEK

RESERVOIR

LONDON BARKING & TILBURY RAILWAY

NORTH WOOLWICH RAILWAY

PLAISTOW MARSH

POPLAR

WEST INDIA DOCKS

COMMERCIAL DOCKS

...THE

...DSEY

...BRANCH

DEPTFORD

ISLE OF DOGS

Greenwich Marshes

VICTORIA DOCKS

THAMES

NORTH WOOLWICH

PLUMSTEAD MARSH.

ORDNANCE

CROSSNESS GROUND LIFT & RESERVOIR

ARTILLERY PRACTICE GROUND

NEW CHARLTON OUTFALL

ROYAL ARSENAL

SOUTHERN OUTFALL SEWER

NORTH KENT RAILWAY

GREENWICH

LIFT

Greenwich Park

WOOLWICH

Barrack Field

CHARLTON

PLUMSTEAD

PLUMSTEAD MARSH

ABBEY WOOD

NEW CROSS

SEWER

BLACKHEATH

UPPER KIDBROOKE

LOWER KIDBROOKE

WOOLWICH COMMON

SHOOTERS HILL

LONDON BRIGHTON & SOUTH COAST RAILWAY

MID KENT RAILWAY

GREENWICH LINE

D. & D. Ry

LEE

LEWISHAM

BROCKLEY

BUSHEY GREEN

BELL GREEN

SOUTH END

...OWER ...DENHAM

MAP
SHEWING THE LINES OF
MAIN INTERCEPTING SEWERS,
OF THE
METROPOLIS.

Scale of Miles.

Mile 1   ¾   ½   ¼   0   1   2   3 Miles

Standidge & Co. Litho. 36, Old Jewry E.C.

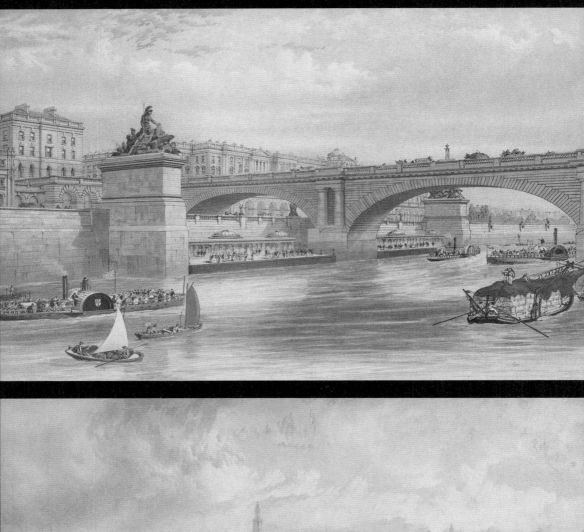

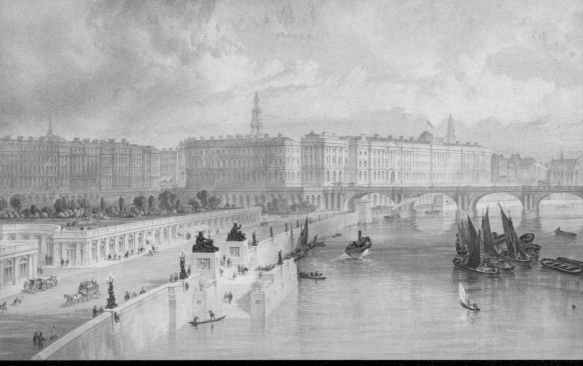

FIGS. 22–25 1863 **PROPOSAL DRAWINGS FOR THE DEVELOPMENT OF THE EMBANKMENT** — LONDON, UK.

BAZALGETTE SUBMITTED THESE PROPOSED PIERS TO THE METROPOLITAN BOARD OF WORKS.

DESPITE THEIR EVIDENT BEAUTY, THE PLANS WERE SCALED BACK DUE TO COSTS.

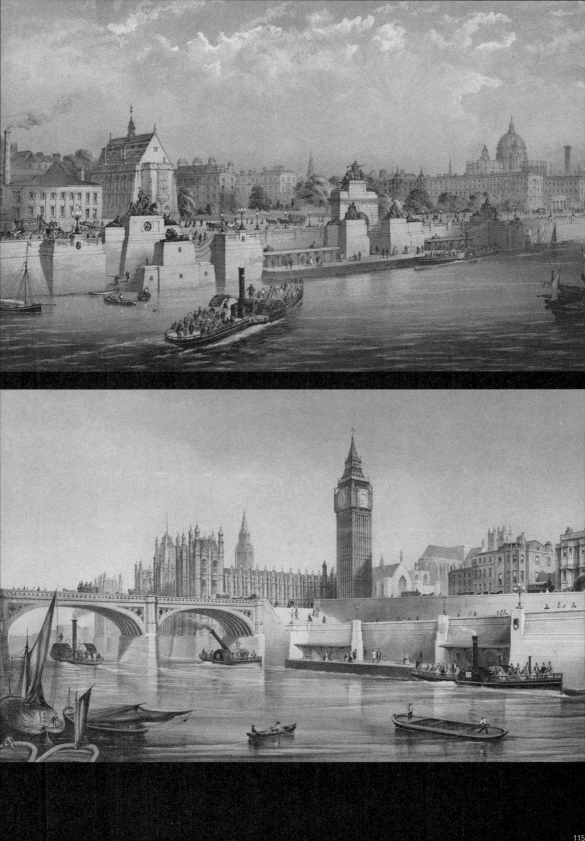

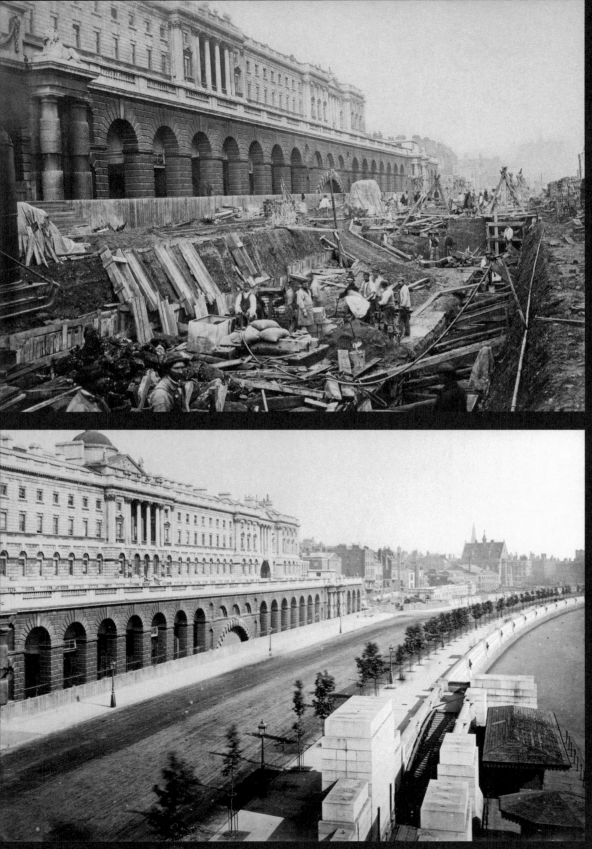

Work began in January 1859 and by 1865 the sewers serving the less populous South Bank were completed, as was the treatment works at Crossness near Abbey Wood in Kent. The official opening of Crossness took place on 4 April 1865 and was performed by Albert Edward the Prince of Wales in the presence of two archbishops, other members of the royal family, MPs and numerous other dignitaries. One of the four great beam engines that lifted the sewage was named after the Prince and switched on by him, the three others bearing the names of other members of the royal family: Queen Victoria, Albert the Prince Consort and the Prince of Wales's wife Alexandra of Denmark. From that time there were no further cholera epidemics south of the river. The pumping station at Crossness has been carefully restored by teams of volunteers working over the past thirty years; one of the great beam engines, 'Prince Consort', has been returned to working order and is opened to the public on 'steaming days', which are advertised on its website. The pumping station, and beam engine (which have now been replaced by modern equipment) are unsurpassed examples of Victorian engineering in its prime. Moreover their lavish use of highly coloured wrought iron is testament to the importance the Victorians attached to the design of public works, as both the pumping stations were in relatively isolated places, their magnificent designs only to be seen by sewage workers. And they are not unique. A similar example is to be found at Leicester City's Museum of Science and Technology and the Cambridge Museum of Technology, both of them – like Crossness – in former sewage pumping stations.

The task north of the river was more complex, since the area was particularly densely populated and digging up busy streets to build huge sewers was unlikely to be acceptable. Bazalgette solved the greatest problem of all, the route for the low level sewer on the north bank of the Thames, by reclaiming almost 16 hectares (40 acres) of land from the Thames to build the Victoria Embankment, running from Westminster Bridge to Blackfriars, with Queen Victoria Street built to complete the link from Westminster to the Bank of England in the heart of the city. The Embankment thus had the further benefits of providing an additional road link between Westminster and the city and a means by which the underground Metropolitan District Railway (now the District Line) could pass from Blackfriars to Westminster. Finally, it also enabled him to create Victoria Embankment Gardens, a much-needed green space in the heart of Westminster. An impression of the scale of the works can even now be gained by standing in these gardens at York Watergate, at the bottom of Buckingham Street, and reflecting that until the 1860s, before the Victoria Embankment was completed, the Dukes of York and Buckingham would step from the Watergate on to their barges. The Watergate is now about 100 metres (328 ft) from the river, which is thus much narrower and faster flowing. The opening of the Embankment was itself a great event, carried out by the Prince of Wales (Queen Victoria had a headache) and attended by royalty, twenty-four ambassadors, virtually all Members of both Houses of Parliament and 10,000 ticket holders who were entertained by the bands of the Grenadier and Coldstream Guards.

Another great challenge was the completion of the northern sewers between Abbey Mills, in West Ham and Beckton. Having been conveyed, mostly by gravity, to Abbey Mills, the sewage was lifted 10.9 m (36 ft) there by pumps into the outfall sewers, which took it across 8 km (5 miles) of marshy

○———————➤ 122

FIGS. 26–27 **CONSTRUCTION OF THE VICTORIA EMBANKMENT** —
LONDON, UK. SOMERSET HOUSE, ORIGINALLY BUILT
ON THE RIVERSIDE, BECAME SET BACK FROM THE THAMES
WITH THE CONSTRUCTION OF THE VICTORIA EMBANKMENT.

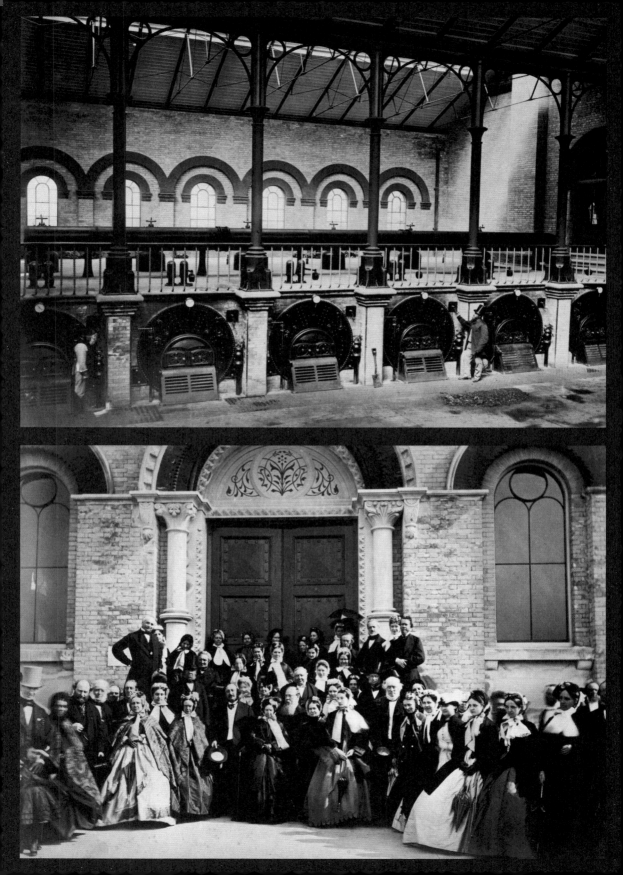

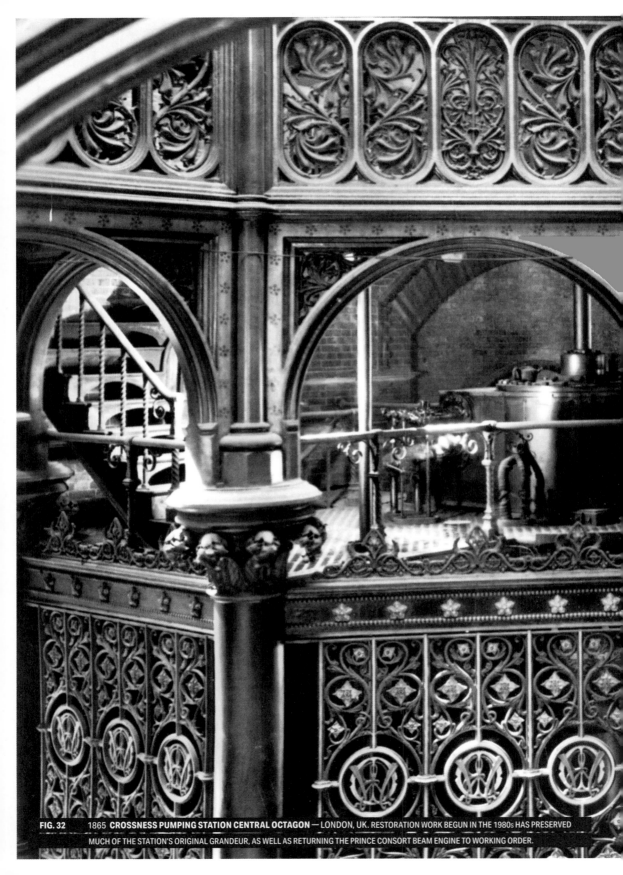

FIG. 32 1865 **CROSSNESS PUMPING STATION CENTRAL OCTAGON** — LONDON, UK. RESTORATION WORK BEGUN IN THE 1980s HAS PRESERVED MUCH OF THE STATION'S ORIGINAL GRANDEUR, AS WELL AS RETURNING THE PRINCE CONSORT BEAM ENGINE TO WORKING ORDER.

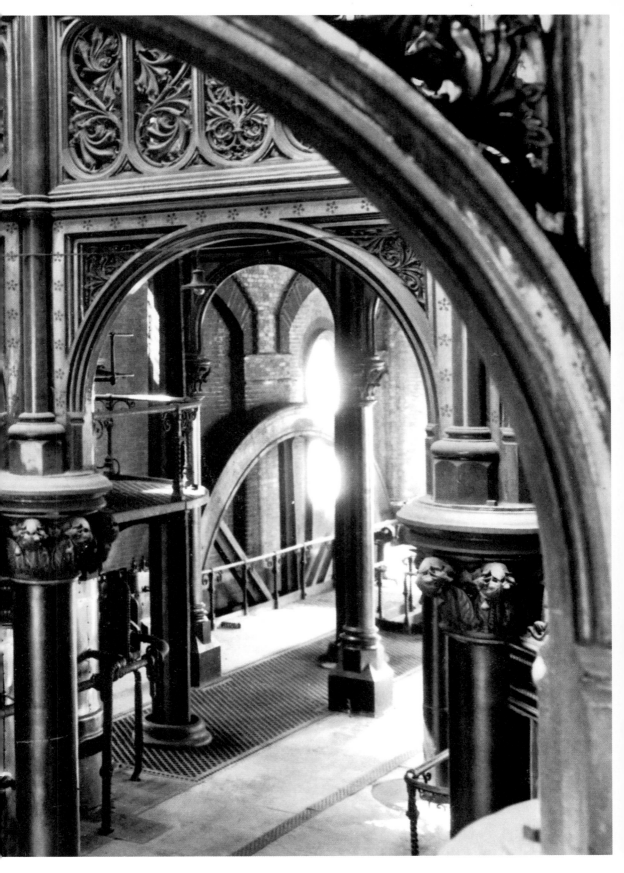

ground, intersected by roads and railways, to the treatment works at Beckton. Massive embankments were built to traverse the unstable terrain, two railway lines had to be lowered and five roads had to be raised 19–52 m (6–16 ft) to enable the outfall sewers to pass over the railways and beneath the roads while maintaining a steady downward gradient. A temporary concrete works was built at Beckton and a temporary railway conveyed the material to Abbey Mills when the construction began. As the sewers advanced the railway retreated until the sewers reached Beckton, the temporary structures were dismantled and taken for use elsewhere.

In the summer of 1866, London suffered its last cholera epidemic, costing 5,596 lives, in about 3 sq km (1 sq mile) of Whitechapel. This was the only part of Bazalgette's system that was not complete and it is hard to imagine how great would have been the death toll if the rest of the city had been lacking sewers. Bazalgette wrote that:

FIGS. 33–35 1867 **DRAWINGS OF ABBEY MILLS PUMPING STATION.**
BAZALGETTE'S ORNATE AND DETAILED DESIGN FOR ONE PUMPING STATION WAS FEATURED WITH AN EXPLANATORY ARTICLE IN THE *ENGINEER* MAGAZINE. THE REPORTER FOR THE JOURNAL PRAISED THE DESIGN AS AN EXAMPLE OF 'HIGH ART IN ENGINEERING'.

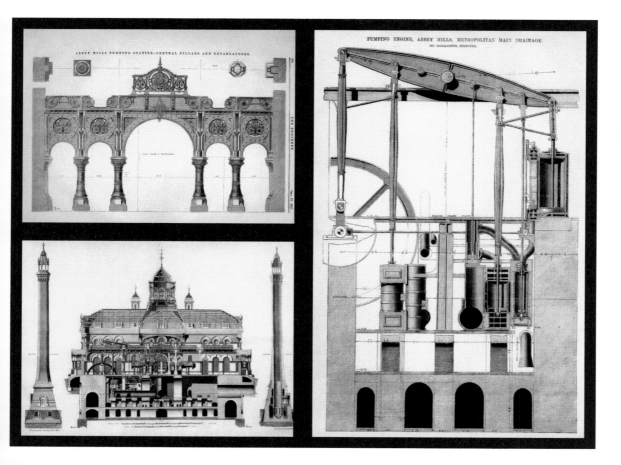

It is unfortunately just the locality where our main drainage works are not complete. The low-level sewer is constructed through the locality but the pumping station at Abbey Mills will not be completed until next summer. I shall recommend the Board to erect a temporary pumping station at Abbey Mills to lift the sewage of this district into the Northern Outfall Sewer. This can be accomplished in about three weeks.

The temporary pumping station was erected, the sewage removed from the water supply and conveyed to Beckton and the cholera outbreak subsided. In 1868, the new, permanent pumping station was opened at Abbey Mills, near West Ham, where it still serves the capital. In 1892 London braced itself for another epidemic as cholera gripped Hamburg, one of London's principal trading partners, but none occurred. In England, 132 deaths were reported in 64 towns, 17 of the deaths in London, probably amongst people who had contracted the disease abroad. Bazalgette had died the previous year, his legacy being a system of sewers that protected London's water supply.

FIG. 36   1891 **MAP FEATURING THE NORTHERN OUTFALL SEWER** —
LONDON, UK. THIS MAP SHOWS THE NORTHERN OUTFALL
SEWER REACHING BECKTON SEWAGE TREATMENT WORKS,
AT GALLIONS REACH, WHERE WASTE WATER WAS DISCHARGED
INTO THE THAMES AT HIGH TIDE.

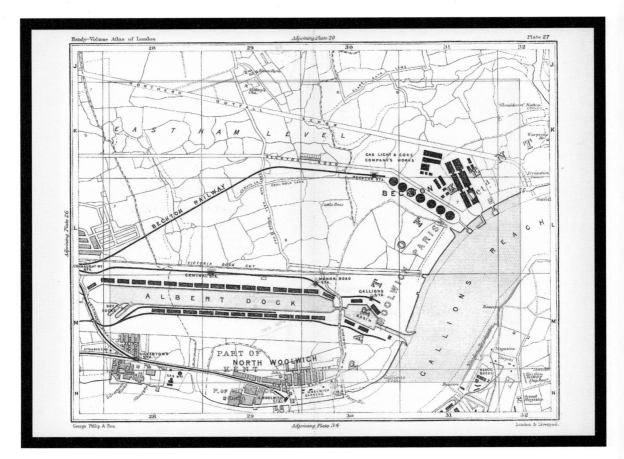

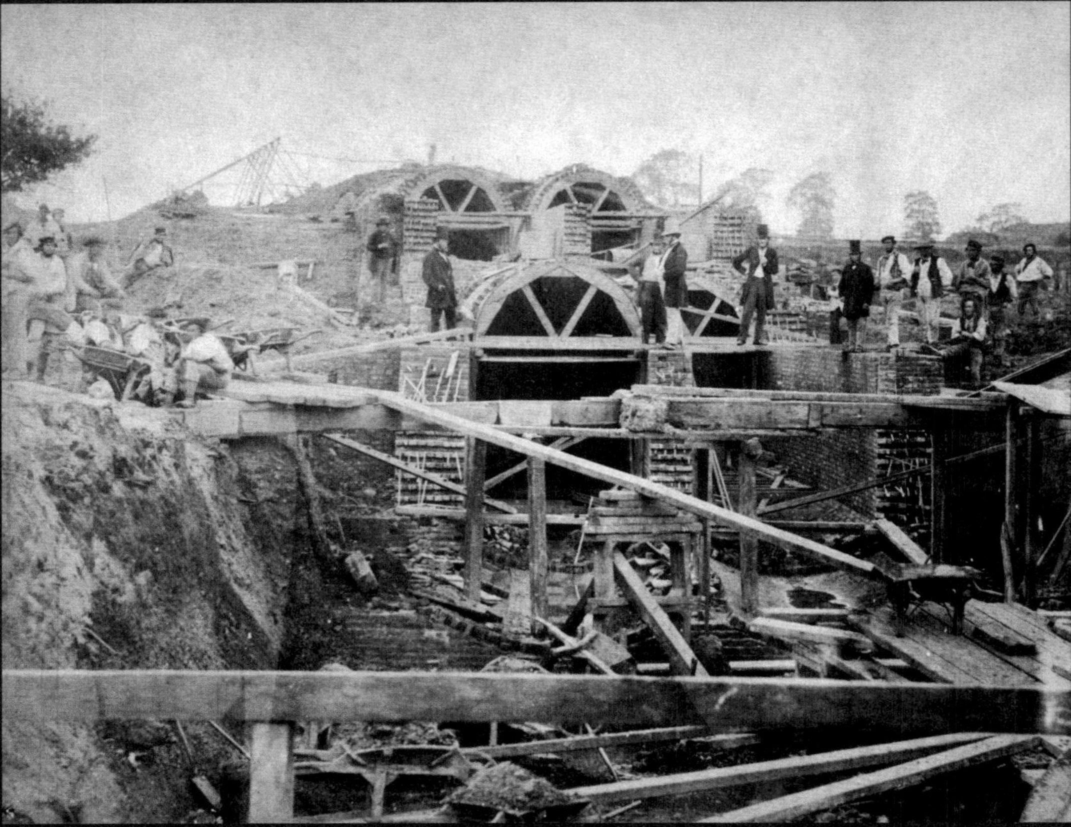

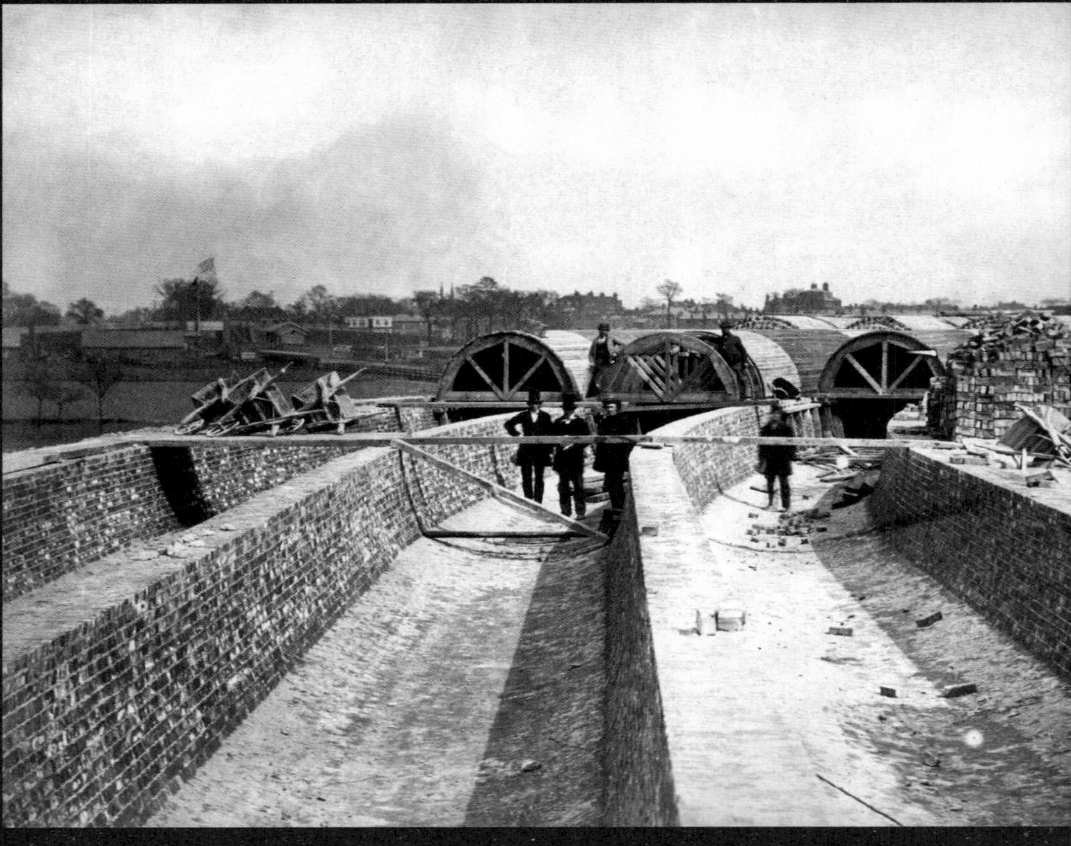

FIGS. 37–40 CONSTRUCTION OF THE NORTHERN OUTFALL SEWER — LONDON, UK. RUNNING 8 KM (5 MILES) FROM ABBEY MILLS PUMPING STATION

TO BECKTON TREATMENT WORKS, THE CONSTRUCTION INCLUDED THE LOWERING OF TWO RAILWAYS AND THE RAISING OF FIVE ROADS.

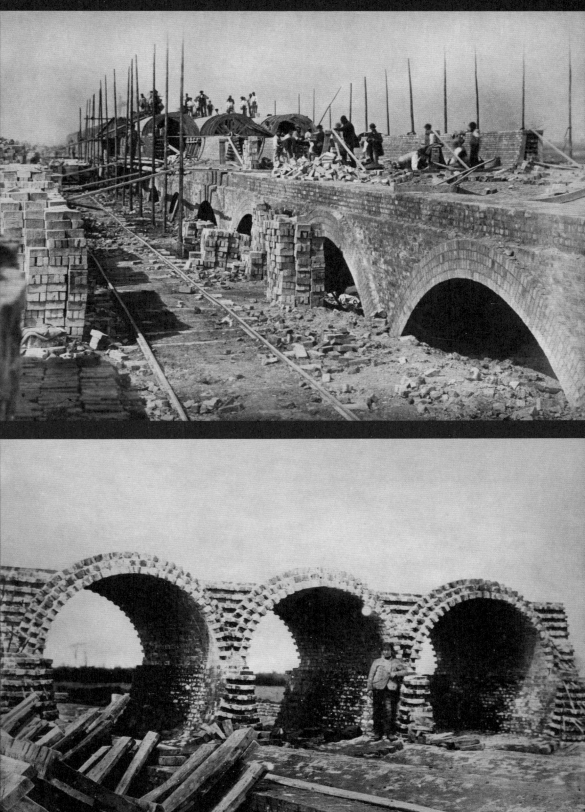

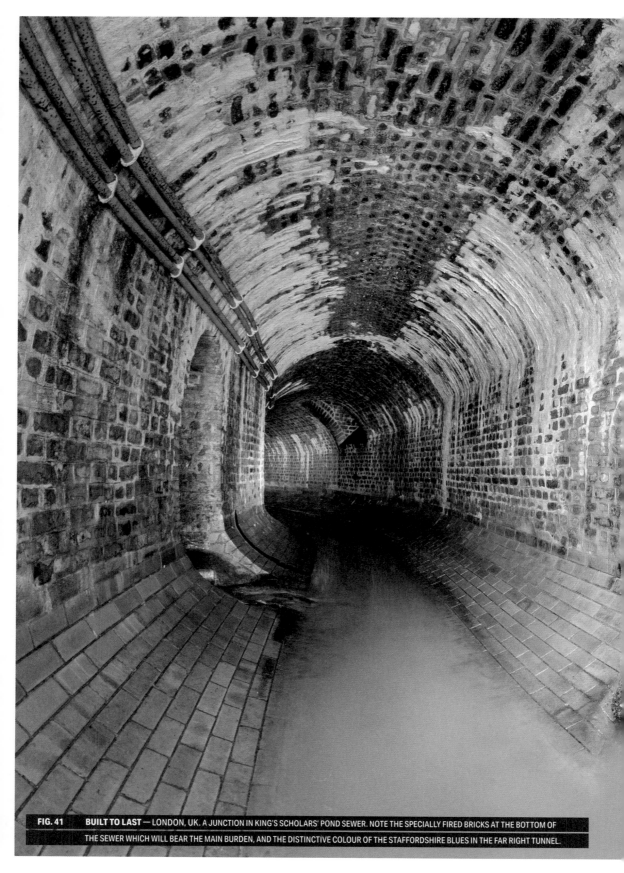

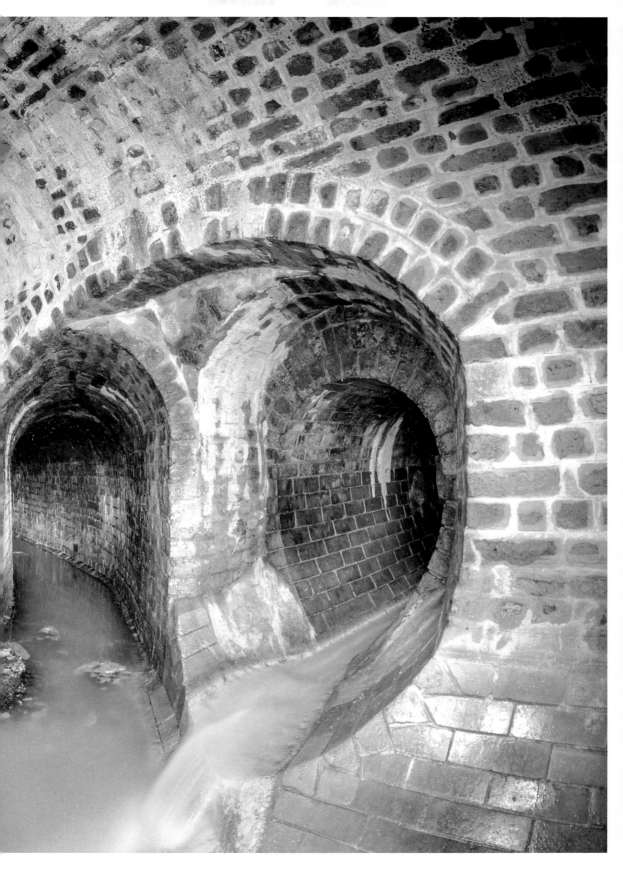

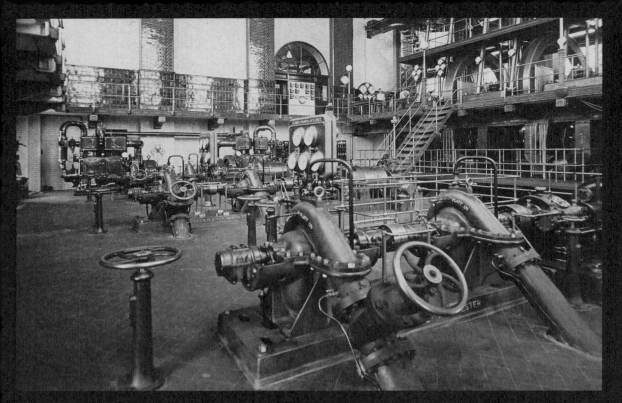

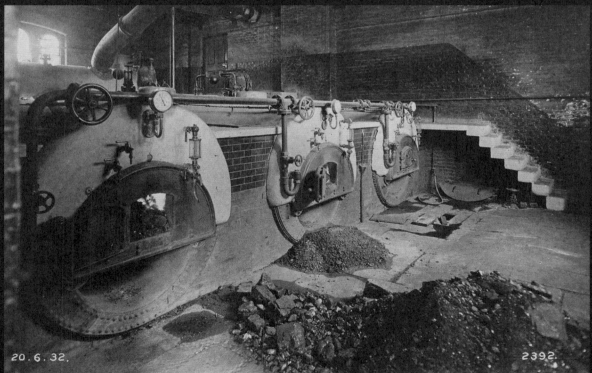

20.6.32.   2392.

FIGS. 42–43 DEPTFORD PUMPING STATION — LONDON, UK. THE PUMPING STATION AT DEPTFORD WAS BUILT TO RAISE
THE SEWAGE OF SOUTH LONDON INTO THE OUTFALL SEWER RUNNING THROUGH WOOLWICH TO CROSSNESS.

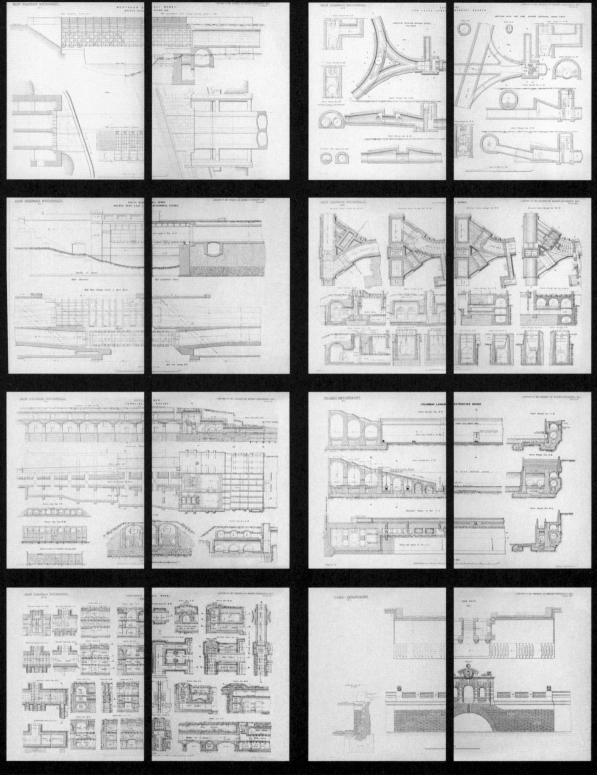

FIGS. 44–51 1865 **MAIN DRAINAGE OF THE METROPOLIS AND THE EMBANKMENT** — LONDON, UK. BAZALGETTE'S DESIGNS FOR THE

NORTHERN LOW LEVEL SEWER, THE LAST LINE OF DEFENCE FOR THE THAMES AS THE SEWER PASSES THROUGH VICTORIA EMBANKMENT.

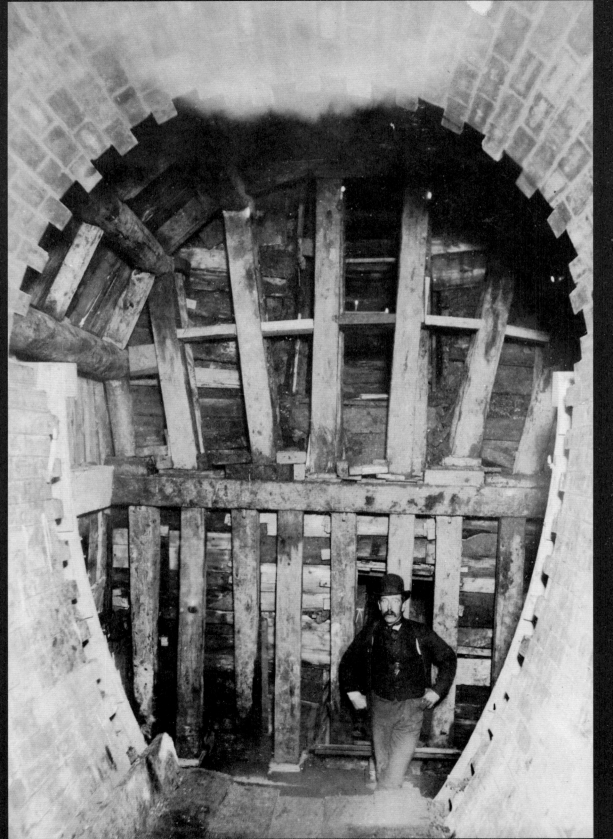

The cost of the whole enterprise was £4.2 million for the sewers and £2.4 million for the Embankments. Haussmann's less comprehensive system for Paris, a much smaller city, cost almost five times as much.

Bazalgette's sewers are a 'combined system', collecting both wastewater from premises and rainwater that falls on the streets. The flow of wastewater can be forecast with some accuracy, almost by the hour, as the engineers know when people will be awake and active and when commercial premises are at work. Rainfall is impossible to forecast in this way and is notoriously subject to peaks and troughs: a sudden summer storm can deposit a month's normal flow in a matter of hours. To accommodate every eventuality would require sewers of unrealistic size, so it was agreed that, on the rare occasions this happened, the sewers could deposit their surplus rain directly into the Thames. The first test of the system fell on 26 July 1867, when one-eighth of the average annual rainfall fell in nine hours. The system, not yet complete, coped. Modern sewerage systems, built in new towns and estates, are usually 'separate systems', in which wastewater and rainwater are collected in separate pipes. This reduces the volume of water going to the treatment works, which makes their job easier, and permits the relatively clean storm water to pass harmlessly into rivers and lakes.

The increasingly widespread belief that 'where there's muck there's brass [i.e. money]' (a phrase popularized in the north of England) meant that there was substantial pressure placed on Joseph Bazalgette to introduce a recycling scheme into his sewerage system so as not to waste such a major source of national wealth. Widespread enthusiasm for the idea was such that in 1860 *The Farmer's Magazine* rhapsodized that 'If the money value of our sewers could be shown to the British farmer in bright and glittering heaps of sovereigns he would gasp at the enormous wealth and make great efforts to obtain the treasure.' This led to an attempt in 1865 to introduce the plan of the Hon. William Napier and Lieutenant-Colonel William Hope, VC, (1834–1909) to send London's sewage to the Dengie Flats and Maplin Sands on the Essex Coast where it could render 81 sq km (20,000 acres) of land reclaimed from the sea fertile. However this fell through following the collapse of the Overend Gurney Bank. Schemes continued to be proposed however: in 1871 the Native Guano Company erected works at Crossness pumping station to manufacture manure, in the 1950s a small operation at the outfall at Barking, near Dagenham, dried and bagged sewage and sold it as 'Dagfert' (Dagenham fertilizer) and as recently as 1987 Thames Water established a pilot plant at its sewage treatment plant at Little Marlow in Buckinghamshire that sold a variety of fertilizers and growbags.

In 1878, a pleasure steamer, the *Princess Alice*, collided with the freighter *Bywell Castle*, causing the former to sink at the cost of many lives. The accident occurred close to Crossness at the time of discharge and it was suggested in some quarters that some fatalities had resulted from poisoning rather than drowning. By this date the areas around Crossness and Beckton had become residential rather than sites of heavy, often polluting, industries as in the past. After much procrastination, it was decided that in future the sewage from Beckton and Crossness, instead of being discharged direct to the 136

FIG. 52   1896 **A LOW-LEVEL DIVERSION SEWER** — LONDON, UK.
BAZALGETTE'S SYSTEM WAS EXPANDED AS LONDON CONTINUED TO
GROW, AND THIS TYPICALLY EGG-SHAPED SEWER WAS ADDED IN 1896.

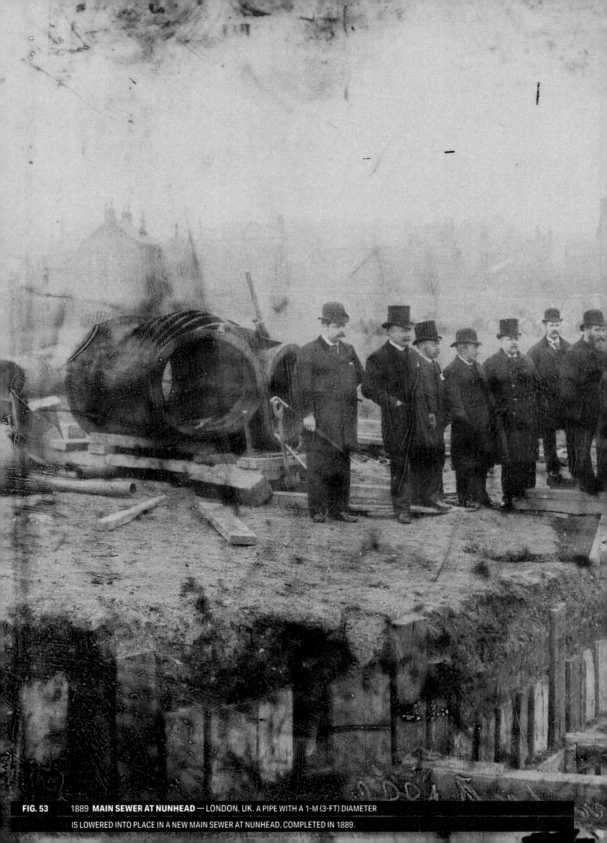

FIG. 53   1889 **MAIN SEWER AT NUNHEAD** — LONDON, UK. A PIPE WITH A 1-M (3-FT) DIAMETER IS LOWERED INTO PLACE IN A NEW MAIN SEWER AT NUNHEAD, COMPLETED IN 1889.

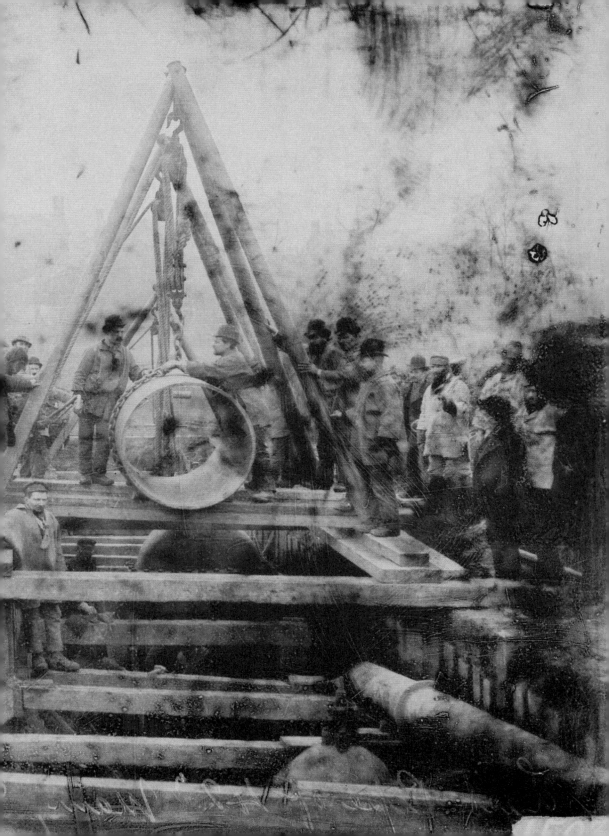

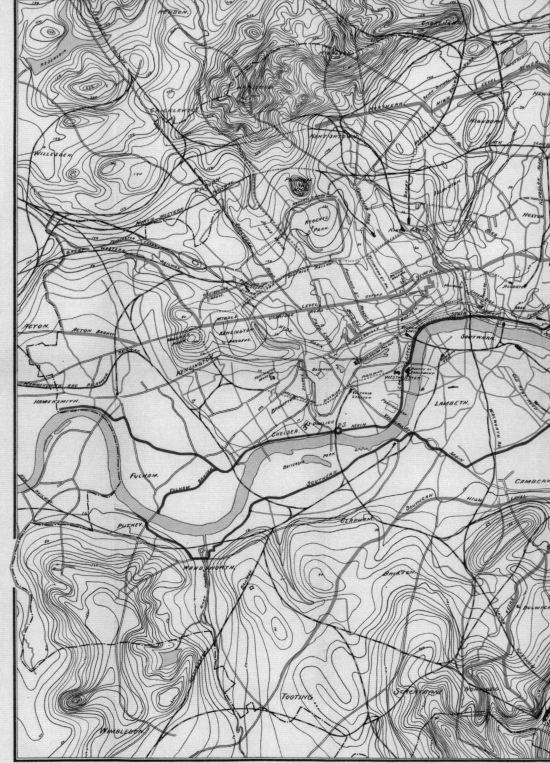

HOUSE EX. DOC. No. 43, 1st SESS., 47th CONG.

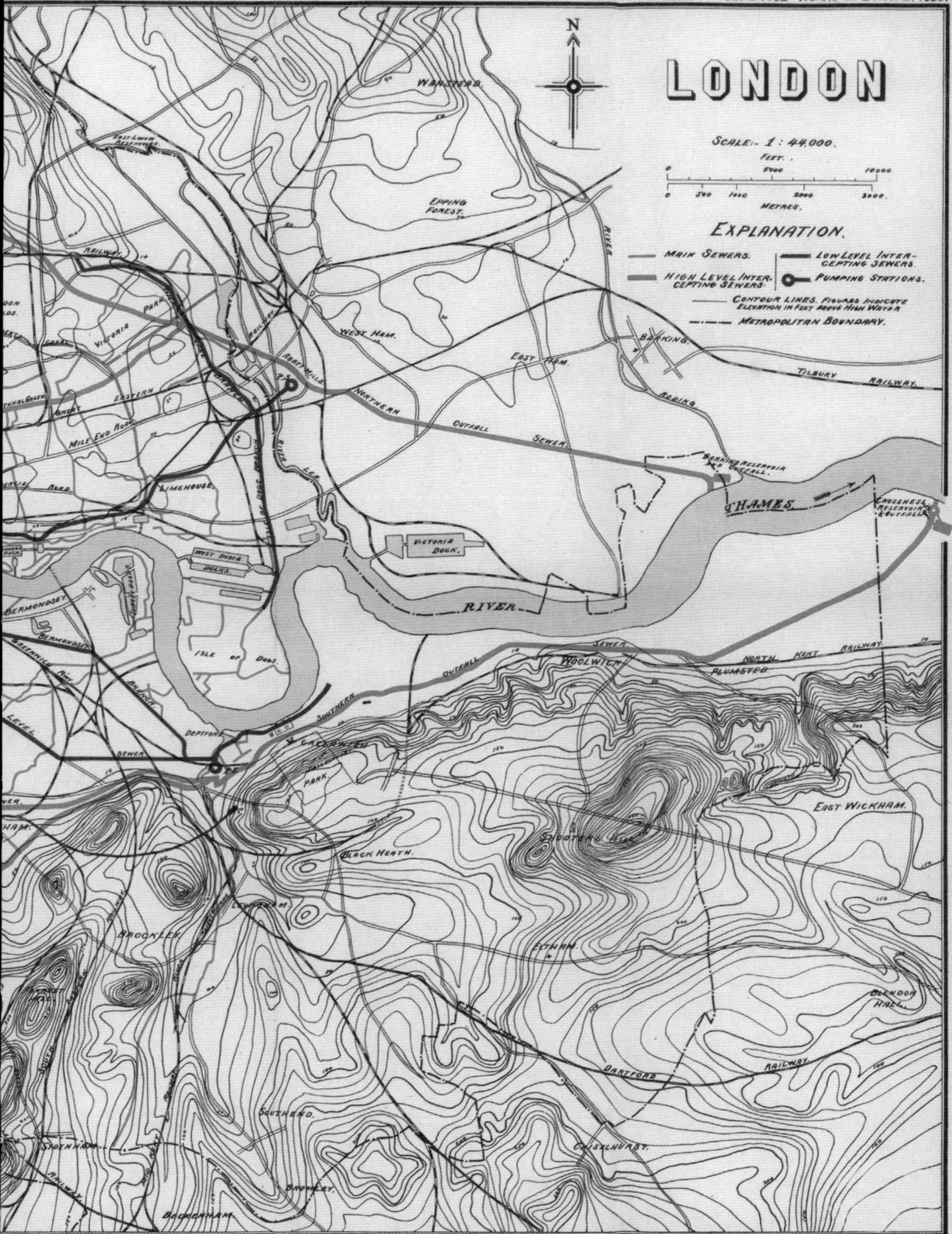

LONDON
N
SCALE:- 1 : 44,000.
FEET.
0
5000
10000
0
500
1000
2000
3000
METRES.
EXPLANATION.
MAIN SEWERS.
HIGH LEVEL INTERCEPTING SEWERS.
LOW LEVEL INTERCEPTING SEWERS.
PUMPING STATIONS.
CONTOUR LINES. FIGURES INDICATE ELEVATION IN FEET ABOVE HIGH WATER
METROPOLITAN BOUNDARY.
WANSTEAD.
EPPING FOREST.
RIVER
WEST HAM.
EAST HAM.
BARKING.
TILBURY RAILWAY.
NORTHERN OUTFALL SEWER.
BARKING RESERVOIR AND OUTFALL.
THAMES.
CROSSNESS RESERVOIR & OUTFALL.
RIVER
VICTORIA DOCK.
WEST INDIA DOCKS.
ISLE OF DOGS.
RIVER LEA
LIMEHOUSE.
MILE END ROAD.
VICTORIA PARK.
CANAL
RAILWAY.
EASTERN
ABBEY MILLS
P.S.
BERMONDSEY
WOOLWICH
PLUMSTED.
NORTH KENT RAILWAY.
SOUTHERN OUTFALL SEWER
DEPTFORD
GREENWICH
PARK.
P.S.
BLACK HEATH.
SHOOTERS HILL
EAST WICKHAM.
LEWISHAM.
BROCKLEY
ELTHAM.
BLENDON HALL.
DARTFORD RAILWAY.
SOUTHEND.
CHISLHURST.
SYDENHAM
BROMLEY.
BECKENHAM.
RAILWAY.

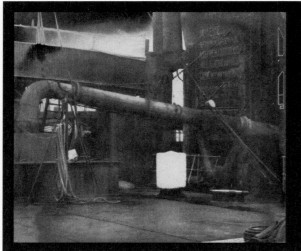

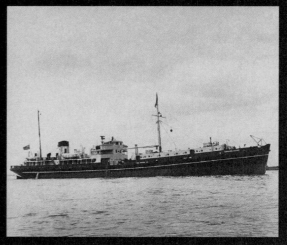

FIG. 55   **SLUDGE LOADING AT BECKTON** — LONDON, UK.
'SOLID' WASTE BEING LOADED ONTO A SLUDGE BOAT AT BECKTON.
ONE OF THE BOATS WAS NAMED *SIR JOSEPH BAZALGETTE*.

FIG. 56   **SLUDGE VESSEL *EDWARD CRUZE*** — LONDON, UK.
A SLUDGE VESSEL SETS SAIL FOR THE NORTH SEA
TODEPOSIT ITS MALODOROUS CARGO.

river, would be pumped into settlement tanks; lime was added to these, aiding the process of settlement and de-odorizing the liquid, which would then be released to the river. The settled sludge would be pumped on to boats (one of them called *Sir Joseph Bazalgette*) and dumped beyond the estuary in the North Sea. This was the system bequeathed by Bazalgette when he retired as Chief Engineer in 1889, dying two years later. And the system survived, virtually unchanged, until 1998, when it was replaced by a modern system described on page 229.

There were other consequences of Bazalgette's work. One was the rapid growth of the firm of Doulton and Watt usually associated with fine china. It was founded by John Doulton (1793–1873) in Lambeth. He had the foresight to buy cheaply, in that poor part of London, land that was exceeded in size only by the grounds of the Archbishop of Canterbury's Lambeth Palace. The business flourished as a manufacturer of large stone jars until 1845, when the ubiquitous Edwin Chadwick 'the Father of sanitary science', persuaded John Doulton's sons and heirs, Henry and Frederick Doulton, that the future lay in a market for glazed earthenware sewers. Doulton built a factory on his land in Lambeth and by 1854, according to the magazine *The Builder*, was producing 16 km (10 miles) of pipe sewers per week, a practice that continued until the 1930s, much of the output being exported. This earthenware was extensively fitted in the street sewers that Bazalgette used to feed the great interceptors though the latter, by virtue of their size, ranging from 1.4 m (4 ft 6 in.) diameter at the western end to 3.3 m (10 ft 9 in.) at Abbey Mills, were built of brick. Many of the bricks installed at the bottom of the sewers were also made by Doulton. These are known as 'Staffordshire Blues' and were made from the 1850s using clay from Staffordshire and fired at very high temperatures to give bricks of exceptional strength, which absorb very little water, and are a deep blue colour. They continue to serve Bazalgette's sewers in the 21st century and are also used in the foundations of modern buildings.

In 1861, as Bazalgette began his work, the population of London was 2.8 million. By 1901, twelve years after his death, it had reached 6.5 million. Fortunately, his designs anticipated a substantial increase in the population of the metropolis, but he cannot have expected that, by the outbreak of World War II in 1939, it would peak at 8.6 million. To accommodate this burgeoning population, huge public housing developments were created. Between 1921 and 1935 the world's largest public housing estate was built at Becontree in east London, accommodating 100,000 people in 26,000 homes, necessitating a major extension to Bazalgette's system – notably additions to the outfall sewers from Abbey Mills to Beckton. This vast structure is now topped by an 8-km (5-mile) long foot-and-cycle path in Tower Hamlets running from Wick Lane in Bow to Beckton. Formerly bearing the accurate but forbidding name 'Sewerbank', it was renovated and landscaped in the 1990s to provide a pleasant route called 'Greenway' with a vista over the landscape below including a fine view of the Olympic Park. It also gives a good impression of the sheer size of the work of Bazalgette and his successors.

The population growth of the interwar period was followed by a slow but relentless decline in the years following the war, falling to less than 6.6 million in 1991 as much of the population was relocated from poor housing, much of it damaged by bombing, to communities in new towns such as Hemel Hempstead, Stevenage and Crawley. Moreover, although the metropolitan population was in decline, in the 1950s the replacement of housing of poor quality within London meant that many families had hot and o———————▶ 140

FIG. 57   **DOULTON SEWER PIPE** — LONDON, UK. A DOULTON SEWER PIPE OF THE KIND USED TO CONNECT BUILDINGS TO STREET SEWERS.

FIG. 58 ↑   **'STAFFORDSHIRE BLUE' DOULTON BRICK** — LONDON, UK. A DOULTON STAFFORDSHIRE BRICK USED TO LINE THE BOTTOM (INVERT) OF SEWERS.

FIG. 59 ↓   1936 **BUILDING A BRICK SEWER**. A NEW SEWER BEING BUILT IN 1936 USING STAFFORDSHIRE BRICKS TO LINE THE INVERT.

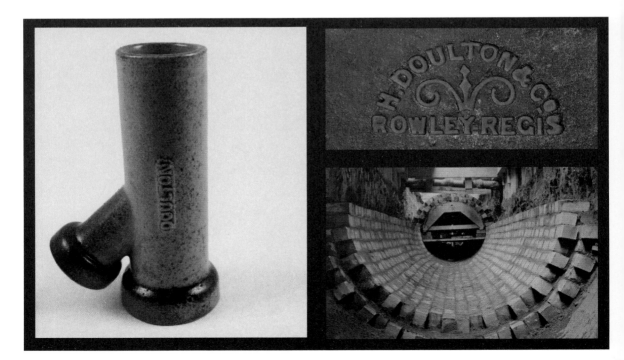

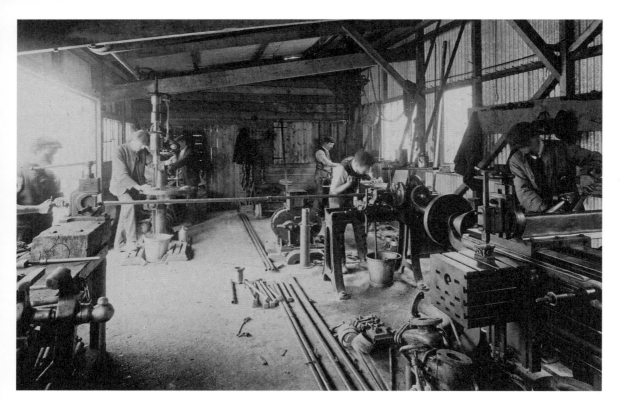

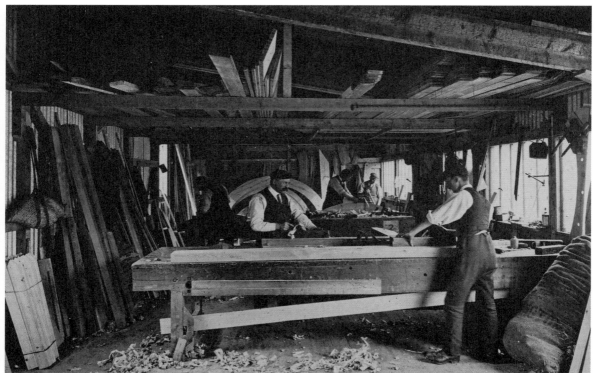

**FIGS. 60–61 COUNCILLOR STREET DEPOT CARPENTERS AND METAL
WORKERS** — LONDON, UK. A LARGE NUMBER OF WORKERS TOOK
PART IN THE EXPANSION OF THE SEWERS IN THE EARLY 20TH CENTURY.

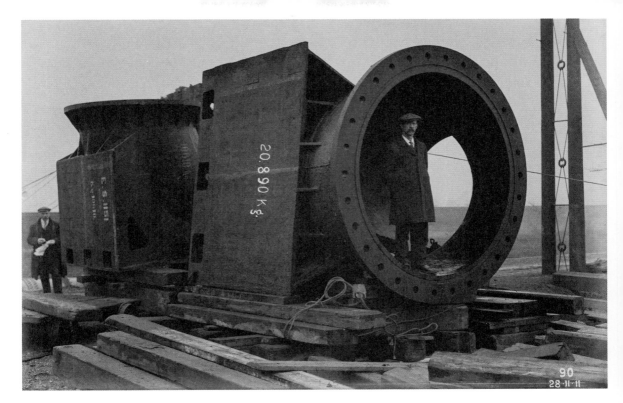

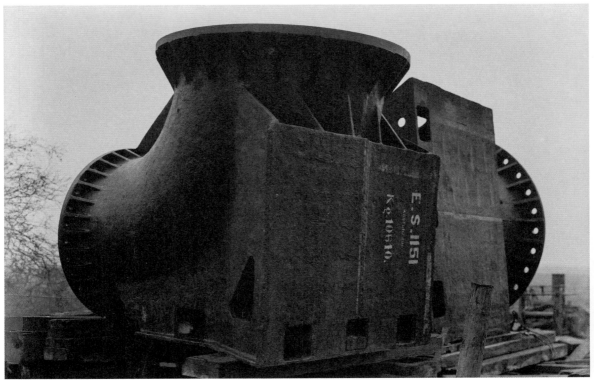

FIGS. 62–63 1911 **SEWERS PRIOR TO INSTALLATION** — LONDON, UK.

THE HUGE SCALE OF SEWERAGE CONSTRUCTION IS EVIDENT FROM

THE ENORMOUS HEIGHT AND WEIGHT OF THESE SEWER JUNCTIONS.

cold running water and water closets for the first time, putting further strains on the system and necessitating more additions to its capacity. Joseph Bazalgette was much admired in his time and the importance of his works recognized by his fellow citizens. His contribution to London was not confined to the creation of its sewerage system and Embankment. He was also responsible for many of London's bridges, including Hammersmith Bridge and Putney Bridge, and worked on many of the capital's most important and famous roads, including Shaftesbury Avenue and Charing Cross Road. His inimitable contribution to the city's development and prosperity led to his being knighted in 1875, and being awarded the Companionship of the Bath and elected President of the Institution of Civil Engineers in 1883. The effects of Bazalgette's revolutionary new sewer designs were reflected in his obituary in *The Times*, published on 16 March 1891. Referring to his most visible work, the Victoria Embankment, the obituarist wrote:

> **Of the great sewer that runs beneath, Londoners as a rule know nothing though the Registrar-General could tell them that it has added some twenty years to their chance of life.**

Bazalgette's work continues to accommodate the needs of a city larger than he could possibly have imagined. London's docks have been transformed into offices and their warehouses have become luxury flats, lavishly equipped with every water-using facility that money can buy. Moreover, in the last decade of the 20th century the population began to recover and has now passed its 1939 peak, reaching 9 million for the first time in the 2nd decade of the century – with consequences for the system Bazalgette created that are examined in the final section of this book, addressing 'the future of waste treatment'.

'JOSEPH BAZALGETTE CREATED A SEWER SYSTEM WHICH HE ORIGINALLY SIZED FOR LONDON'S NEEDS OF THE TIME – HE THEN DOUBLED IT TO ANTICIPATE THE FUTURE BEYOND. THESE ARE THE QUALITIES THAT I ADMIRE.'

Sir Norman Foster, architect of many of London's most famous landmarks including City Hall, the Millennium Bridge and the Gherkin (2008)

FIGS. 64–81 SEWERMEN AT WORK — LONDON, UK. SEWERMEN ARE REQUIRED TO WEAR PROTECTIVE CLOTHING, OCCASIONALLY INCLUDING MASKS, TO GUARD AGAINST INFECTION.

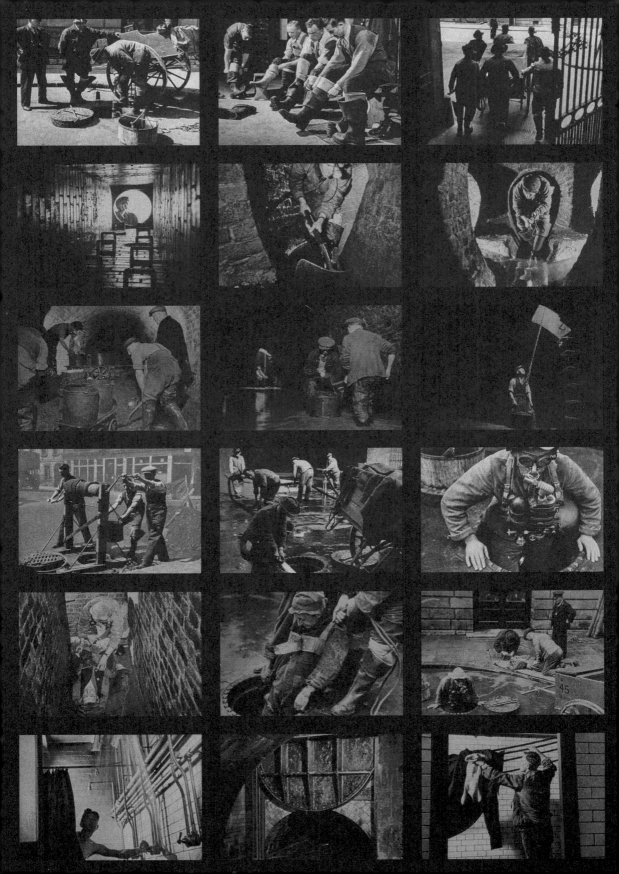

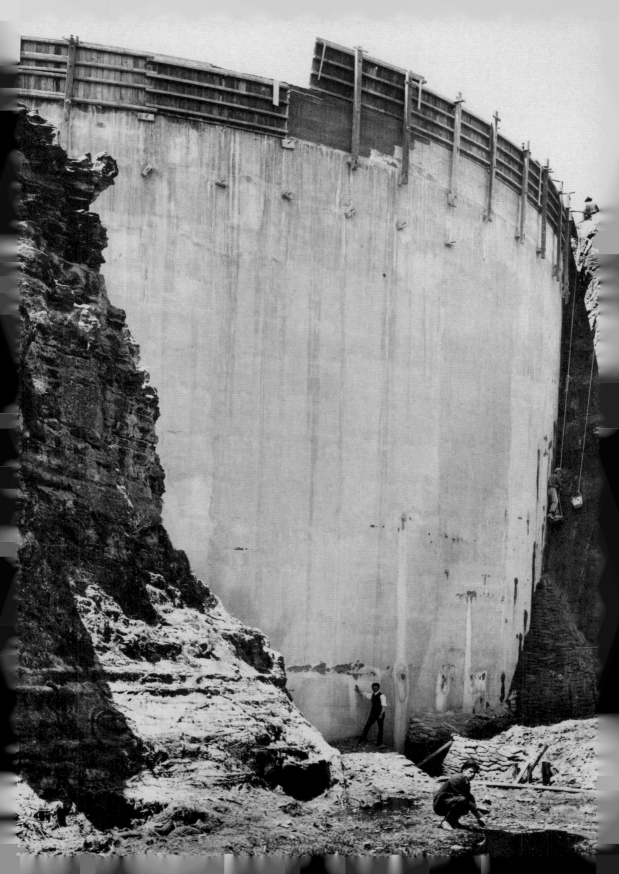

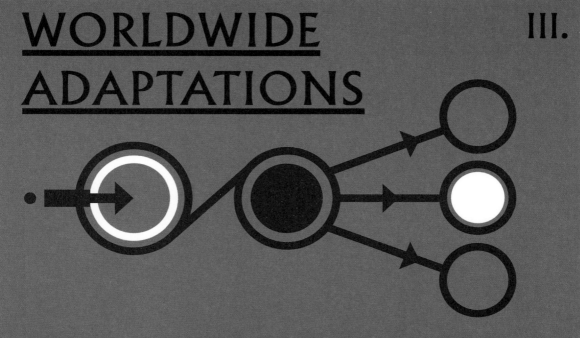

WORLDWIDE ADAPTATIONS

'IT'S THE MAIN SEWER…RUNS RIGHT INTO THE BLUE DANUBE. SMELLS SWEET, DOESN'T IT?'

Sergeant Paine (Bernard Lee) in *The Third Man* (1949)

The late 19th century witnessed the introduction of effective sewerage systems to central Europe, Australia and Japan as the growth of their urban populations, together with the threat of waterborne disease, encouraged the residents to undertake great engineering works similar to those already described in France and Britain. Some new techniques were added, however, and there was a move towards the integration of collection and treatment of sewage that provided a model for the future. There were also new concepts of sewage movement involving techniques such as vacuums, now used in trains and aircraft as well as in Norway, Sweden and Hong Kong, and the use of sand filters to purify drinking water.

The development of systems in Germany and much of central Europe at that time is inseparable from the names of the English engineers William Lindley (1808–1900) and his son Sir William Heerlein Lindley (1853–1917). They left their mark on many towns on the European continent, especially Germany. The elder William Lindley was born in London, his father dying when William was an infant. At the age of sixteen, he went to study in Hamburg for ten months and became fluent in German 146

FIG. 1   1909–28 **WATER DAM** — NEW SOUTH WALES, AUSTRALIA.
ONE OF MANY DAMS IN NEW SOUTH WALES WHERE WATER IS STORED
AND CLEANED FOR HUMAN USE IN THIS DRIEST OF CONTINENTS.

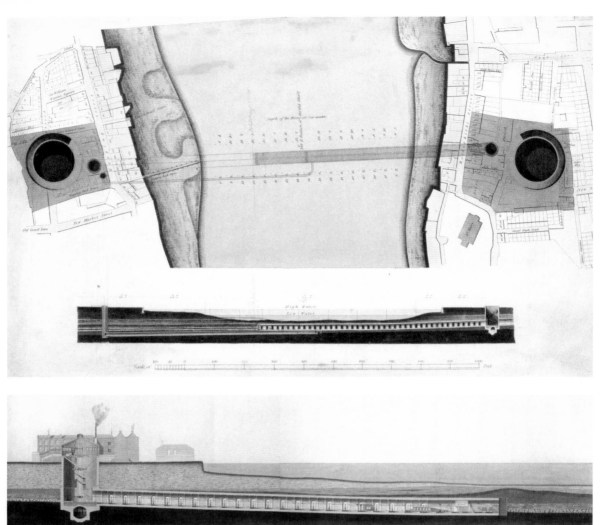

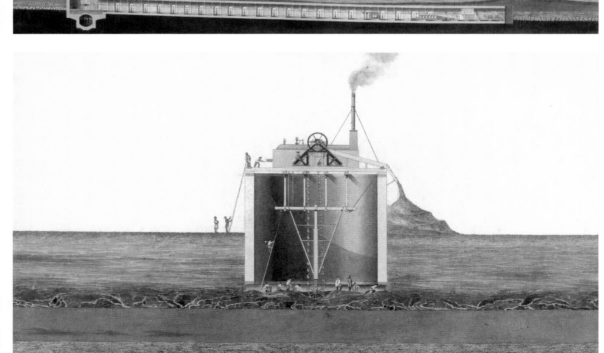

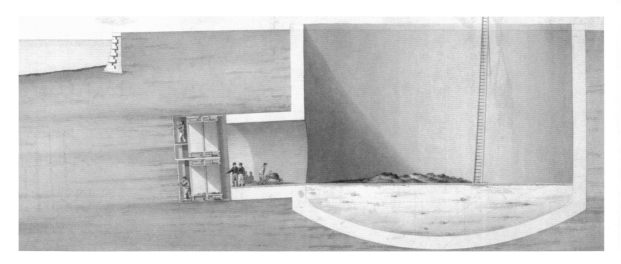

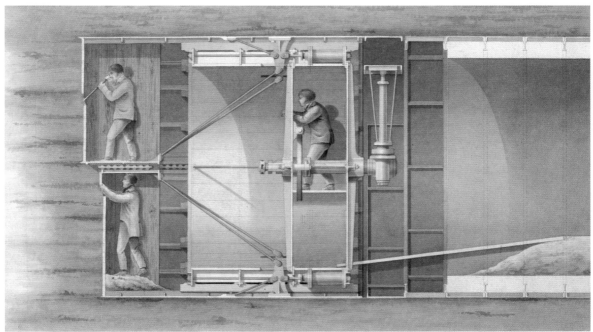

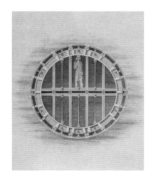

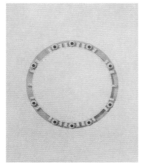

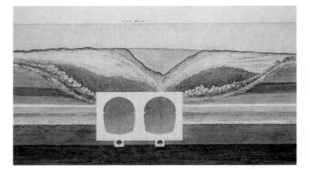

FIGS. 2–9   1827 **MARC ISAMBARD BRUNEL'S WATERCOLOURS FOR THE THAMES TUNNEL** — LONDON, UK. THE WORLD'S FIRST TUNNEL BENEATH A RIVER, FROM WAPPING TO ROTHERHITHE, WAS DESIGNED BY MARC BRUNEL AND BUILT WITH THE ASSISTANCE OF HIS SON ISAMBARD KINGDOM BRUNEL AND WILLIAM LINDLEY. IT TOOK EIGHTEEN YEARS TO BUILD AND WAS OPENED IN 1843.

before returning to England to become an engineering pupil, working with Isambard Kingdom Brunel on the Thames Tunnel designed by Isambard's father Marc and using the latter's tunnelling shield to build a tunnel beneath the Thames between Wapping and Rotherhithe.

In 1837, William returned to the continent to work on railway projects and in 1839, at the age of thirty-one, he was recommended by Isambard Brunel and Robert Stephenson to create Hamburg's first railway. By 1842, it was ready to enter service but its opening, due to take place on 7 May, was interrupted by the great Hamburg fire, which broke out on 5 May and burned for three days, destroying one-third of the city. Lindley earned the gratitude of the burgomeister and council by using the new railway to bring in firefighters and to evacuate people from the burning city and by using explosives to create fire breaks to slow the path of the blaze. He was then engaged as a consulting engineer to plan

FIG. 10   1864 **THE WATER SUPPLY OF HAMBURG** — HAMBURG,
GERMANY. A MAP SHOWING THE WATER SUPPLY NETWORK OF
HAMBURG, DESIGNED BY THE ENGLISH ENGINEER WILLIAM LINDLEY.

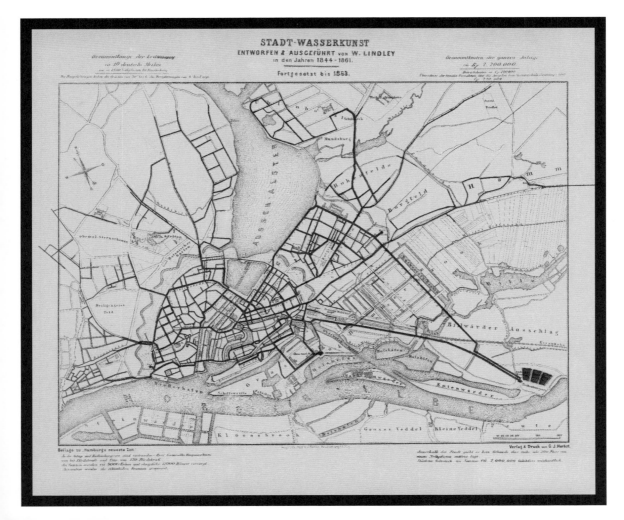

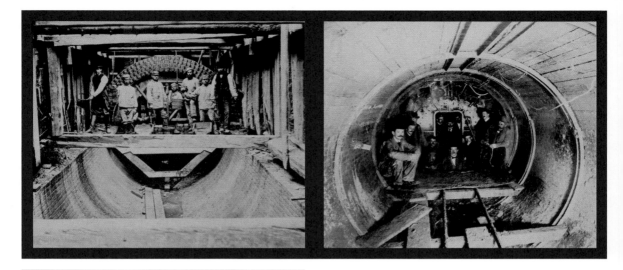

FIGS. 11–12 CONSTRUCTION OF THE HAMBURG SEWERS — HAMBURG,
GERMANY. CONSTRUCTION OF THE HAMBURG SEWERS; DESIGNED
BY WILLIAM LINDLEY AND BUILT BETWEEN 1848 AND 1860.
THE SYSTEM WAS FLUSHED BY THE RIVER ELBE WHICH
UNFORTUNATELY CARRIED CHOLERA INTO THE CITY IN 1892.

the rebuilding of the city. Between 1842 and 1847 he drained Hammerbrook, a marshy area of almost
607 hectares (1,500 acres) to the east of Hambug's centre, by creating an intricate system of canals
and locks that drained into the Elbe. Between 1844 and 1848, Lindley designed a system for supplying
water to the city and recommended the use of sand filters to help ensure the purity of the drinking water,
although these were not adopted for almost fifty years. Finally, he proposed a comprehensive plan
for a system of sewers, which he began to build in 1848, the first such system for any city in Germany.
By 1860, he had constructed 64 km (40 miles) of main sewers of a size designed to cope with the
widespread use of the increasingly fashionable water closets. The sewage was discharged, in its
raw state, into the Elbe, while the system was flushed by rainwater collected from the roofs of houses.
Provision was also made for it to be flushed by tidal waters from the Elbe at times of low rainfall.
This was a clever engineering solution that kept the sewers clear of debris but proved to be a
weakness when the city was struck by cholera in 1892.

Lindley also undertook a rather unusual task for Hamburg, which, with Bremen and Lübeck, was one
of the leading members of the Hanseatic League of a hundred European cities that had dominated
continental trading from the 13th to the 16th centuries. One of the relics of the League was the
'Steelyard' a warehousing and trading complex in the heart of the City of London for which Hamburg,
Bremen and Lübeck had no further use. Lindley arranged its sale in 1852 to the South-Eastern
Railway and it became the site of Cannon Street Station.

Many German cities were stuck by cholera in 1867–68 and although there was disagreement in
Germany, as in England, over whether the epidemics were caused by polluted water or foul smells,
it was accepted that one of the remedies was a sewerage system to remove waste and, in the
process, remove the smells that accompanied it. William Lindley was appointed as consulting
engineer to Frankfurt in 1863 and in 1867, following the cholera epidemic, began its construction, 152

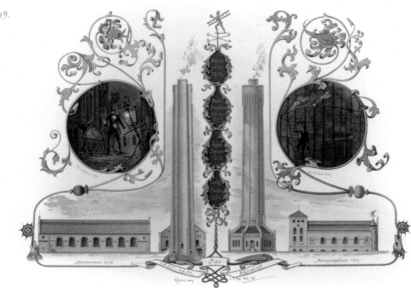

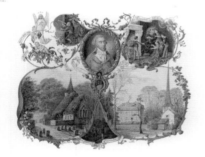

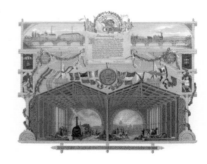

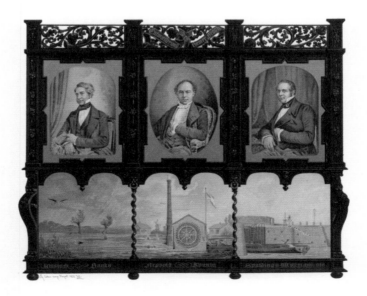

FIGS. 13–20 1852 ALBUM CELEBRATING THE WORKS OF WILLIAM LINDLEY IN HAMBURG. CREATED BY GERMAN ILLUSTRATOR HERMANN WILHELM SOLTAU, THIS BEAUTIFUL ALBUM WAS

COMMISSIONED BY WILLIAM LINDLEY'S SON, WILLIAM HEERLEIN LINDLEY, TO COMMEMORATE THE NUMEROUS EXCEPTIONAL PUBLIC WORKS CREATED BY HIS FATHER IN HAMBURG.

№ 5.

№ 8.

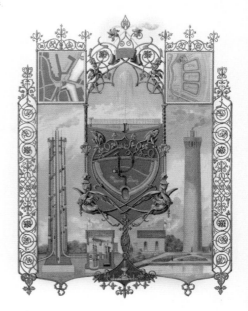

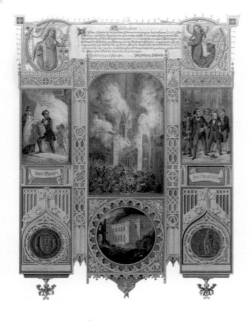

№ 10.

№ 11.

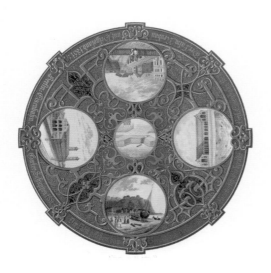

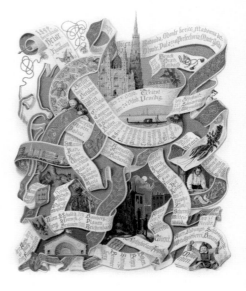

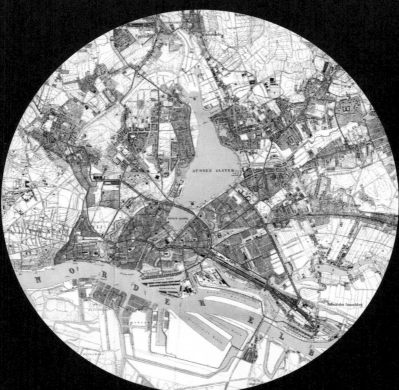

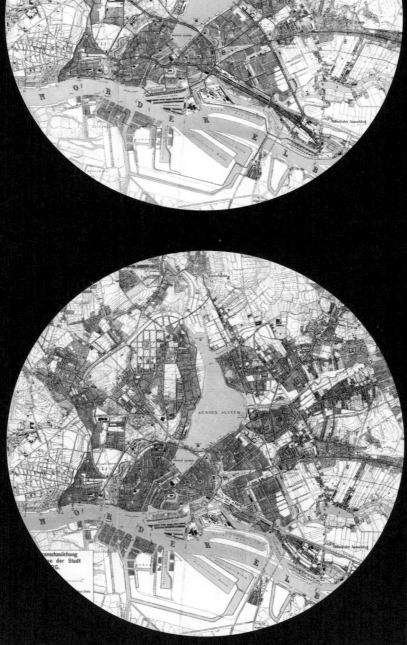

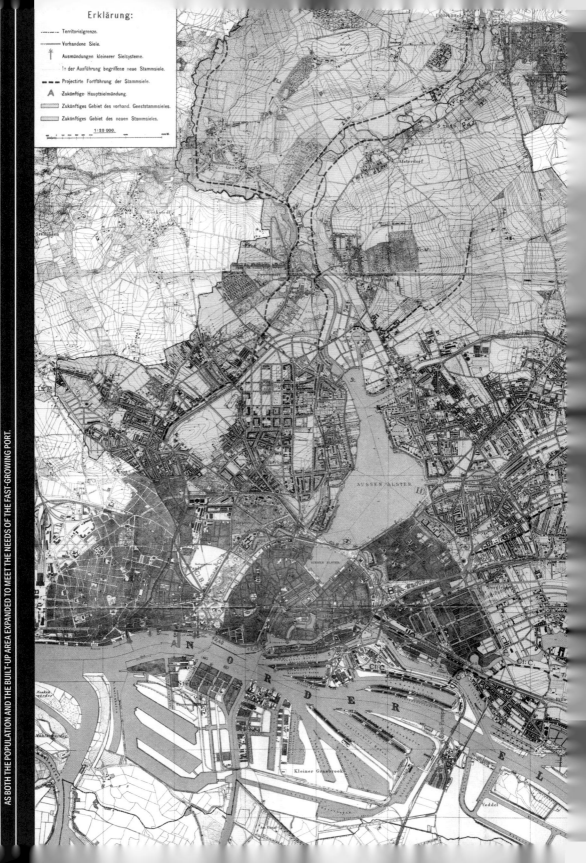

FIG. 23 · 1904 **HAMBURG SEWER SYSTEM** — HAMBURG, GERMANY. BY 1904 THE SYSTEM WAS MORE DENSE AND WIDESPREAD

AS BOTH THE POPULATION AND THE BUILT-UP AREA EXPANDED TO MEET THE NEEDS OF THE FAST-GROWING PORT.

Erklärung:

Territorialgrenze.

Vorhandene Siele.

Ausmündungen kleinerer Sielsysteme.

In der Ausführung begriffene neue Stammsiele.

Projectirte Fortführung der Stammsiele.

Zukünftige Hauptsielmündung.

Zukünftiges Gebiet des vorhand. Geeststammsieles.

Zukünftiges Gebiet des neuen Stammsieles.

1:120 000.

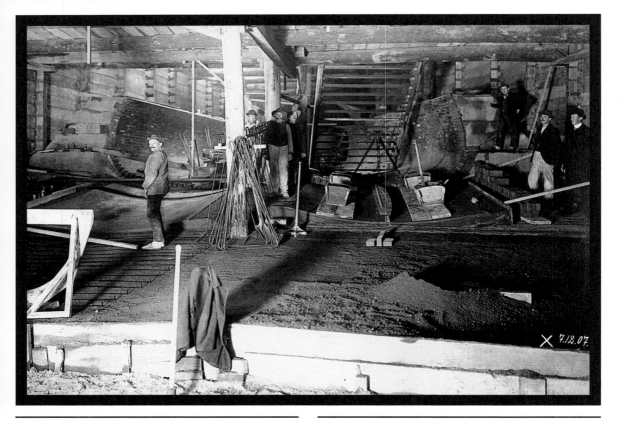

FIG. 24 1907 **BERLIN SEWER** — BERLIN, GERMANY. THE SEWER SYSTEM WAS BUILT IN THE LATE 19TH CENTURY AND USED IN THE 20TH CENTURY TO SMUGGLE PEOPLE FROM EAST TO WEST BERLIN.

FIGS. 25–26 → 1949 **SCENES FROM *THE THIRD MAN*** — VIENNA, AUSTRIA. HARRY LIME (ORSON WELLS) ATTEMPTS TO EVADE HIS PURSUERS BY TAKING TO THE SEWER.

with 129 km (80 miles) of street sewers of sufficient capacity to handle the waste from 19,000 water closets. Germany's first sewage treatment works followed in the city in 1887. He installed egg-shaped sewers in Frankfurt – probably the first in Germany, although they had been used earlier in the century in London and Liverpool. He was also involved in the design of systems for Düsseldorf and Leipzig. Between 1868 and 1883, the death rate from typhoid, another waterborne disease, fell eightfold in these cities.

In Vienna, Lindley designed a drainage system to prevent flooding from the Danube, though not the sewers, dating from the 1850s, through which 'Harry Lime' (Orson Wells) fled in the climax of the film *The Third Man* (1949). An invitation to visit Australia to design a sewerage system for Sydney was declined as Lindley was too busy designing a system for Warsaw, for which he also designed a filtration plant for drinking water from the Vistula that incorporated slow sand filters and began to supply clean water to the citizens in 1886. It still bears his name, 'Filtry Lindleya' ('Lindley's Filters') as does a street in Warsaw. The system was later modernised by his son Sir William Heerlein Lindley, who also designed the system for Prague.

Berlin, the capital of Prussia and later of the German Reich, was already Germany's largest city in 1850. It is situated on the flat, marshy lands of the North European Plain in the valley of the Spree river and surrounded by relatively infertile soil. In 1859, the land surveyor James Hobrecht (1825–1902) was appointed to head a commission to determine a land-use plan for the city and its surroundings. He devised a scheme that envisaged the city growing to accommodate a population of 2 million and later designed a programme for sewerage of the city. It consists of twelve radial sewers, seven to the north and five to the south of the Spree, with rainwater and wastewater flowing together, partly by gravity and partly by pumping, to irrigate fields on the outskirts of the city. Having been passed through the soil, and thereby cleansed, the water flows via drainage channels to canals and rivers. The work was begun in 1873 and completed in 1893. The system survived two world wars and much of it is still in use.

In 1961 the impenetrable Berlin Wall divided the east and west of Berlin. However beneath the surface, the sewer network connected the whole city, irrespective of the political boundaries above. It thus became a highly useful conduit for those wishing to smuggle goods – or people – across the border. Even before the erection of the Wall the sewers had been used to transport goods such as cigarettes between East and West Berlin, an illegal activity that meant by the time of the Wall many of the sewers had already been shut off. However, some daring students found a sewer running from Kreuzberg in the East through to the West – the perfect escape route. Once the thick sewer grille had been sawed through at least 134 students were able to use the sewer to escape to West Berlin. ○———————➤ 160

'THE CHIEF CHARACTERISTICS OF MR. LINDLEY'S WORKS WERE THE THOROUGHNESS AND FAR SIGHTEDNESS OF HIS DESIGNS WHICH WERE ALWAYS BASED ON THE DEMANDS OF A FAR FUTURE, THE CARE SPENT ON DETAILS OF CONSTRUCTION, AND THEIR CONSCIENTIOUS EXECUTION.'

William Lindley's obituary from the Institution of Civil Engineers (1900)

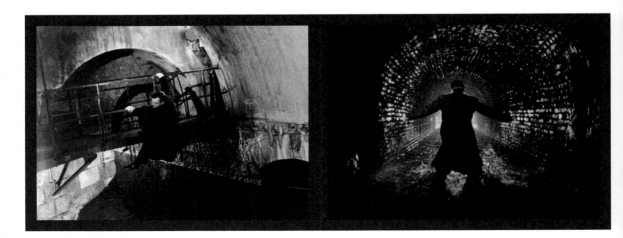

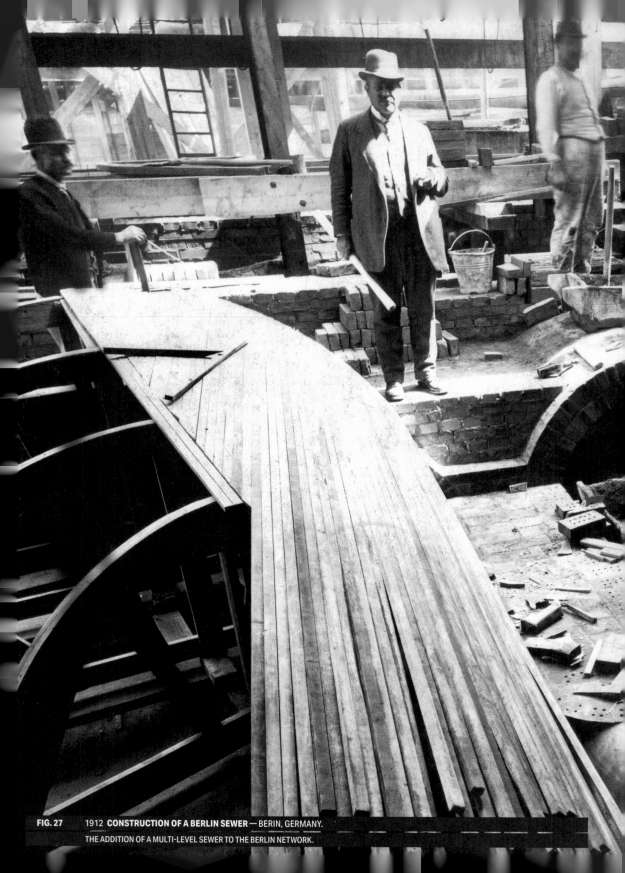

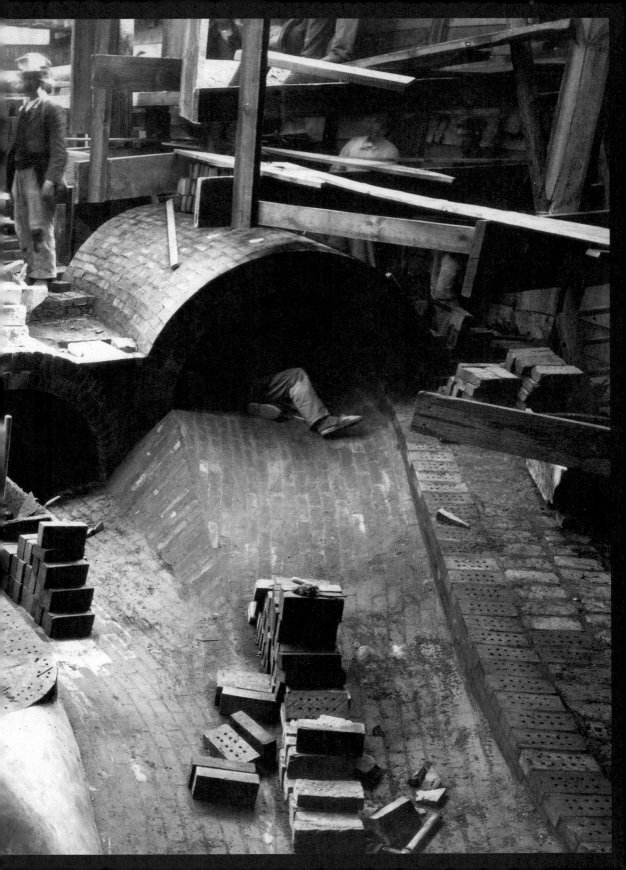

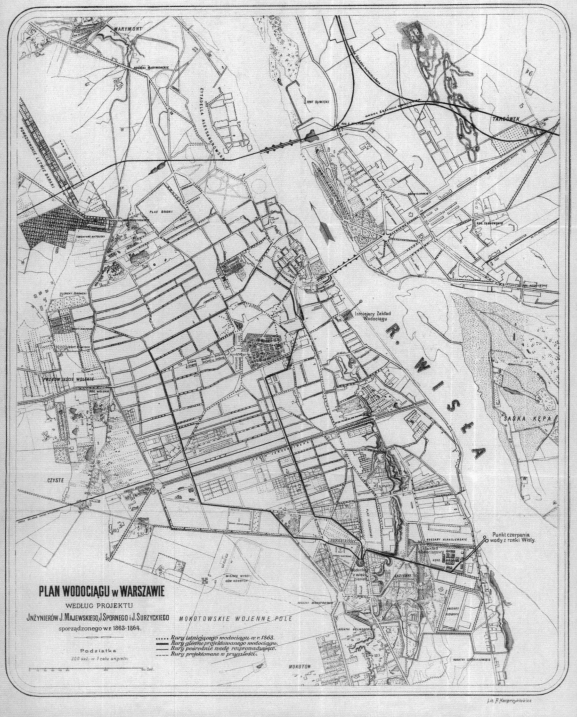

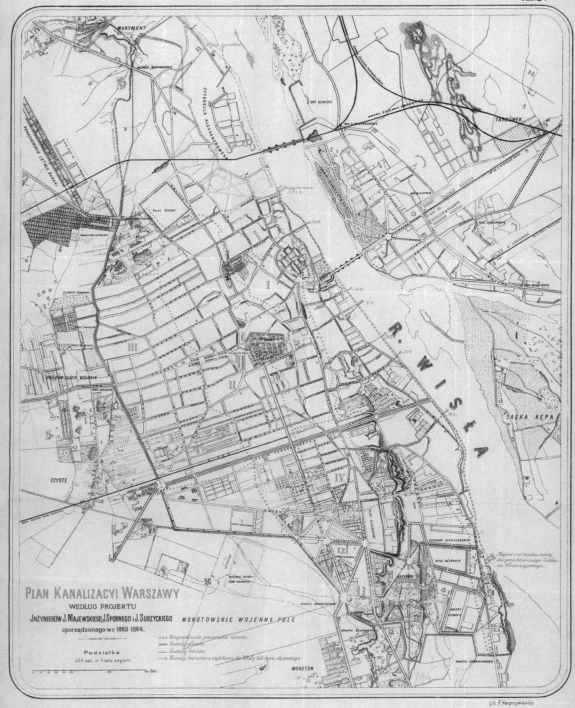

Tab. II.

Lit. F. Kasprzykiewicz

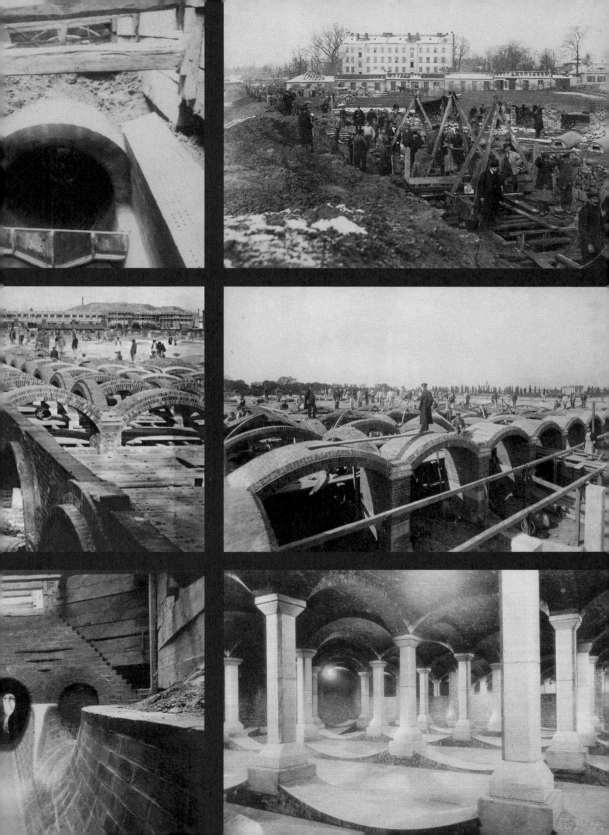

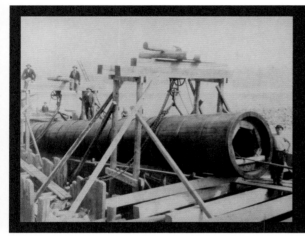

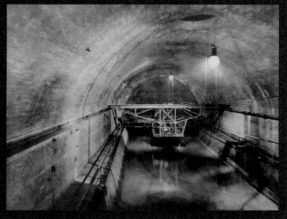

The sewers that William Lindley senior designed for Warsaw were also to assume a heroic role in the 20th century. In 1943 the Jewish population of the Warsaw ghetto took refuge in the sewers during their uprising against the Nazis. And in August 1944, with the Red Army at the gates, the Polish Home Army rose in a vain attempt to liberate the city, again seeking refuge in the sewers as the Nazi occupiers destroyed the city. Unusually, the survivors of the uprising were treated as prisoners of war rather than massacred as the Nazi generals, faced with the advance of the Russians from the East and the Allies from the West, pondered the fate that could await them at the hands of the Allies if they perpetuated further atrocities. The sewers of the Polish city of Lvov also sheltered Jewish families, led by the Chiger family, and supported by the generosity of a gentile sewerman called Leopold Socha (1909–46), thereby saving their lives. When the Nazis left and the families emerged from their subterranean refuge where they had lived from June 1943 to July 1944, Socha announced 'This is my work, all my work. These are my Jews.' The story of Lvov's Jews hiding in the city's sewers was made into a film called *In Darkness* (2011).

The first modern sewers in Prague were found in a Jesuit seminary, its latrines flushed by water from fountains and kitchen waste into the Vltava, a tributary of the Elbe. By the 1820s, about 44 km (27 miles) of sewers had been added to the system, which still discharged untreated sewage into the river. Charles Liernur (1828–93), a former captain of Dutch descent in the US army, proposed a system of pneumatic sewers through which waste would be drawn by a partial vacuum, removing the need for a steady flow of water. The system was patented in Britain and the Netherlands in the 1880s and installed on a small scale in the Netherlands, in a barracks in Prague and the town of Trouville in France, where it continued in use until 1980. It has been adopted for aircraft and some trains. Doubts about the effectiveness and safety of the system in the Prague barracks led to its rejection and two rival schemes were devised by Czech engineers, one of them proposing to conduct the sewage to create an island in the river called Holesovicky, an idea redolent of the 'gold from sewage' schemes proposed in Britain and France (see page 67) and equally chimerical. Lindley was called in to judge between the merits of the two rival schemes and used them as the basis of a design of his own that extended the system to a wider area and incorporated a treatment plant using sedimentation and sludge processing to remove the solids from the sewage and take them by barges to fields beyond the city. At this point rivalries became

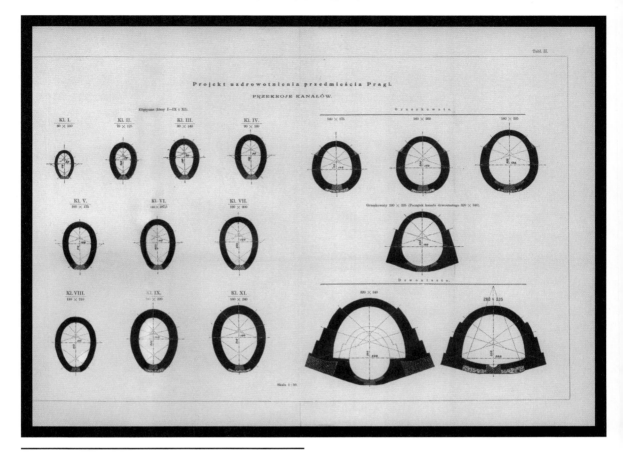

FIG. 41   1903 **SEWER DESIGNS** — PRAGUE, THE CZECH REPUBLIC.
ENTITLED 'HEALING PROJECT FOR THE SUBURBS OF PRAGUE', THIS
SHEET SHOWS THE VARIETY IN SIZE OF OVOID SEWER PIPES USED.

personal, with a representative of the mayor of Prague having to assure the citizens that 'Aspersions have been cast regarding Mr Lindley that he is a German and a Jew but he is in fact a Dane, his wife is English and he is of Anglican faith'! Hindley's system was built between 1895 and 1906. The sewers are still in use and the treatment plant continued to serve the city until 1967.

One of William Lindley senior's most challenging assignments was for the Russian city of St Petersburg. Founded in 1703 by Tsar Peter the Great (1672–1725) it was, in effect, carved out of the Gulf of Finland to realize the Tsar's ambition of a seaport that would provide an outlet to the Baltic Sea and the West. Much of the City is at or below sea level and about 10% of it consists of water, from the river Neva and the city's lakes. During the reign of Catherine the Great (1729–96), an elaborate system of subterranean channels and pipes, made of bricks or drilled out logs, was installed to provide drainage to the Baltic while drinking water was drawn from the Neva. Cesspits, unfortunately, drained to the rivers despite prohibitions (which were, admittedly, rarely enforced) so when cholera reached St Petersburg in 1831 the city was particularly vulnerable. Many other epidemics followed, the most famous victim of the disease being the composer Pyotr Ilyich Tchaikovsky (1840–93), whose death was attributed to drinking water from the city's polluted supply eight days before he died.

166

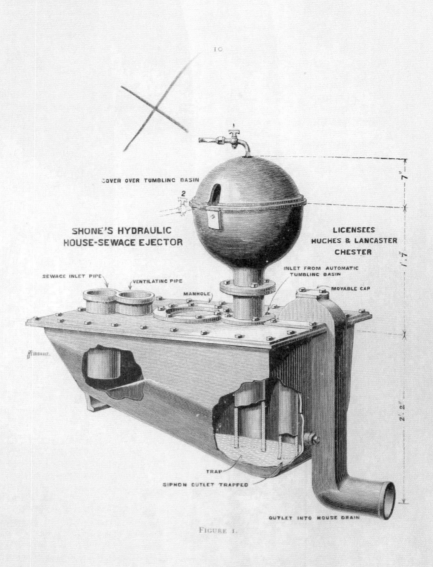

IO

COVER OVER TUMBLING BASIN

2

SHONE'S HYDRAULIC
HOUSE-SEWAGE EJECTOR

LICENSEES
HUGHES & LANCASTER
CHESTER

7"

1.7"

INLET FROM AUTOMATIC
TUMBLING BASIN

SEWAGE INLET PIPE   VENTILATING PIPE

MOVABLE CAP

MANHOLE

2.2"

TRAP

SIPHON OUTLET TRAPPED

OUTLET INTO HOUSE DRAIN

FIGURE I.

FIG. 42 1887 **SHONE'S HYDRAULIC HOUSE-SEWAGE EJECTOR**. FIXED IN THE HOUSE, THE HYDRAULIC EJECTOR

WAS DESIGNED TO DISCHARGE WASTE COLLECTED FROM THE HOUSE INTO A PIPE CONNECTING IT TO THE CITY

SEWERAGE SYSTEM TEN TIMES A DAY.

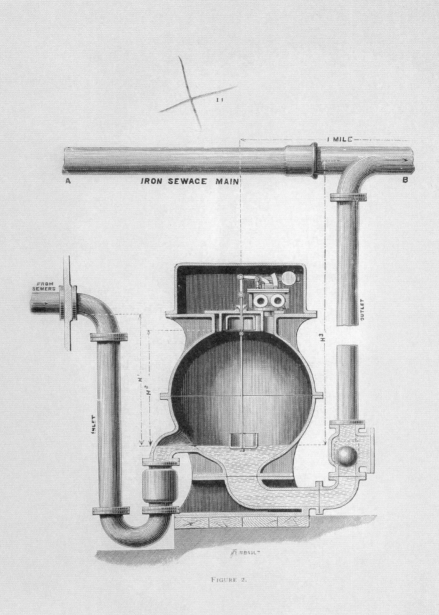

FIGURE 2.

FIG. 43   **1887**   **SHONE'S PNEUMATIC SEWAGE EJECTOR**. FIXED AT REGULAR INTERVALS ALONG A STREET'S SEWAGE PIPE,

THE PNEUMATIC EJECTOR WAS DESIGNED TO RECEIVE SEWAGE FROM SEVERAL HOUSE-SEWAGE EJECTORS AND

FORCE IT INTO THE MAINS SEWAGE PIPE.

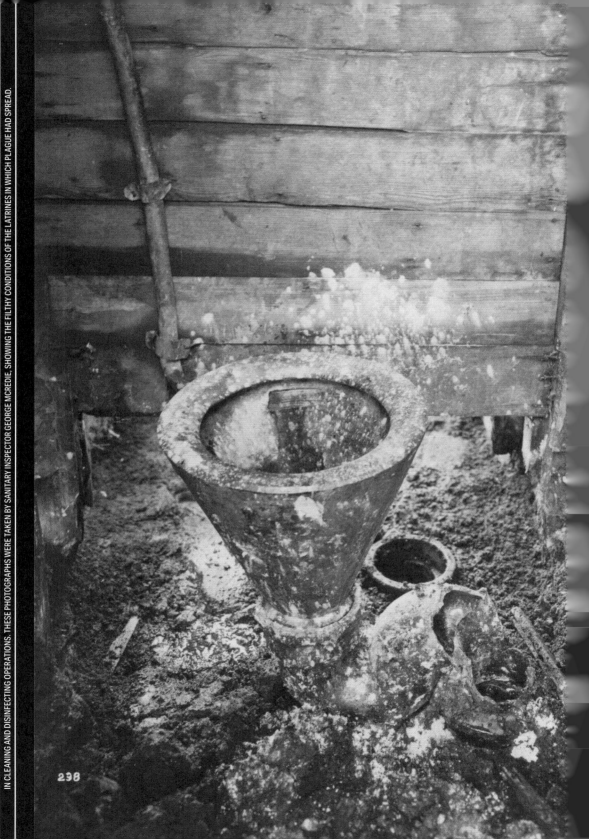

FIGS. 44–45 1900 **DUNNIES** —SYDNEY, AUSTRALIA. IN 1900 BUBONIC PLAGUE STRUCK SYDNEY, KILLING 103 PEOPLE IN EIGHT MONTHS. QUARANTINE AREAS WERE ESTABLISHED AND RESIDENTS WERE EMPLOYED IN CLEANING AND DISINFECTING OPERATIONS. THESE PHOTOGRAPHS WERE TAKEN BY SANITARY INSPECTOR GEORGE MCREDIE, SHOWING THE FILTHY CONDITIONS OF THE LATRINES IN WHICH PLAGUE HAD SPREAD.

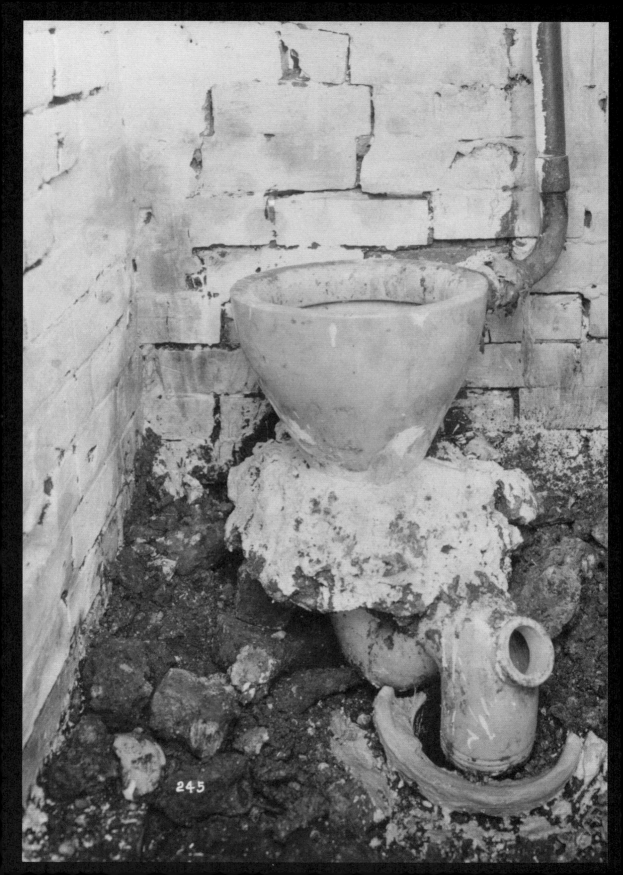

A new sewerage system was designed by William Lindley from 1876 but little was done until after World War I and the October Revolution, when a new system was finally installed, the last serious cholera epidemic occurring in St Petersburg in 1908.

In Australia, as in Europe, modern water supply and sewerage systems were developed in response to the growth of its major cities in the 19th century. Sydney, the site of the first European settlements in Australia and the destination of many of the convict ships between 1788 and 1868, owes its location to its famous harbour and to one of the early captains, Arthur Phillip (1738–1814), the first Governor of New South Wales, who chose the site because of a freshwater supply called the Tank Stream. The stream was of great symbolic importance to the local Aboriginal people, but within forty years it had become so polluted by sewage, garbage and farmyard effluent that a fresh source had to be found. These were the Lachlan Swamps, now the Centennial Park near the Sydney Cricket Ground, 'Busby's Bore' being constructed in 1858 to bring water to Hyde Park, closer to the harbour, whence it was taken by water carts to homes and businesses. The Tank Stream then became a sewer, emptying its contents into the harbour and it was shortly joined by five new sewage outfalls, all draining into its once pristine waters. This arrangement prevailed until the late 19th century, with sewage also being discharged at Botany Bay, the site of Captain Cook's landfall in 1770, and at a further discharge point at Bondi Beach – now noted for its surfing, volleyball and occasional visiting sharks but then one of the least salubrious beaches in New South Wales. In 1885, Botany sewage farm was built; which processed the sewage before sending it to the bay; two further treatment works were added and now handle about 80% of Sydney's sewage.

At the outset of World War II, half of Sydney's households were not connected to the sewerage system, being dependent upon 'dunny carts', also known as Honey Wagons, for the weekly collection of excrement from metal containers, a slightly more advanced version of the Revd Henry Moule's device described on page 67. This led to occasional disasters when a dunny man lost his grip – as recorded in the Australian Clive James's *Unreliable Memoirs* (1980), an account of his early years in his native

FIG. 46   1788 **SETTLEMENT AT SYDNEY COVE, PORT JACKSON** — SYDNEY, AUSTRALIA. DURING THE EARLY YEARS OF SYDNEY'S SETTLEMENT THE WATER SUPPLY WAS PRISTINE.

FIG. 47   1832 **IMPROVEMENTS MADE TO SYDNEY COVE** — SYDNEY, AUSTRALIA. AS THE SHORELINE BECAME MORE BUILT UP, THE WATER SUPPLY BECAME SEVERELY POLLUTED.

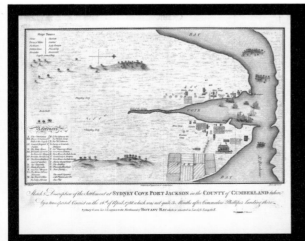

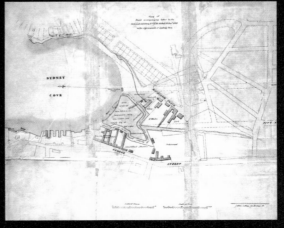

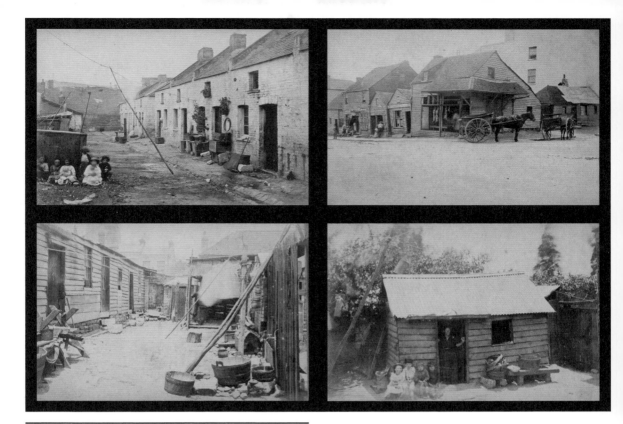

FIGS. 48–51 1875 **REPORT INTO THE STATE OF SYDNEY DWELLINGS** —
SYDNEY, AUSTRALIA. PRIMITIVE DWELLINGS IN SYDNEY,
EACH WITH POOR SANITATION, REPORTED IN AN INQUIRY
INTO CROWDING AND ITS AFFECT ON PUBLIC HEALTH.

land. As late as the 1950s, Bondi Beach was notorious for water and sand polluted by grease and sewage. Finally, in the 1960s, new facilities were proposed and completed in 1990. There are now thirty treatment and water recycling plants that clean the wastewater of pollutants to the point where it can safely be used before discharge to water gardens, flush toilets, feed carwashes and fight fires while almost 200,000 tonnes of fertilizer is recovered from the sewage to supply to farmers and methane gas is used to fuel the plants. Some of the drinking water upon which Sydney depends is drawn from sources fed by the Warragamba Dam, which itself receives water from rivers into which upstream communities have discharged their sewage. Fortunately, the sewage treatment is of a high order!

The city of Adelaide in South Australia was first settled in the 1830s and depended for its water upon the River Torrens; this, like so many other rivers of the time, became both a source of drinking water and a means of waste disposal, leading to epidemics of waterborne diseases such as dysentery. In the 1860s, fresh supplies were channelled to the city and by 1903, with the population reaching 200,000, five reservoirs were in use. But in the late 19th century citizens still used several thousand cesspits, which were flushed into the River Torrens (then still used for washing, drinking and cooking), with a consequent death rate of 24 per 1,000 people, twice the rate of the rest of South Australia. The local authority engaged the services of the English civil engineer William Clark (1821–80) to design a sewerage system for the city and in 1879 passed an 'Act for the Better Sewerage and 170

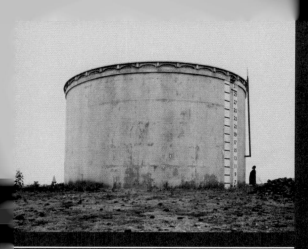

FIG. 52   1909–28 **COUNTRY TOWNS' WATER SUPPLY —**
SYDNEY, AUSTRALIA.

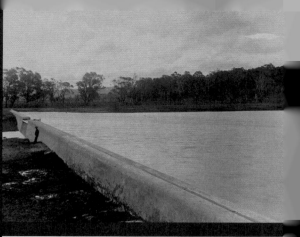

FIG. 53   1909–28 **COUNTRY TOWNS' WATER SUPPLY —**
SYDNEY, AUSTRALIA.

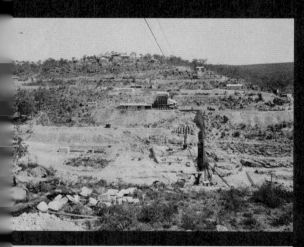

FIG. 54   1927 **WORONORA DAM, PHASE I —**
SYDNEY, AUSTRALIA.

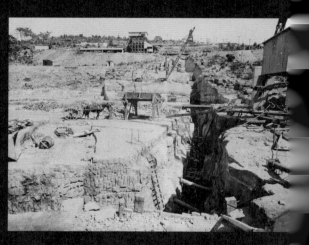

FIG. 55   1927 **WORONORA DAM, PHASE II —**
SYDNEY, AUSTRALIA.

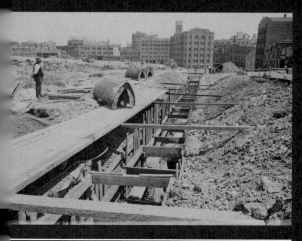

FIG. 56   1921–35 **STORM WATER CHANNEL OF SEWER —**
SYDNEY, AUSTRALIA.

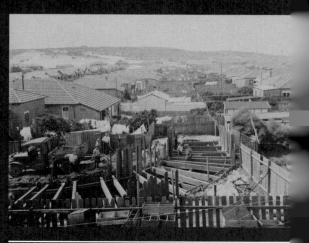

FIG. 57   1929 **ROSE BAY STORM WATER CHANNEL —**
SYDNEY, AUSTRALIA.

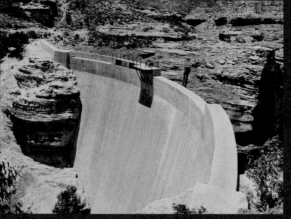
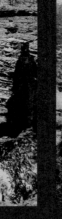

FIG. 58 1909–28 **COUNTRY TOWNS' WATER SUPPLY —** SYDNEY, AUSTRALIA.

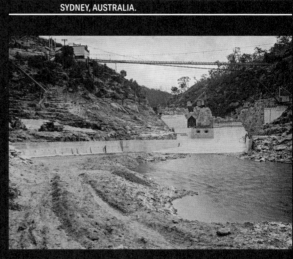

FIG. 59 1909–28 **COUNTRY TOWNS' WATER SUPPLY —** SYDNEY, AUSTRALIA.

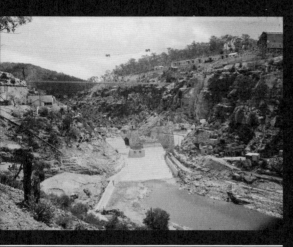

FIG. 60 1927–29 **WORONORA DAM, PHASE III —** SYDNEY, AUSTRALIA.

FIG. 61 1927–29 **WORONORA DAM, PHASE IV —** SYDNEY, AUSTRALIA.

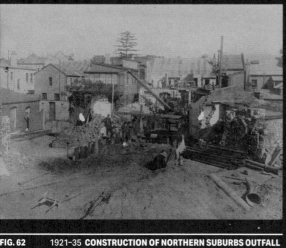

FIG. 62 1921–35 **CONSTRUCTION OF NORTHERN SUBURBS OUTFALL SEWER —** SYDNEY, AUSTRALIA.

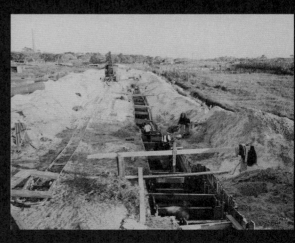

FIG. 63 1921–35 **CONSTRUCTION OF RIFLE RANGE SUB MAIN SEWER —** SYDNEY, AUSTRALIA.

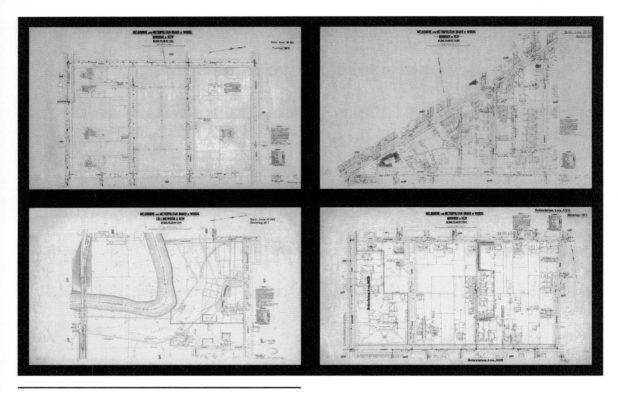

FIGS. 64–71 1905 **DETAILS OF THE MELBOURNE SEWER PLANS —** MELBOURNE, AUSTRALIA. THE ORIGINAL SURVEY PLAN WAS ISSUED BY THE MELBOURE AND METROPOLITAN BOARD OF WORKS TO A CONTRACTOR CONSTRUCTING SEWERS IN THE BOROUGH OF KEW.

Cleansing of Adelaide and Suburbs Thereof' which, following Clark's designs, had by 1885 installed a system of drainage and a sewage farm built at Tam O'Shanter Belt to the north of Adelaide.

The first European settlers visited Melbourne in 1802, but it was not until 1851 that the state of Victoria was established as a separate colony, by which time the population of Melbourne itself was a little over 20,000. The discovery of gold in that year led to a sudden and massive increase in population. By the 1880s, it was Australia's most populous city, with almost 500,000 residents. There was no effective provision for waste disposal, with waste of all kinds, from homes, farms and businesses, being thrown into open channels and washed into the Yarra and Hobson rivers. These supplied much of Melbourne's water. Consequently, epidemics of typhoid and dysentery resulted, though strict quarantine regulations kept Australia largely free of cholera epidemics. Toilets, like those in Sydney, would have been recognized by the Revd Henry Moule and comprised little more than a bucket with a wooden seat, the device being referred to as a 'Thunderbox', like that which brings about the humiliation of Lieutenant Apthorpe in Evelyn Waugh's wartime novel *Men at Arms* (1952). The hot climate and prevalence of flies often made householders reluctant to await the weekly call of the 'nightman' with his 'dunny cart', leading to the practice of simply emptying the contents into street channels.

In 1888, a Royal Commission examined the problems arising from Melbourne's sewage problem and the following year engaged an English engineer, James Mansergh (1835–1905), to design a system. In 1892, construction started, with a system of underground sewers taking the city's waste to a sewage

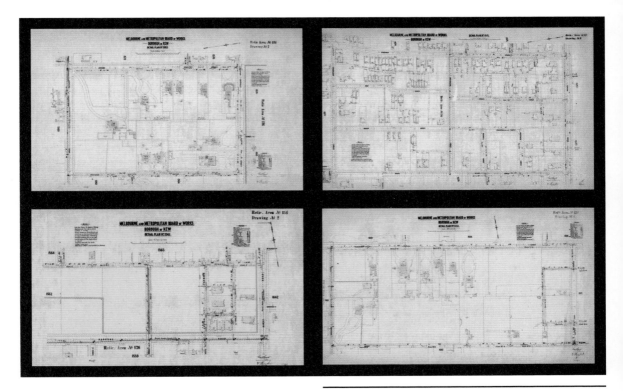

PP. 172–73 **CONSTRUCTING A SEWERAGE SYSTEM** — MELBOURNE, AUSTRALIA. ALL PHOTOGRAPHS ARE TAKEN FROM *THE MELBOURNE & METROPOLITAN BOARD OF WORKS – WATER SUPPLY, SEWERAGE ETC. PHOTOGRAPHIC VIEWS* (1908).

farm at Werribee beyond the city boundary. The first homes were connected to the system in 1897. The sewage was filtered through paddocks, in effect sewage farms. The effluent, having been filtered and cleaned by the soil, passing into earthenware drains, which took it to Port Phillip Bay where it was discharged into the Bass Strait separating Victoria from Tasmania. Once this process had been completed and the paddock was free of sewage, sheep and cattle grazed there while another paddock was used for the filtration. The Werribee plant is still in use, now known as the Western Treatment Plant and occupying 10,500 hectares (40.5 sq miles). Like other treatment plants in Melbourne, it now makes use of 'treatment lagoons' covered with huge plastic covers – about 20 hectares (49 acres) in size – that provide anaerobic (oxygen-free) conditions in which bacteria thrive to consume pathogens in the sewage while producing methane which is captured to provide energy for electricity generation. The sewage then flows to aerobic (oxygen-rich) lagoons into which air is pumped to stimulate the appetites of other bacteria that consume the remaining pathogens. The plant has earned recognition for its wetland habitat, notably for waterfowl.

Australia is the world's driest inhabited continent, with less rainfall than any other and a growing population. Canberra, its most populous inland city, is in one of the driest locations of any city. Consequently, water conservation and re-use is a major concern for its inhabitants. It was chosen as the federal capital in 1908, its site, known as the Australian Capital Territory, situated between the two most populous states of New South Wales and Victoria. Planning for Canberra's sewerage system began in 1915 and led to the creation of a 5-km (3-mile) tunnel from the city to Weston Creek, where a 174

CONSTRUCTING A SEWERAGE SYSTEM

BOARD OF WORKS ESTABLISHED

1

IN 1891 THE MELBOURNE AND METROPOLITAN BOARD OF WORKS WAS FORMED, TASKED WITH CREATING A SYSTEM FOR THE CITY'S WATER SUPPLY AND WASTE REMOVAL. THEY HAD THE AUTHORITY TO RAISE MONEY, DRAW UP PLANS AND EXECUTE THEM.

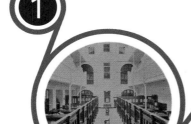

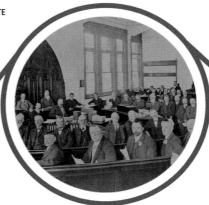

CONSTRUCTING THE SEWERS

3

IN 1892 THE BOARD'S FIRST ENGINEER-IN-CHIEF, MR WILLIAM THWAITES, BEGAN CONSTRUCTION ON MELBOURNE'S SEWERAGE SYSTEM, DESIGNED TO COLLECT AND CHANNEL WASTE FROM BUILDINGS AND STREETS. THE FIRST HOMES WERE CONNECTED TO THE SYSTEM IN 1897.

PUMPING STATION

4

A PUMPING STATION WAS BUILT AT SPOTSWOOD, WHICH WOULD CARRY THE CITY'S WASTE TO THE TREATMENT PLANT AT WERRIBEE.

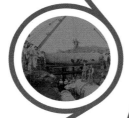

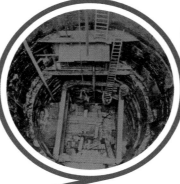

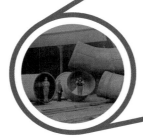

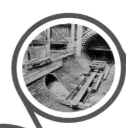

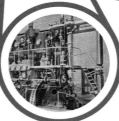

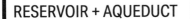

RESERVOIR + AQUEDUCT

BY THE SECOND HALF OF THE 19TH CENTURY MELBOURNE'S POPULATION HAD GROWN TO 500,000. WATER FROM THE EXISTING YAN YEAN RESERVOIR WAS INCREASINGLY POLLUTED AND SO THE WATTS RIVER WAS TAPPED TO CREATE A NEW SUPPLY, TRANSPORTING WATER TO THE CITY VIA THE MAROONDAH AQUEDUCT.

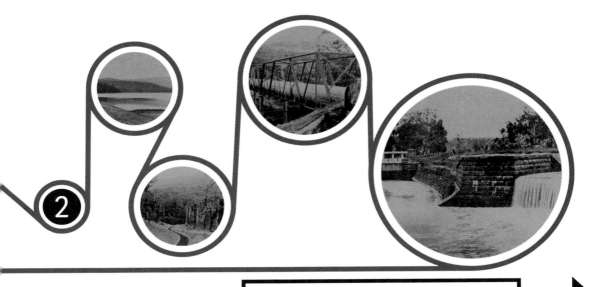

2

SEWAGE FARM + TREATMENT WORKS

THE MAIN OUTFALL SEWER CARRIED THE WASTE 25 KM (15.5 MILES) TO THE WERRIBEE SEWAGE FARM, WHERE THE WASTE WAS MADE FIT FOR DISCHARGE. FLOODING PADDOCKS WITH THE SEWAGE ALLOWED IT TO BE NATURALLY FILTERED BY THE LAND.

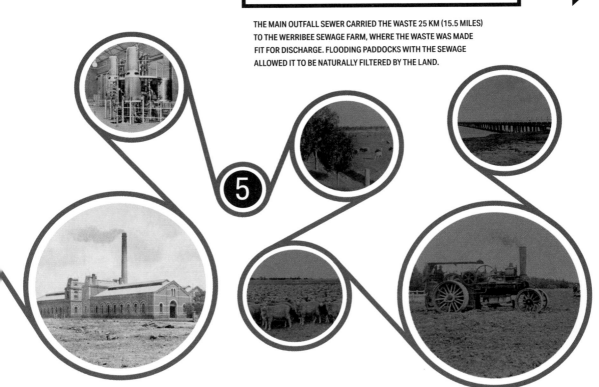

5

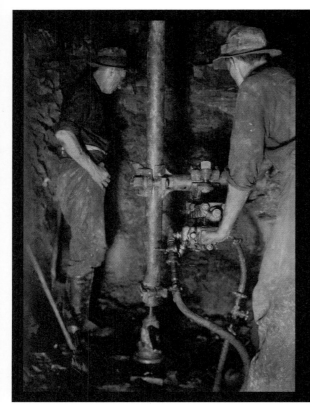
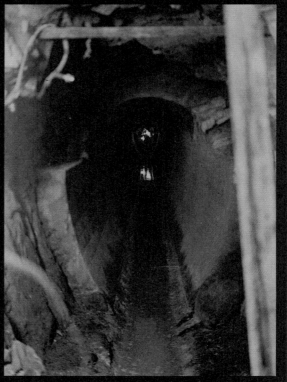

FIG. 72   1921–35 **CONSTRUCTING CANBERRA SEWERS** — CANBERRA, AUSTRALIA. A 5-KM (3-MILE) TUNNEL WAS BUILT TO TAKE THE EFFLUENT TO WESTON CREEK TREATMENT PLANT.

FIG. 73   1921–35 **CONSTRUCTION OF CANBERRA MAIN OUTFALL SEWER** — CANBERRA, AUSTRALIA. WASTE IS TAKEN FOR TREATMENT AND THEN USED FOR IRRIGATION.

treatment works was built and the treated effluent released for irrigation of farmland. The construction work was halted by the outbreak of World War I but resumed in 1922. The treatment works was completed in 1927 to a high standard of effluent treatment, its output eventually reaching the Molonglo River. The plant remained in use until the 1970s. Canberra has introduced means of collecting wastewater that distinguishes between grey water (from surface water, baths and domestic appliances) that can be recycled for irrigation and car washes with little further treatment, and black water (from toilets) that is subjected to more elaborate treatment for use as fertilizer and release to rivers and lakes.

Although the Japanese came rather late to modern sewerage systems, the story of a growth in sewerage systems in concurrence with increasing populations and industrialisation can be seen here too. Although there are traces of drainage systems in earlier periods, the first modern system was built in the Kanda district of Tokyo in 1884, which used brick-lined culverts and both circular and oval pipes. In Osaka the theme common to this period – outbreaks of cholera – led to the construction of the Honda Pumping Station in 1895, making it the first in Japan. Mikawashima Sewer Treatment Plant followed as the first treatment plant in the 1920s but it was the American administration following World War II that led to a burst of activity in the construction of sewerage systems on a large scale: in 1948 the first public sewerage system was begun in Fukai City, in 1958 the New Sewerage Law came into force aiming to conserve the quality of public water, in 1963 the first Five Year Program for Sewerage Construction was launched and in 1964 the Japan Sewage Works Association was established. However this rapid growth of industry and construction led to an increase in water demand, and a simultaneous deterioration in the water quality of rivers and oceans. The water quality of Dokai Bay (on the south-west coast of Japan) was so polluted by 1963 from the effluent of the city of Kitakyushu that it was known as the 'Dead Sea'. Thus In the 1970s, a major effort was mounted to improve the sanitation of Japanese cities, with the emphasis on the treatment and recycling of wastewater and the recovery of incinerated ash from treatment works to make bricks, tiles and cement. These measures were so successful that one can now find up to 100 species of fish and marine life in Dokai Bay. In the 20th and 21st centuries the Japanese have shown innovation and flair in the construction of their sewers. In the Tokyo area some sewage treatment works, with their high-tech appearance, have been used to stage exhibition and even fashion shows, while the skills of artists have been applied to the design of manhole covers, cities and towns having their own designs like a coat of arms. And although they came late to modern sewerage systems, the Japanese have shown characteristic enterprise in the invention of new domestic toilets, integrating, among other features, heated seats, hands-free use and air de-odorization!

FIGS. 74–77   PLANS FOR THE MIKAWASHIMA SEWAGE DISPOSAL PLANT —
TOKYO, JAPAN. JAPAN'S FIRST SEWAGE TREATMENT PLANT WAS
BUILT IN 1922. IN 2007 IT WAS RECOGNIZED AS A CULTRAL ASSET
OF NATIONAL IMPORTANCE.

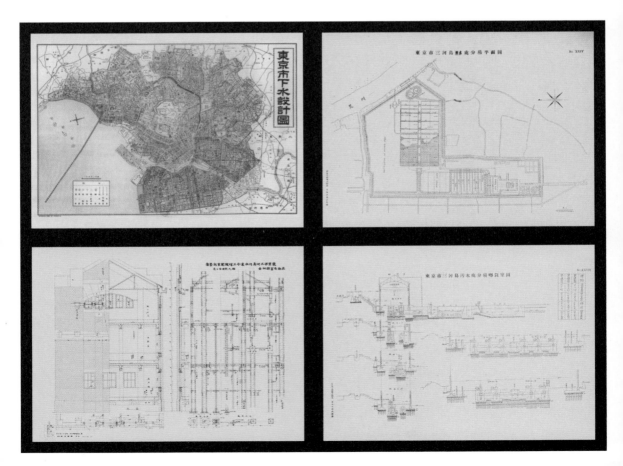

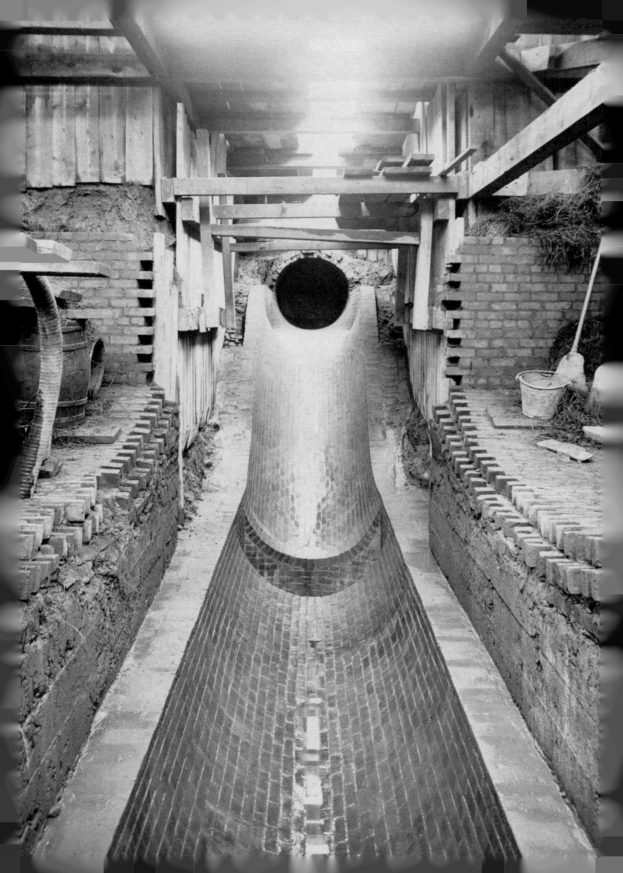

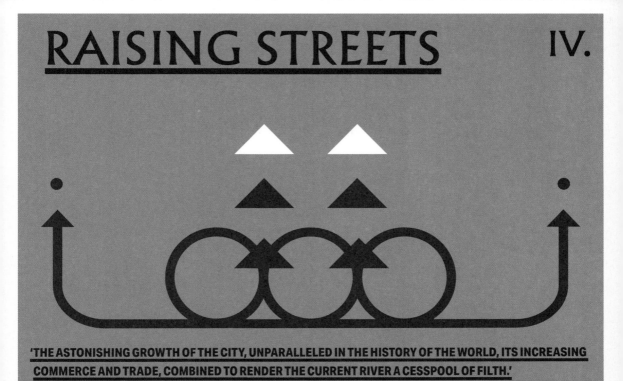

RAISING STREETS IV.

'THE ASTONISHING GROWTH OF THE CITY, UNPARALLELED IN THE HISTORY OF THE WORLD, ITS INCREASING COMMERCE AND TRADE, COMBINED TO RENDER THE CURRENT RIVER A CESSPOOL OF FILTH.'

The Great Chicago Lake Tunnel, 1867

As in Europe the expansion of American cities and their populations placed strain on existing systems, leading to polluted water supplies and outbreaks of diseases such as typhoid and cholera throughout the 19th century. This resulted in the construction of modern sewerage systems throughout America, although in several cases it occurred relatively late in the 19th century and some cities did not upgrade their systems until well into the 20th century. American engineers faced a wide range of natural obstacles, including earthquake-prone rock and arid plains; they remained admirably undeterred by the prospect of elevating cities, reversing rivers or draining swamps.

The colony (later state) of Massachusetts had water-pollution-control regulations in place as early as 1647, twenty-seven years after the Pilgrim Fathers first set foot on Plymouth Rock. Its principal city, Boston, had sewers made of hollowed-out logs by the 18th century, though these were replaced in the 1840s by a more comprehensive system of cast-iron pipes following a design by the civil engineer John Jervis (1795–1885). Boston's early example was followed by Philadelphia which, with a legacy from Benjamin Franklin (1706–90), in 1801 installed a system designed by an English immigrant named Benjamin Latrobe (1764–1820). This brought water from the Schuylkill River through a 72-km (45-mile) long network of wooden pipes made of oak, pine and spruce. ⊙———————▶ 186

FIG. 1 1880–89 **BOSTON SEWER SIPHON** — BOSTON, USA.
A SEWER SIPHON REPLACED ONE OF THE ORIGNAL HOLLOWED
OUT LOGS INSTALLED BY EARLY SETTLERS.

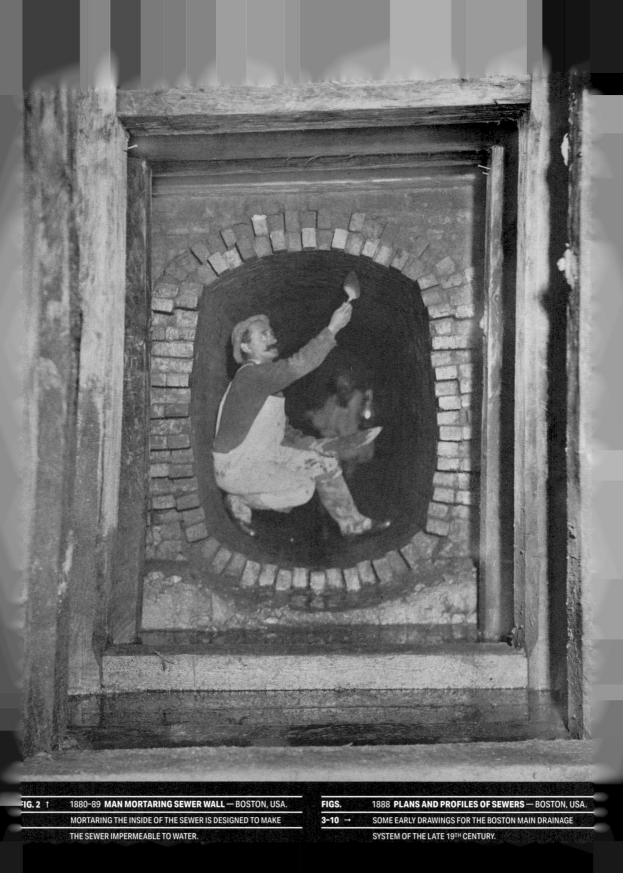

FIG. 2 ↑   1880–89 **MAN MORTARING SEWER WALL** — BOSTON, USA.
MORTARING THE INSIDE OF THE SEWER IS DESIGNED TO MAKE
THE SEWER IMPERMEABLE TO WATER.

FIGS.   1888 **PLANS AND PROFILES OF SEWERS** — BOSTON, USA.
3–10 →   SOME EARLY DRAWINGS FOR THE BOSTON MAIN DRAINAGE
SYSTEM OF THE LATE 19TH CENTURY.

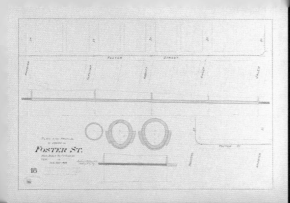

FOSTER ST.

18

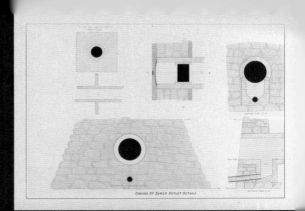

OSGOOD ST. SEWER OUTLET DETAIL

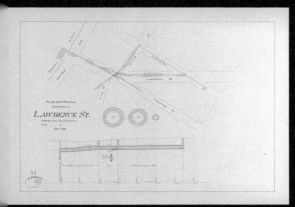

PLAN AND PROFILE
OF SEWER IN
LAWRENCE ST.

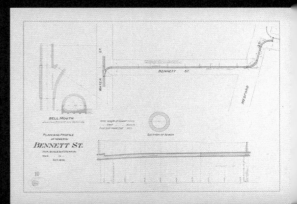

BELL MOUTH

PLAN AND PROFILE
OF SEWER IN
BENNETT ST.

10

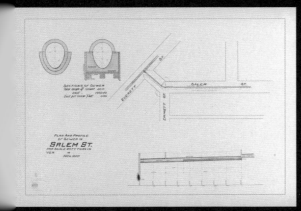

SECTION OF SEWER

PLAN AND PROFILE
OF SEWER IN
SALEM ST.

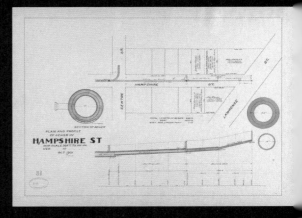

SECTION OF SEWER

PLAN AND PROFILE
OF SEWER IN
HAMPSHIRE ST
OCT 1901

31

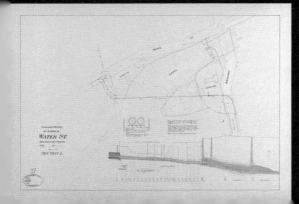

PLAN AND PROFILE
OF SEWER IN
WATER ST.

SECTION 1.

27

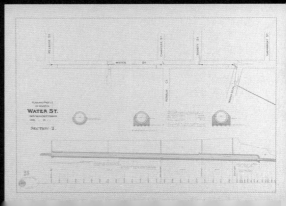

WATER ST.

SECTION 2.

28

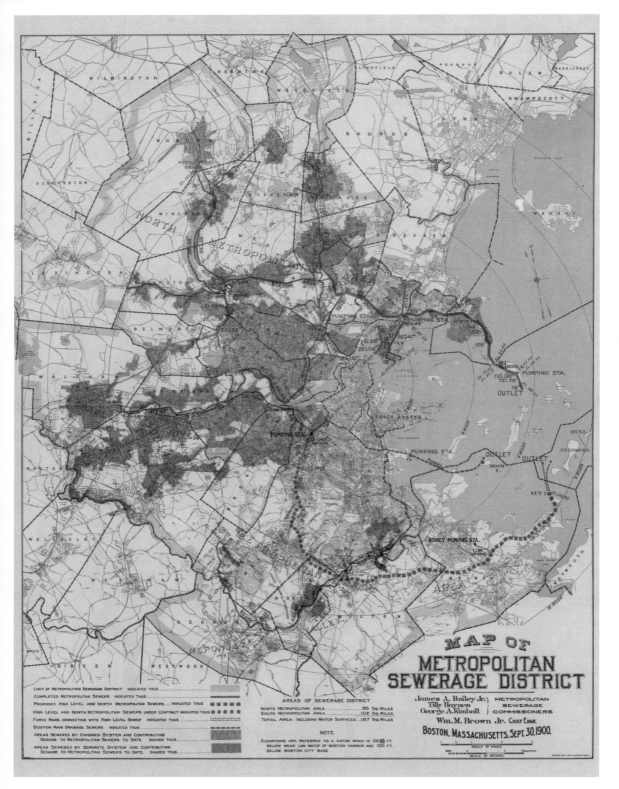

FIG. 11   1900 **MAP OF METROPOLITAN SEWERAGE DISTRICT** — BOSTON, USA. THIS PLAN ILLUSTRATES HOW BOSTON'S WASTE WAS CARRIED

IN SEWERS – INDICATED BY RED LINES – TO MOON, DEER AND NUT ISLANDS IN BOSTON HARBOUR WHERE IT WAS HELD IN SEWAGE RESERVOIRS

BEFORE BEING RELEASED INTO THE BAY ON THE OUTGOING TIDE.

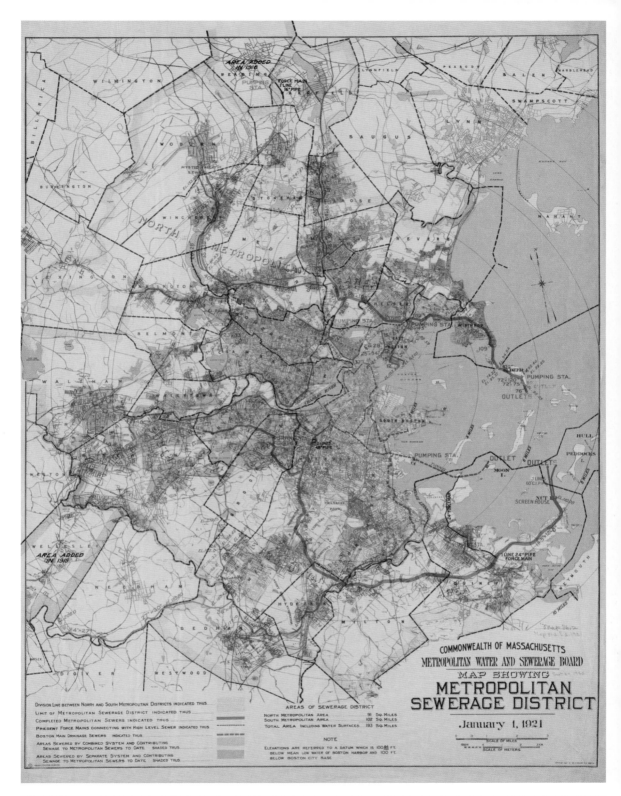

FIG. 12   1921 **MAP OF METROPOLITAN SEWERAGE DISTRICT** — BOSTON, USA. BY 1921 THE BAY HAD BECOME SEVERELY POLLUTED FROM THE CITY'S

SEWAGE. IN 1952 A TREATMENT PLANT WAS CONSTRUCTED ON NUT ISLAND. HOWEVER, THIS MADE AN INSUFFICIENT DIFFERENCE AND IT WAS NOT

UNTIL THE BOSTON HARBOUR CLEAN UP DURING THE 1980s THAT THE HARBOUR WATER WAS RESCUED.

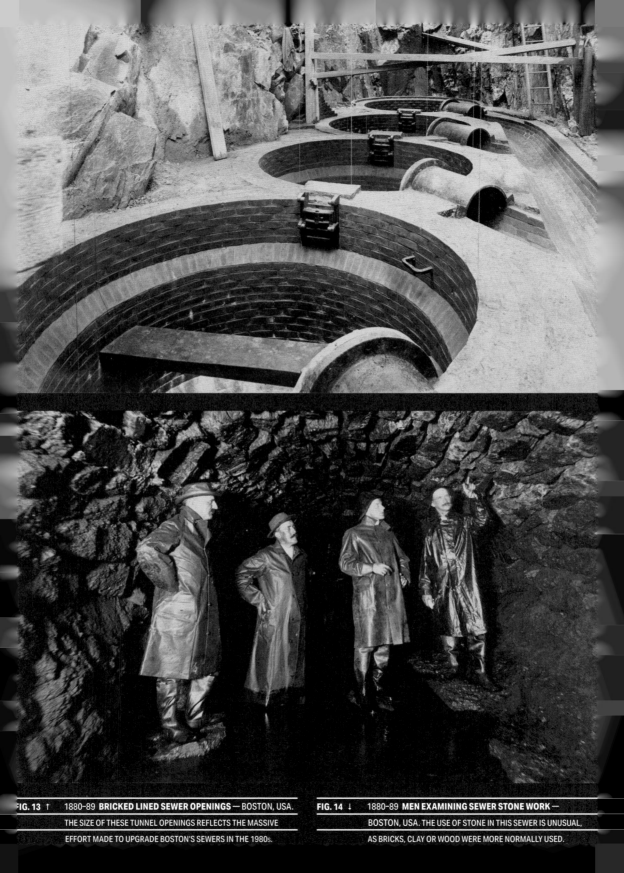

FIG. 13 ↑   1880-89 **BRICKED LINED SEWER OPENINGS** — BOSTON, USA.
THE SIZE OF THESE TUNNEL OPENINGS REFLECTS THE MASSIVE
EFFORT MADE TO UPGRADE BOSTON'S SEWERS IN THE 1980s.

FIG. 14 ↓   1880-89 **MEN EXAMINING SEWER STONE WORK** —
BOSTON, USA. THE USE OF STONE IN THIS SEWER IS UNUSUAL,
AS BRICKS, CLAY OR WOOD WERE MORE NORMALLY USED.

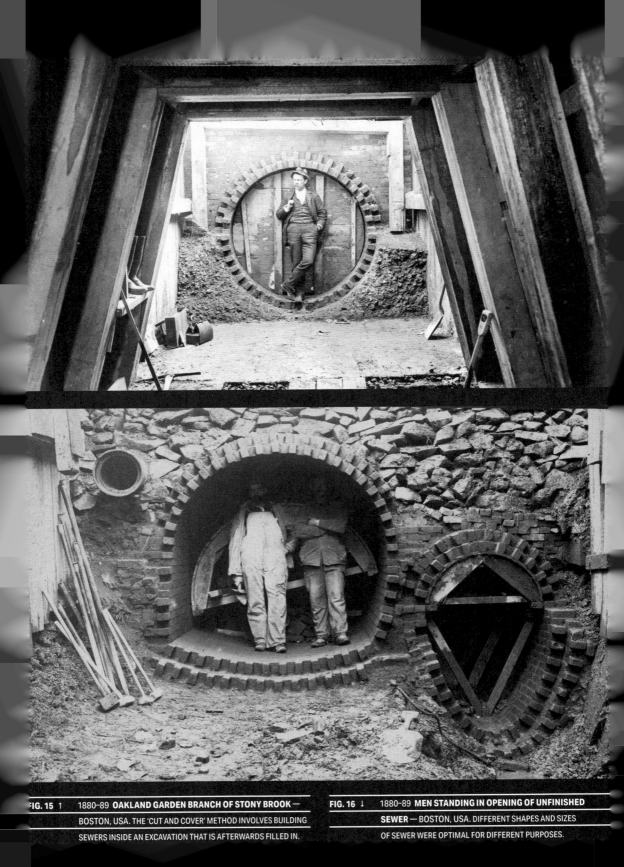

FIG. 15 ↑ 1880–89 **OAKLAND GARDEN BRANCH OF STONY BROOK** — BOSTON, USA. THE 'CUT AND COVER' METHOD INVOLVES BUILDING SEWERS INSIDE AN EXCAVATION THAT IS AFTERWARDS FILLED IN.

FIG. 16 ↓ 1880–89 **MEN STANDING IN OPENING OF UNFINISHED SEWER** — BOSTON, USA. DIFFERENT SHAPES AND SIZES OF SEWER WERE OPTIMAL FOR DIFFERENT PURPOSES.

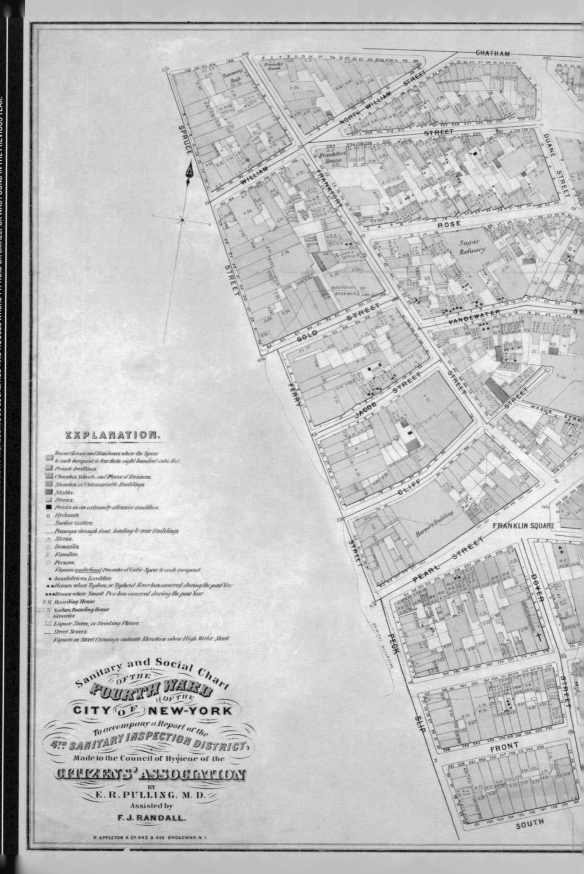

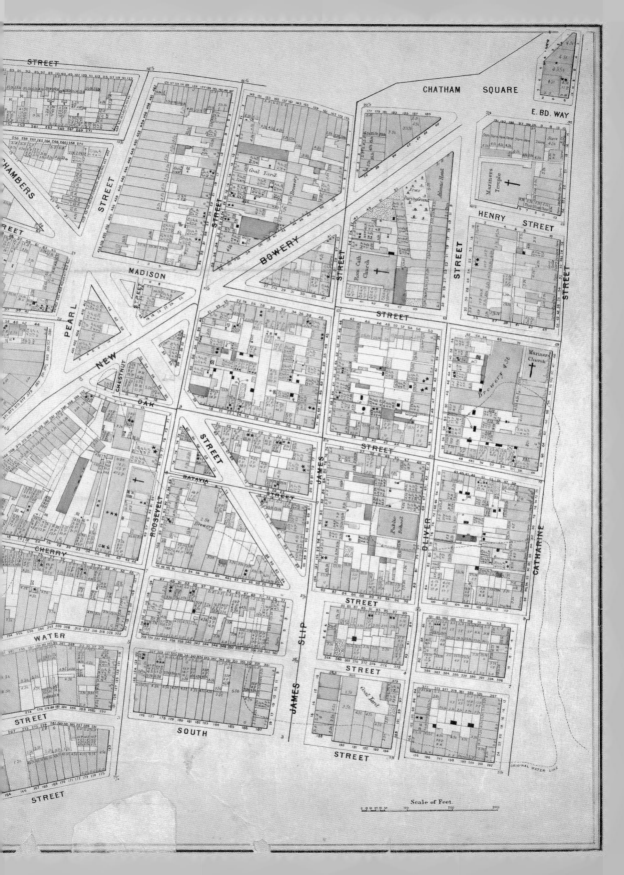

Some of Philadelphia's pipes remained in service until 1858, when the last ones were substituted by cast-iron replacements. The faint taste of timber in the water drawn from standpipes was preferred to the dangers of epidemic disease from polluted wells. Boston's early sewers were mostly privately owned and were used to drain water from cellars and low-lying areas into nearby rivers and lakes and in 1709 the Massachusetts General Court passed regulations governing the ways in which sewers should be constructed, the system at this point being concerned, as in London, with the drainage of surface water. In 1833, recalling the situation in London, it was permitted to discharge sanitary waste into the sewers and rainwater was used to flush the waste into rivers and other sources of drinking water that led, as in Europe, to outbreaks of waterborne diseases, including cholera, typhoid and dysentery.

As in Europe, the arrival of epidemic disease galvanized the city fathers into action and from 1877 to 1884 the Boston Main Drainage System was built. It included 40 km (25 miles) of intercepting sewers that collected sewage from buildings and streets and took it to Moon Island in Boston Harbor, where it was discharged. In 1889, as the city grew, the drainage area was increased and as the volume of sewage increased the harbour became polluted (see maps on pages 180–81). Wastewater treatment plants were built there, one at Nut Island in 1952 and a second at Deer Island in 1968, the latter being upgraded in 2000 to give more effective treatment to the waste before it is discharged into the harbour.

FIG. 18   1865 **TOPOGRAPHICAL MAP OF THE CITY OF NEW YORK** —
NEW YORK, USA. MARSHLAND IS TURQUOISE, MADE LAND IS PALE
PINK AND MEADOW LAND IS PALE BLUE IN THIS ILLUSTRATION OF
THE CHALLENGES PRESENTED TO ENGINEERS BY THE LANDSCAPE.

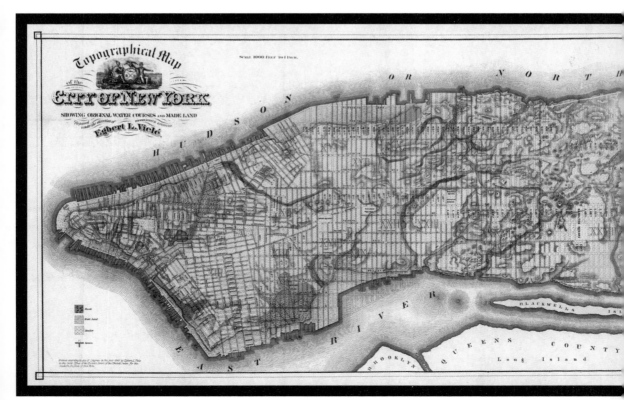

By 1840, New York was already the USA's most populous city with more than 300,000 citizens, thrice the size of Baltimore, the second largest. Most New Yorkers lived on the island of Manhattan, which is surrounded by the East River and Hudson River, both containing salty Atlantic water, leaving the residents dependent upon wells for their sometimes brackish drinking water. In 1842, the Croton Aqueduct was completed, designed by John Jervis, who later produced a water system for Boston. The aqueduct brought fresh water 67.5 km (42 miles) from the Croton River in Westchester County. The wells fell into disuse, leading to a rise in the water table that caused cellars to become flooded. Sewers already existed for rainwater and they were usually open, running along the middle of the street like the kennels of London (see page 38), though often much larger, such as the one on 9th Street, which was reported to be 6 m (20 ft) wide. Following a cholera epidemic, in 1845 the city's authorities permitted residents to dump human, animal and food waste in the sewers and in 1857 this prompted the New York State legislature to set up a Board of Sewers 'to devise and carry into effect a plan of drainage and sewerage for the whole city, upon a regular system, for the purpose of carrying off the water and filth to be carried off in sewers for the health and convenience of the inhabitants.' Between 1850 and 1855, the city laid about 113 km (70 miles) of sewers and by 1900 virtually all the city's buildings were connected to public sewers. Treatment plants followed in the 20th century but until the 1980s much of Manhattan's sewage flowed untreated into the Hudson River. The city continues to suffer from sewage overflows when heavy rain causes sewage, swollen by rain, to overflow into the rivers, the remedy being huge underground reservoirs where the overflow can be stored until the rain subsides and the contents of the reservoirs can be pumped to treatment works.

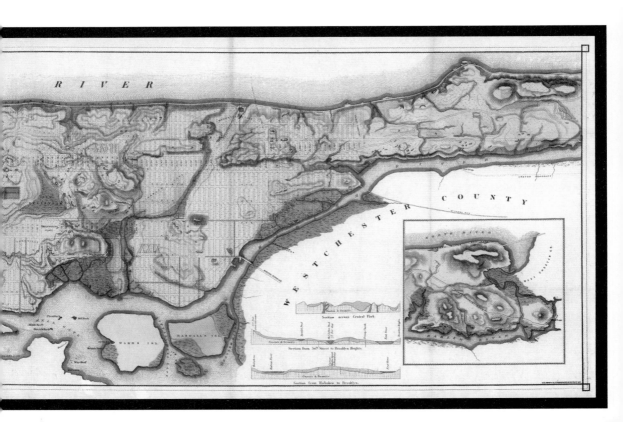

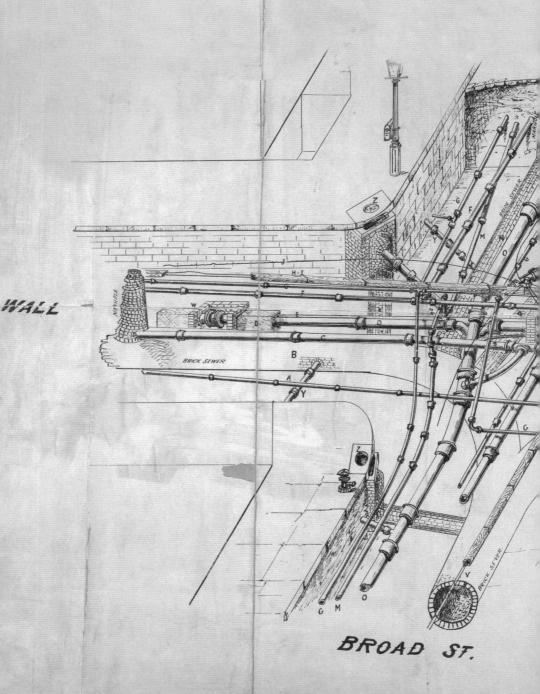

WALL

BROAD ST.

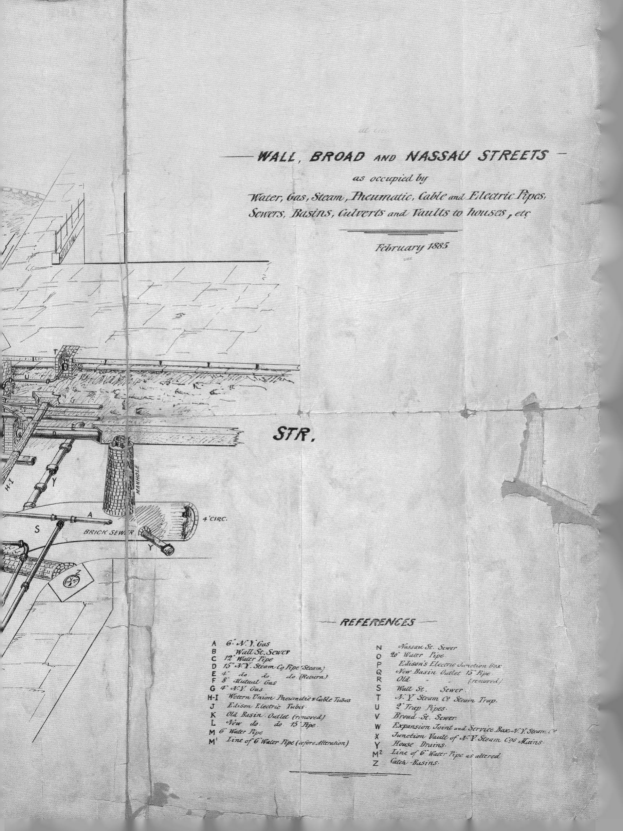

— WALL, BROAD AND NASSAU STREETS —

as occupied by

Water, Gas, Steam, Pneumatic, Cable and Electric Pipes, Sewers, Basins, Culverts and Vaults to houses, etc

February 1885

STR.

MANHOLE

4'CIRC.

BRICK SEWER

— REFERENCES —

A	6" N.Y. Gas	N	Nassau St. Sewer
B	Wall St. Sewer	O	20" Water Pipe
C	12" Water Pipe	P	Edison's Electric Junction Box
D	15" N.Y. Steam Co Pipe (Steam)	Q	New Basin Outlet 15" Pipe
E	4" do. do. do (Return)	R	Old do. (removed)
F	8" Mutual Gas	S	Wall St. Sewer
G	4" N.Y. Gas	T	N.Y. Steam Co. Steam Trap.
H-I	Western Union Pneumatic & Cable Tubes	U	2" Trap Pipes.
J	Edison Electric Tubes.	V	Broad St. Sewer
K	Old Basin Outlet (removed)	W	Expansion Joint and Service Box. N.Y. Steam Co
L	New do. do 15" Pipe.	X	Junction Vault of N.Y. Steam Co's Mains.
M	6" Water Pipe	Y	House Drains.
M¹	Line of 6" Water Pipe (before Alteration)	M²	Line of 6" Water Pipe as altered
		Z	Catch Basins.

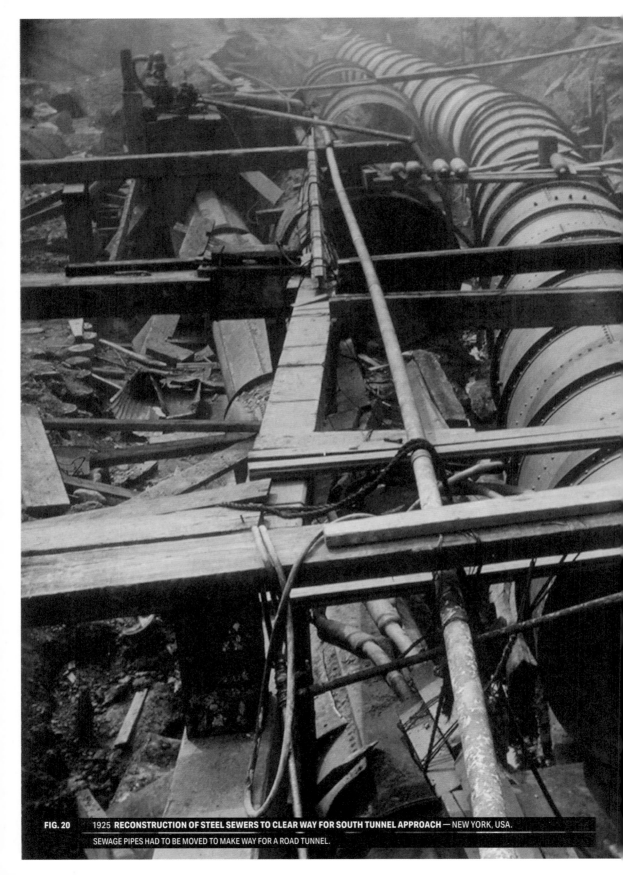

FIG. 20   1925 **RECONSTRUCTION OF STEEL SEWERS TO CLEAR WAY FOR SOUTH TUNNEL APPROACH** — NEW YORK, USA.

SEWAGE PIPES HAD TO BE MOVED TO MAKE WAY FOR A ROAD TUNNEL.

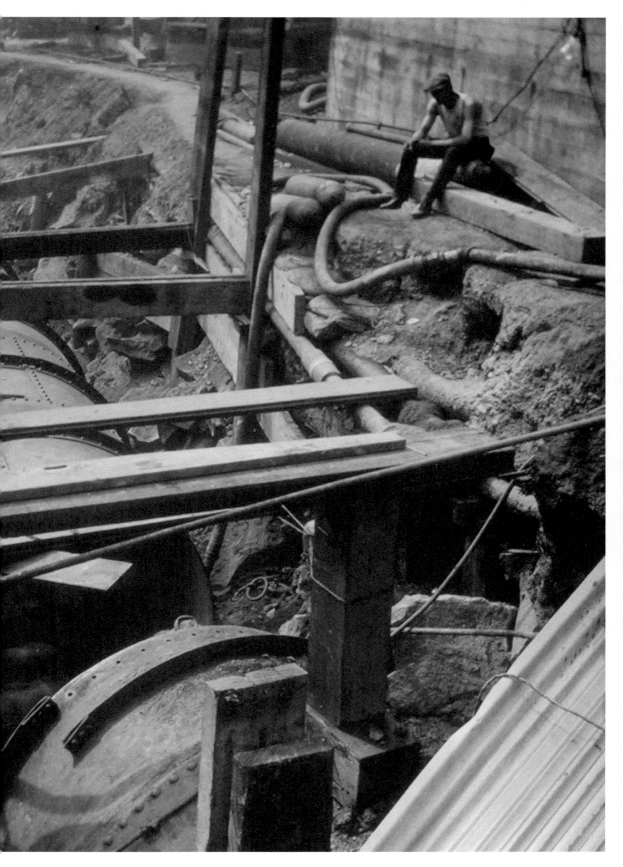

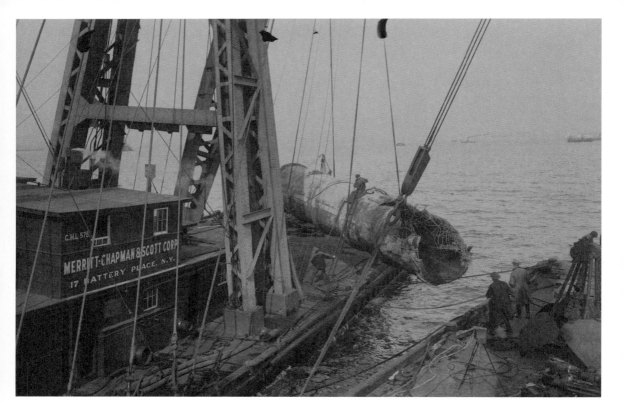

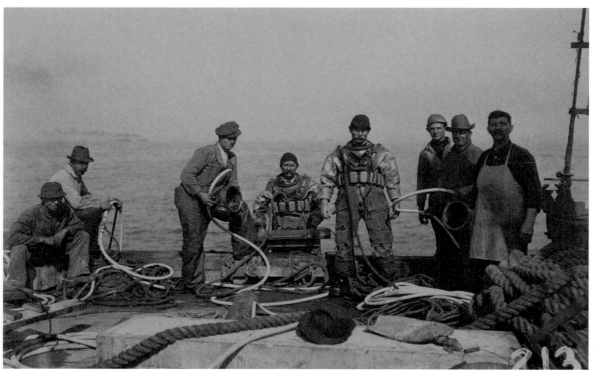

FIG. 21 ↑ 1923 **A DAMAGED SEWER PIPE** — NEW JERSEY, USA.
THE GROUNDING OF THE SS *LEVIATHON* OFF ROBBINS REEF
CAUSED SEVERE DAMAGE TO A SEWER PIPE.

FIG. 22 ↓ 1920s **CONSTRUCTION OF OUTFALL PIPE** — NEW JERSEY, USA.
DIVERS ABOUT TO PLUNGE INTO THE HUDSON RIVER IN ORDER TO
CONSTRUCT AN OUTFALL PIPE.

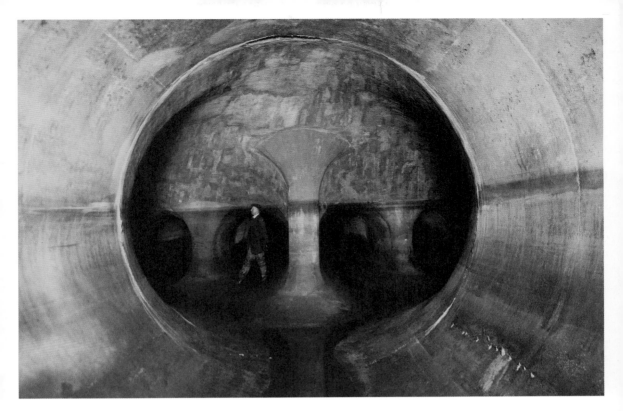

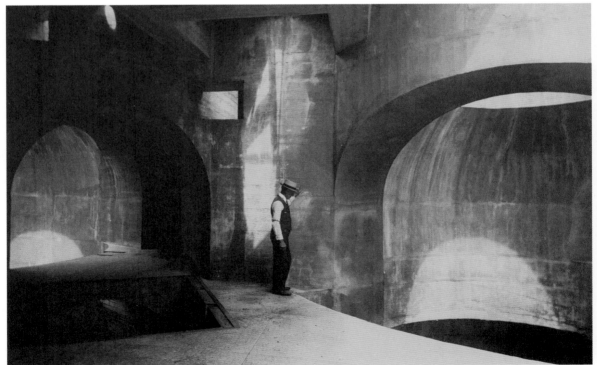

FIG. 23 ↑   1920s **CONSTRUCTION OF INTERCEPTOR SEWERS** —
NEW JERSEY, USA. THE MAIN INTERCEPTOR IS 35 KM (22 MILES)
LONG AND CONNECTS TO 29 KM (18 MILES) OF BRANCH SEWERS.

FIG. 24 ↓   1920s **WET WEATHER PUMP STATION** — NEW JERSEY, USA.
THE WET WEATHER PUMP STATION WAS REQUIRED TO RELIEVE
THE SEWERS AT TIMES OF HEAVY RAINFALL.

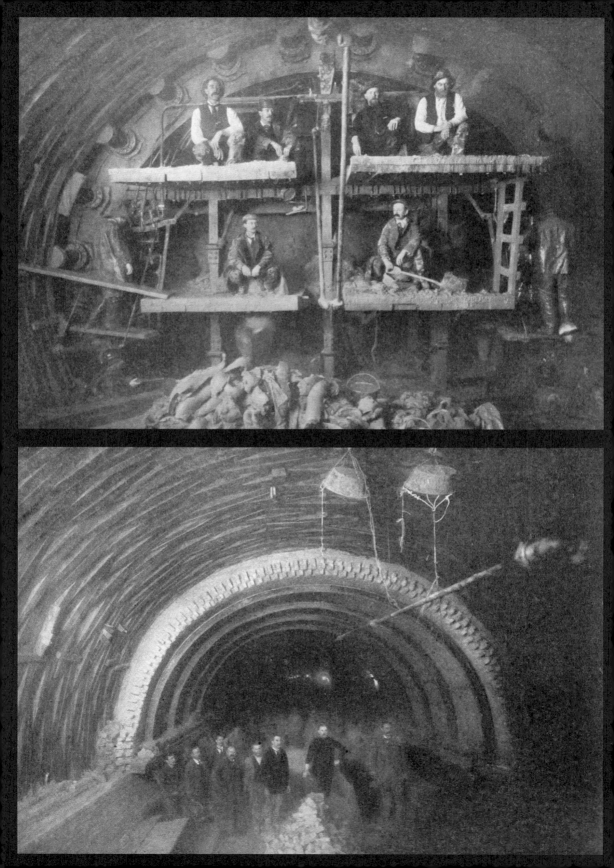

New York's sewers have been more subject than most to the growth of legends. One concerns the supposed tendency of New Yorkers to return from their holidays in Florida with baby alligators, only to dispose of them in the sewers when they become unmanageably large. This legend appears to owe its origins to the memories of a former sewer inspector. A further myth concerns the supposed existence in the sewers of 'New York White' marijuana flushed down water closets by citizens, the plant then flourishing in the nutrient-rich environment of the sewers. There is as much evidence to support these legends as there is for that of the Loch Ness Monster.

That said, the sewers of New York have provided potent imagery that has been effectively drawn on by artists, writers and filmmakers. In 1952 Gordon Parks interpreted Ralph Ellison's novel *The Invisible Man* (1952) into a surreal and haunting photo series. Particularly arresting images are those of the unnamed narrator emerging from a sewer onto a Harlem Street. The sewers symbolised both his ostracism from society, but also his sanctuary from the virulent racism that nearly destroyed him. Though perhaps a better-known example of the New York sewers permeating popular consciousness is their use as the home for the Mutant Ninja Turtles!

Chicago presented unusual problems for sanitary engineers, owing to the fact that the city sits just a few feet above the level of the water in Lake Michigan, making it difficult to channel wastewater to the lake by gravity, from which, in any case, drinking water was drawn. In 1855, therefore, the Chicago Board of Sewerage Commissioners decide to raise the level of the streets close to the lake, and the buildings on them, by 1.2–4.2 m (4–14 ft). One of the engineers employed to execute this amazing task was George Pullman (1831–97), who is more often remembered for his invention of the sleeping and restaurant cars on trains, from which he made his fortune and which bear his name. He was assigned the task of raising the buildings on Lake Street; he did so by installing 6,000 jackscrews beneath the buildings, manned by teams of men who, on a signal, would raise the buildings by a fraction of an inch. This was repeated over several days while new foundations were inserted beneath the buildings (which remained occupied while this was going on). In other places, logs were slid beneath the buildings, which were then rolled to new sites. The sewerage system was designed by the city engineer Ellis Chesbrough (1813–86), who laid the sewers above ground while the buildings were raised and then buried the sewers when the city had been raised to the required level.

Much of the sewage was despatched to the Chicago River, which carried it into Lake Michigan, but to protect the drinking water supply a tunnel was driven beneath the lake 3 km (2 miles) offshore in the hope that the water drawn through it from the lake would be free of pollution. This was only partially and temporarily successful. As Chicago expanded, the tunnel was extended farther into the lake, but eventually the decision was taken to reverse the flow of the river so that it took the city's sewage away from Lake Michigan towards the Mississippi, this work being completed after Chesbrough had died. Finally, in the early 20th century, Chicago constructed its first sewage treatment works. It now has six, the largest being the Stickney Plant in the city's Cicero district, where the wastewater is cleaned and, when the pollutants have been removed, returned to local rivers.

o———————➤ 198

FIGS. 25–26 1912 **CONSTRUCTING THE 39TH STREET INTERCEPTING SEWER** — CHICAGO, USA. MEN AT WORK CONSTRUCTING WHAT WAS, IN 1905, THE LARGEST SEWER IN THE WORLD.

FIGS. 27–34 | 1913 BLUEPRINTS FOR SEWER SYSTEMS IN ILLINOIS — ILLINOIS, USA. THESE PLANS WERE SUBMITTED AS PART OF A UNIVERSITY DEGREE THESIS AT THE ARMOUR INSTITUTE OF TECHNOLOGY, ILLINOIS.

FIG. 35 | | 1912 DEFLECTOR RING AND HUB OF SCREW PUMP IN 39TH STREET PUMPING STATION — CHICAGO, USA. THE SCREW PUMP DESIGN WAS REUSED FROM A MODEL USED TO FLUSH THE MILWAUKEE RIVER.

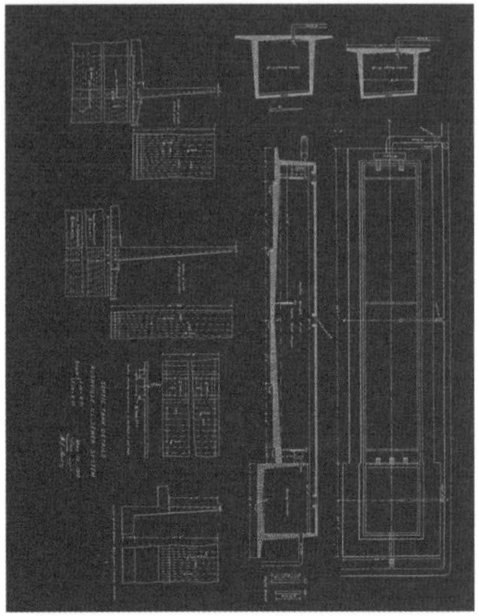

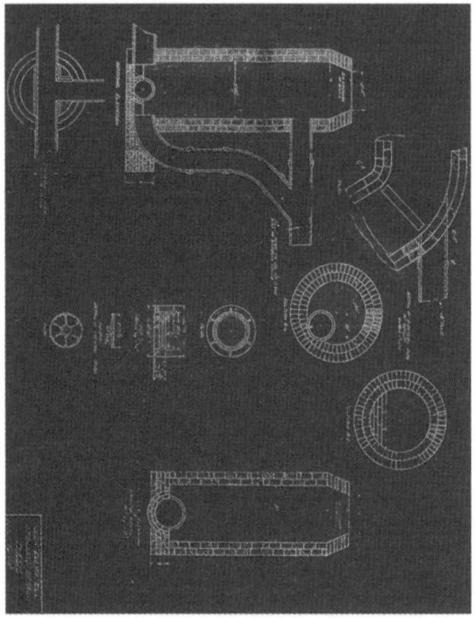

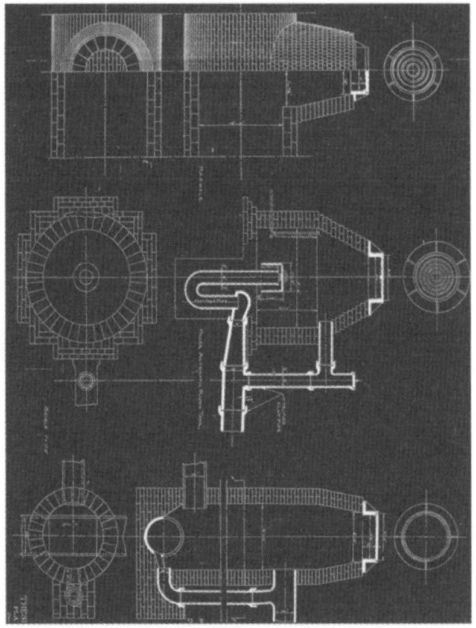

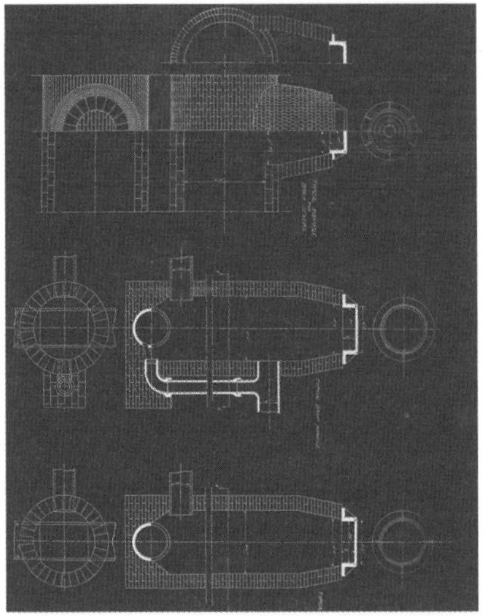

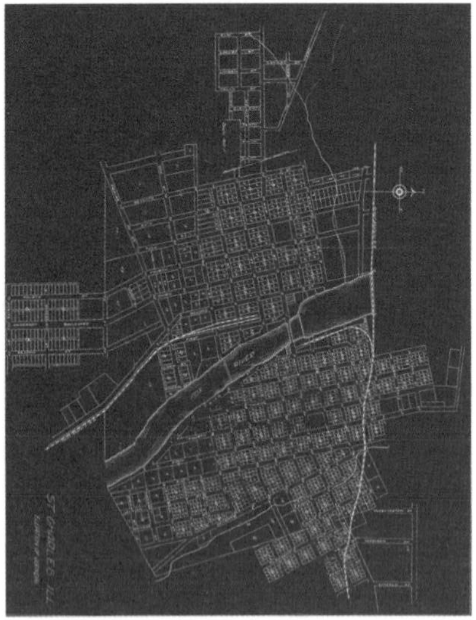

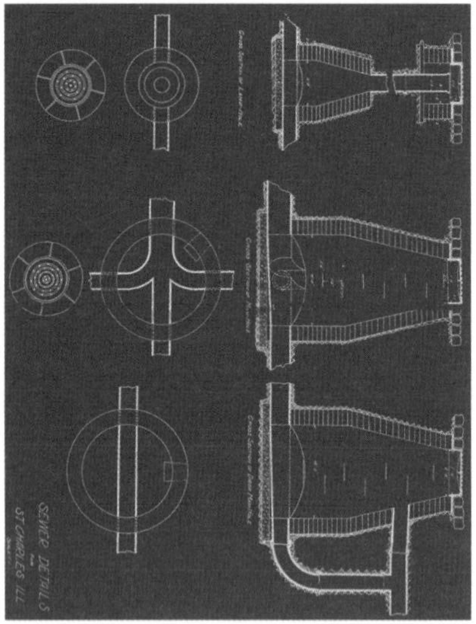

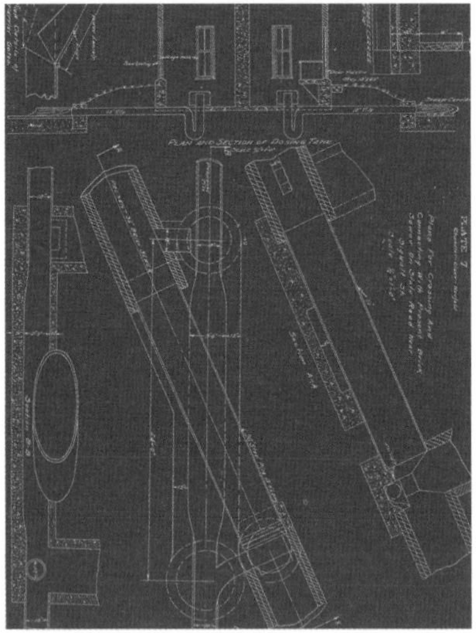

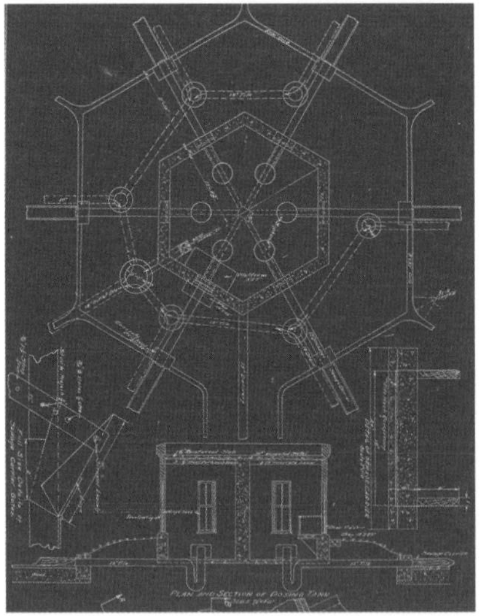

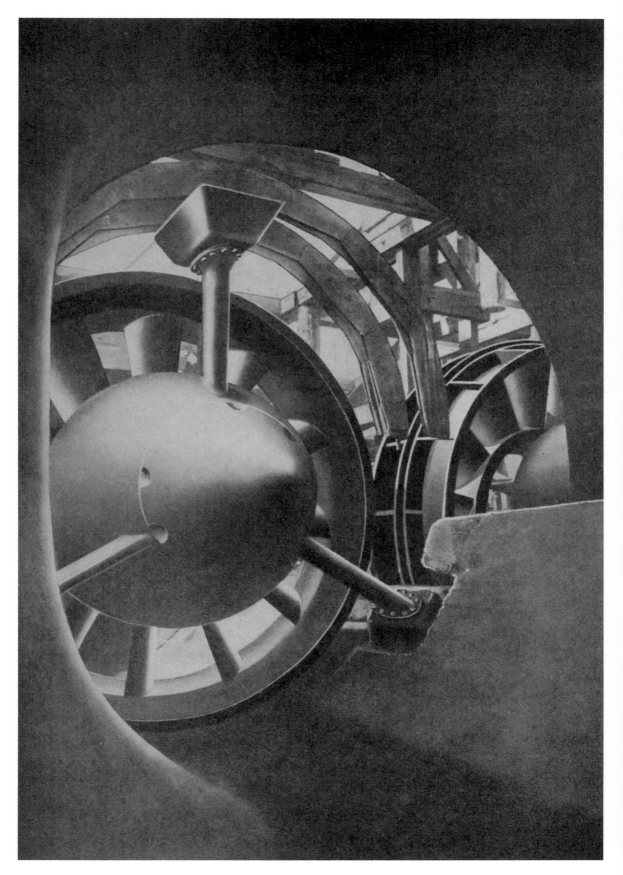

Washington, DC came late to the adoption of modern sewage treatment processes but it eventually installed particularly effective technology to clean its waste. In the early years of the 19th century, the first sewers were built to drain storm water from the low-lying, swampy site that had been carved from the borderland between Virginia and Maryland as a home for the Federal government. These drainage channels were not linked to a coherent system and, in the absence of any treatment works, simply discharged sewage into the Potomac and Anacostia rivers. In 1852, the US Army Corps of Engineers began to build the Washington aqueduct to bring fresh water to the capital but still no sewer system was built and in their absence the increase in population that occurred during the Civil War led to epidemics of typhoid and malaria that cost thousands of lives. In the 1870s, some 129 km (80 miles) of sewers were built to collect both wastewater and rainwater and conducted them to the Potomac – which, downstream of the capital, became heavily polluted. It was in 1938 that a treatment plant was finally built, at Blue Plains, on the fringe of the District of Columbia. In 2015, as part of a scheme to restore the ecology of Chesapeake Bay, the world's largest thermal hydrolysis treatment plant was installed at Blue Plains to ensure an exceptionally high level of water purity before discharge into the Potomac and hence to the bay (the thermal hydrolysis process is described on page 228).

FIG. 36   1937 **RAW SEWAGE BEING DISCHARGED INTO SANTA MONICA BAY** — LOS ANGELES, USA. PRIOR TO THE CONSTRUCTION OF THE HYPERION TREATMENT PLANT IN 1950 RAW SEWAGE WAS DUMPED INTO THE BAY.

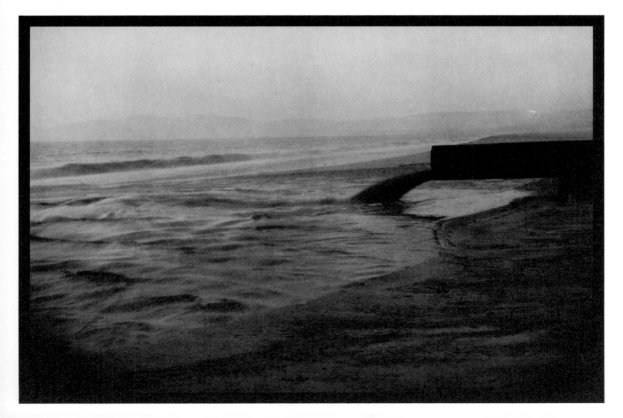

In 1870, Los Angeles had fewer than 6,000 residents, little more than a large village, and even in 1900, with just over 100,000, it was only the 36th US city in population size. In 2017, however, it was second only to New York, its inhabitants numbering almost 4 million. In the circumstances it is not surprising that, well into the 20th century, its sewerage was primitive. It had started well when, in 1781, the Spanish settlers had dug a brick ditch – the 'Zanja Madre' or 'Mother Ditch' – to bring water from the nearby Los Angeles River to the settlement. The ditch was covered over in the 19th century and from time to time building and excavation work reveals traces of it. The first major attempt to prepare a sewerage plan for the city was made by a civil engineer called Fred Eaton while he was working as city surveyor in 1887, by which time the population was approaching 50,000. Eaton's scheme collected waste from street sewers and conducted it by outfalls, in its raw state, to the Santa Monica Bay so by 1925 that part of the Pacific Ocean was seriously polluted. It was not until 1950, with the population close to 2 million, that a modern treatment plant named 'Hyperion' was built close to Santa Monica Bay; by 1957 the growth of the city was such that Hyperion could not fully treat the effluent that continued to flow through a pipe 8 km (5 miles) long into the ocean. Monitoring of the ocean floor revealed that the only creatures able to survive among the effluent, which included tampons, condoms and used syringes, were worms and some species of clam.

○————▶ 204

FIG. 37 1935 **WORKERS INSTALLING STORM DRAIN PIPE** — LOS ANGELES, USA. THESE PIPES WERE USED TO DIVERT HEAVY RAINFALL INTO THE SANTA MONICA BAY.

FIGS. 38–39 1935 **A SEWER MAINTENANCE YARD** — LOS ANGELES, USA. SEWER WORKERS WERE SUITABLY EQUIPPED WITH APPARATUS AND PROTECTIVE CLOTHING.

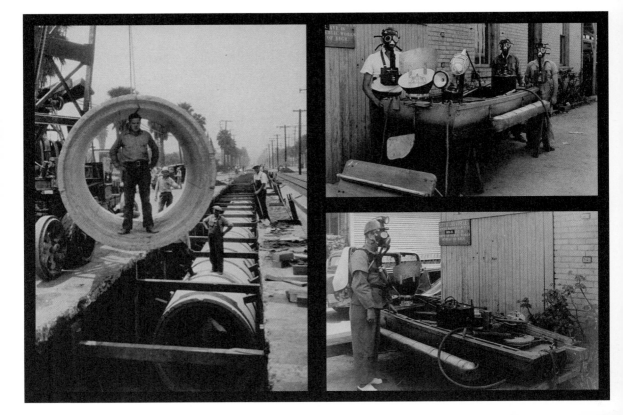

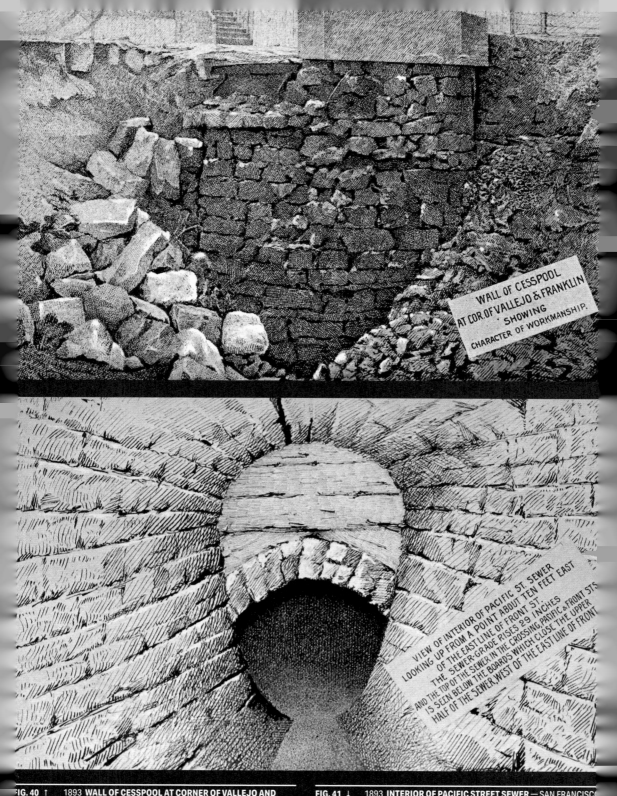

WALL OF CESSPOOL
AT COR. OF VALLEJO & FRANKLIN
SHOWING
CHARACTER OF WORKMANSHIP.

VIEW OF INTERIOR OF PACIFIC ST SEWER
LOOKING UP FROM A POINT ABOUT TEN FEET EAST
OF THE EAST LINE OF FRONT ST
THE SEWER-GRADE RISES 29 INCHES
AND THE TOP OF THE SEWER IN THE CROSSING PACIFIC & FRONT STS
IS SEEN BELOW THE BOARDS WHICH CLOSE THE UPPER
HALF OF THE SEWER, WEST OF THE EAST LINE OF FRONT

FIG. 40 ↑   1893 **WALL OF CESSPOOL AT CORNER OF VALLEJO AND FRANKLIN STREETS** — SAN FRANCISCO, USA. THIS CESSPOOL HAS BEEN RECORDED AS AN EXAMPLE OF POOR WORKMANSHIP.

FIG. 41 ↓   1893 **INTERIOR OF PACIFIC STREET SEWER** — SAN FRANCISCO, USA. THIS SHOWS THE CLASSIC EGG-SHAPED SEWER THAT BECAME A STAPLE FEATURE OF 19TH-CENTURY SEWER CONSTRUCTION.

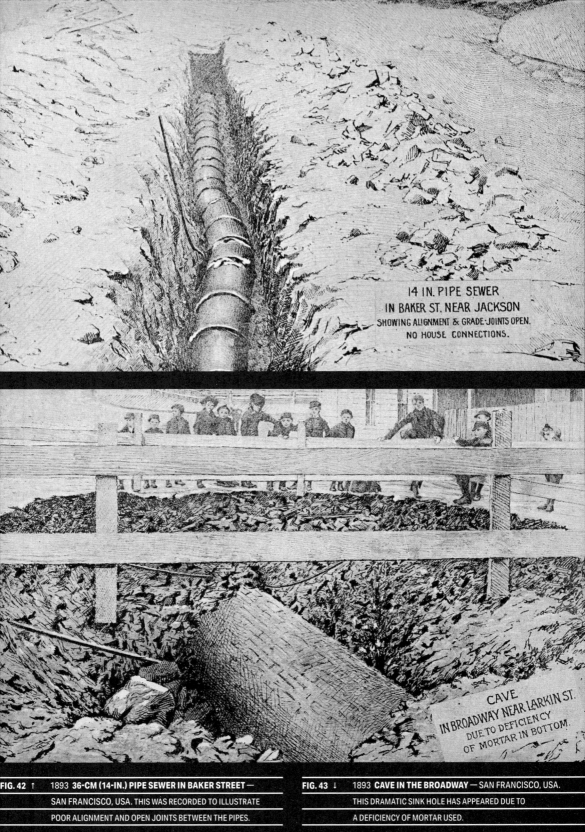

14 IN. PIPE SEWER
IN BAKER ST. NEAR JACKSON
SHOWING ALIGNMENT & GRADE-JOINTS OPEN.
NO HOUSE CONNECTIONS.

CAVE
IN BROADWAY NEAR LARKIN ST.
DUE TO DEFICIENCY
OF MORTAR IN BOTTOM.

FIG. 42 ↑   1893 **36-CM (14-IN.) PIPE SEWER IN BAKER STREET** —
SAN FRANCISCO, USA. THIS WAS RECORDED TO ILLUSTRATE
POOR ALIGNMENT AND OPEN JOINTS BETWEEN THE PIPES.

FIG. 43 ↓   1893 **CAVE IN THE BROADWAY** — SAN FRANCISCO, USA.
THIS DRAMATIC SINK HOLE HAS APPEARED DUE TO
A DEFICIENCY OF MORTAR USED.

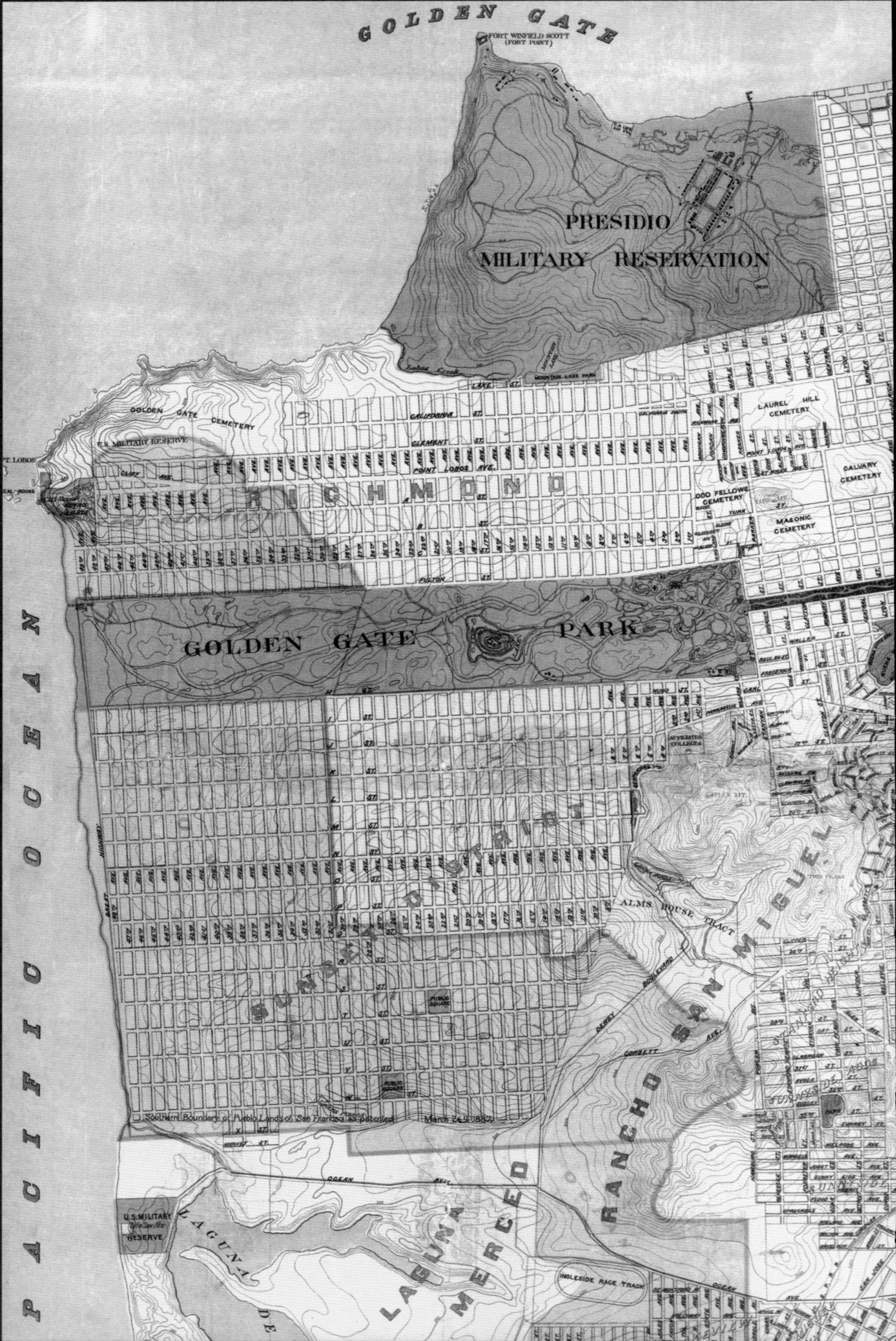

FIG. 44   1899   SYSTEM OF SEWERAGE FOR SAN FRANCISCO — SAN FRANCISCO, USA. IN THIS MAP SOLID RED LINES REPRESENT THE SEWERS

RECOMMENDED FOR IMMEDIATE CONSTRUCTION AND RED CIRCLES INDICATE THE SUGGESTED LOCATIONS OF PUMPING STATIONS.

PACIFIC OCEAN

GOLDEN GATE

FORT WINFIELD SCOTT
(FORT POINT)

PRESIDIO
MILITARY   RESERVATION

GOLDEN GATE CEMETERY

U.S. MILITARY RESERVE

PT. LOBOS

RICHMOND

LAUREL HILL
CEMETERY

ODD FELLOWS
CEMETERY

CALVARY
CEMETERY

MASONIC
CEMETERY

GOLDEN   GATE   PARK

SUNSET DISTRICT

RANCHO SAN MIGUEL

ALMS HOUSE TRACT

PUBLIC SQUARE

PUBLIC SQUARE

Southern Boundary of Pueblo Lands of San Francisco as established   March 24, 1887

U.S. MILITARY
RESERVE

LAGUNA   DE   LA   MERCED

INGLESIDE RACE TRACK

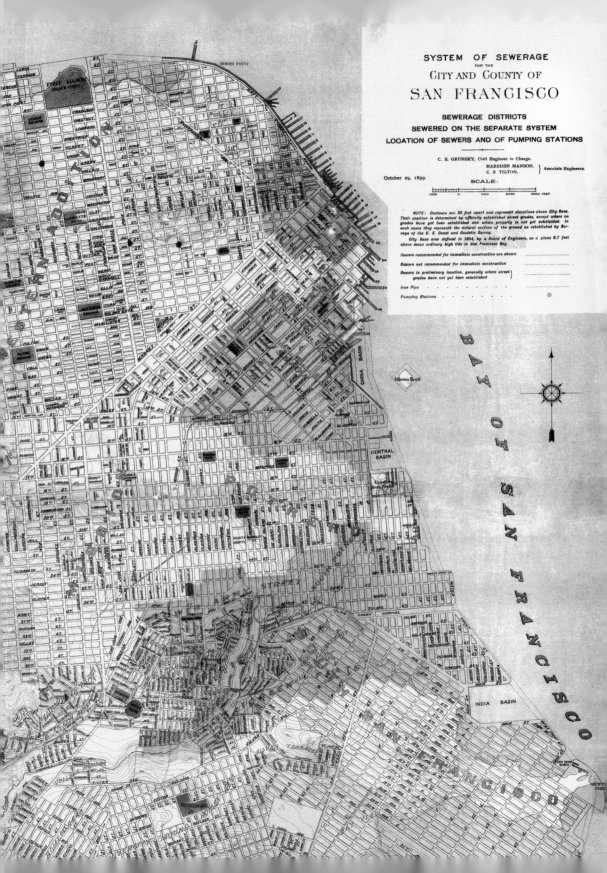

SYSTEM OF SEWERAGE
FOR THE
CITY AND COUNTY OF
SAN FRANCISCO

SEWERAGE DISTRICTS
SEWERED ON THE SEPARATE SYSTEM
LOCATION OF SEWERS AND OF PUMPING STATIONS

C. E. GRUNSKY, Civil Engineer in Charge.

MARSDEN MANSON,
C. S TILTON, } Associate Engineers.

October 29, 1899.

SCALE:

1000   0   1000   2000   3000 FEET

NOTE: Contours are 20 feet apart and represent elevations above City Base. Their position is determined by officially established street grades, except where no grades have yet been established and where property is not yet subdivided. In such cases they represent the natural surface of the ground as established by Surveys of the U. S. Coast and Geodetic Survey.

City Base was defined in 1854, by a Board of Engineers, as a plane 6.7 feet above mean ordinary high tide in San Francisco Bay.

Sewers recommended for immediate construction are shown ——————

Sewers not recommended for immediate construction ————————

Sewers in preliminary location, generally where street grades have not yet been established ————————

Iron Pipe . . . .

Pumping Stations . . . . ●

Under pressure from the Environmental Protection Agency and an organization called 'Heal the Bay', the plant was upgraded in the 1980s in what became called the 'sludge-out' project. The Hyperion plant thus reached the standards required by the State of California but scares continue to occur as when, in 2017, it had to undergo maintenance, with unwelcome consequences for local beaches. The scale and high-tech appearance of Hyperion has gained it a different kind of notoriety: it has featured in films produced by the nearby motion-picture industry including *Battle for the Planet of the Apes* (1973) and *The Terminator* (1984).

The city of Baltimore, Maryland, dates its foundation to the year 1729, but Chesapeake Bay, on which Baltimore stands, has a history stretching back into the previous century and the first European settlement on the East Coast. Captain John Smith (1580–1631) is usually remembered as the husband of the Native American Princess Pocahontas, but in 1608 he explored and mapped Chesapeake Bay and, impressed by the abundant fish, freshwater rivers (including the Potomac and Susquehanna), forests and grasses, later declared that 'Heaven and earth never agreed better to frame a place for man's habitation.' The bay became the site of the first English colony in North America, at Jamestown, and thrived, though as tobacco farms and cornfields replaced forests and the area became more heavily populated, the soil was washed into the bay and the multitude of streams and rivers were used to dispose of the rubbish of Baltimore and the other settlements that overlooked the bay. By the late 19th century, many of the streams and rivers that touched Baltimore had been encased in concrete and brick channels and massive pipes in metal or wood. Sanitary arrangements were primitive, depending mostly upon cesspits. It was estimated that in 1880, when the population of the city had reached 350,000, approximately 80,000 cesspits were in use, much of the content draining into the sandy soil and leaking into watercourses, which helped to explain the exceptionally high incidence of typhoid in Baltimore.

In 1904, a great fire destroyed much of Baltimore and the opportunity was taken to rebuild the city and, in the process, install an effective sewerage system. Construction began in 1907 and was completed with the opening of a sewage treatment plant in 1915. Showing considerable foresight, the opportunity was taken to install one system for wastewater, including sewage, and a separate system of storm-water drains to carry away rainwater. This reduced the burden on the treatment works and enabled overflows from these drains to pass directly into rivers at times of very heavy rain, unpolluted by human waste. Baltimore now has more than 1,600 km (1,000 miles) of storm drains and over 4,800 km (3,000 miles) of sewers, many of them showing their age and sometimes rupturing. An agreement between the local authorities and the Environmental Protection Agency, drawn up in 2002, requires the repair or renewal of the ageing infrastructure by 2019.

FIG. 45   1869 **DESIGN FOR THE IMPROVEMENT OF THE CHANNEL OF JONES FALLS** — BALTIMORE, USA. DURING THE 19TH CENTURY THE JONES FALLS RIVER BECAME IN ESSENCE AN OPEN SEWER. CHANNELLING IT BENEATH THE CITY IN A SERIES OF TUNNELS WAS PROPOSED TO COMBAT THE POLLUTION, DISEASE AND FLOODS THAT IT CAUSED.

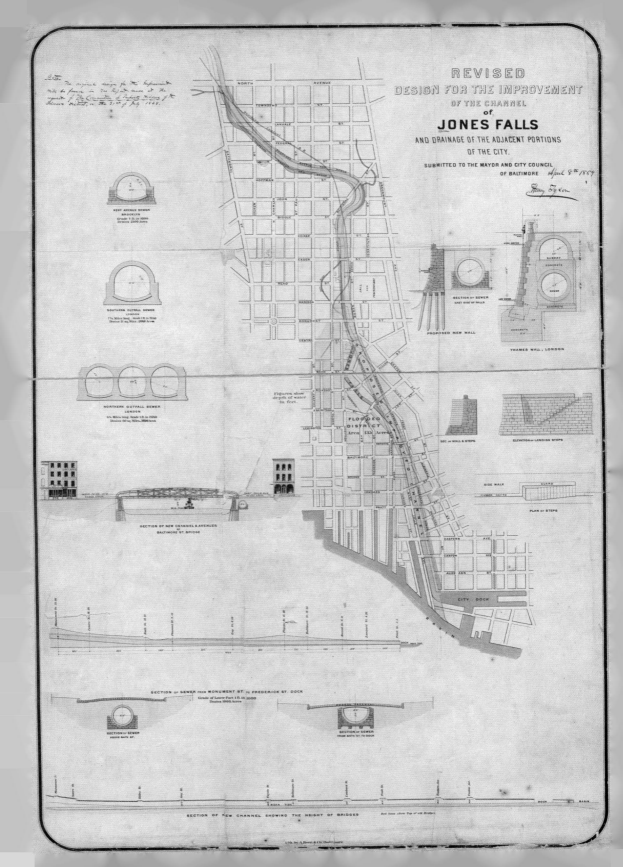

REVISED
DESIGN FOR THE IMPROVEMENT
OF THE CHANNEL
of
JONES FALLS
AND DRAINAGE OF THE ADJACENT PORTIONS
OF THE CITY.

SUBMITTED TO THE MAYOR AND CITY COUNCIL
OF BALTIMORE
April 8th 1859

REVOLUTIONS OF PURITY

3

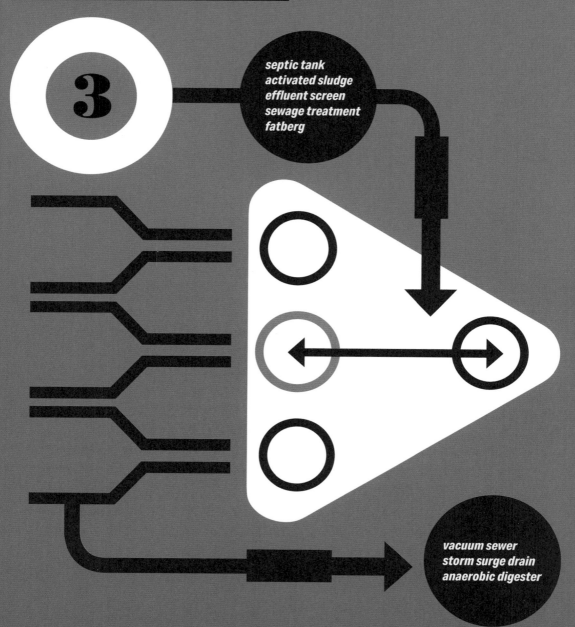

septic tank
activated sludge
effluent screen
sewage treatment
fatberg

vacuum sewer
storm surge drain
anaerobic digester

[I. PROCESSING & TREATING SEWAGE]

[II. THE FUTURE OF WASTE TREATMENT]

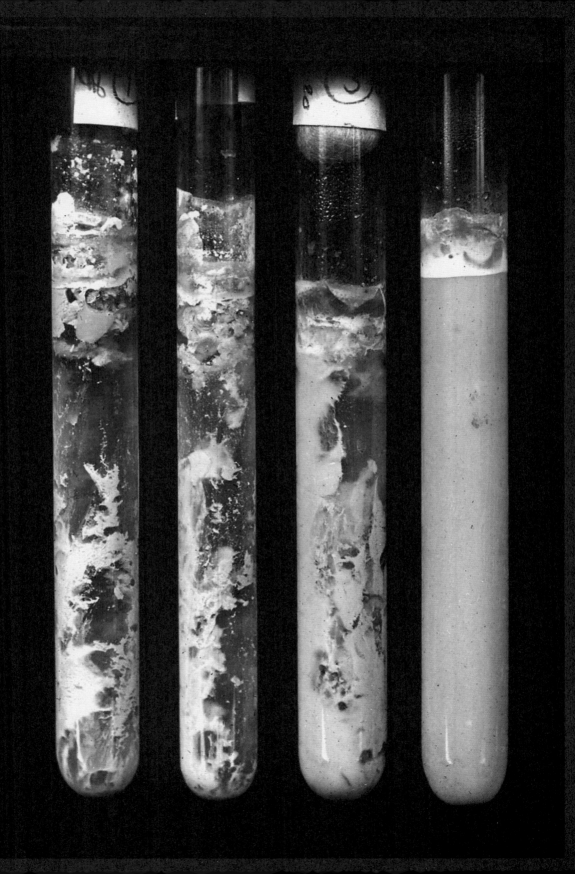

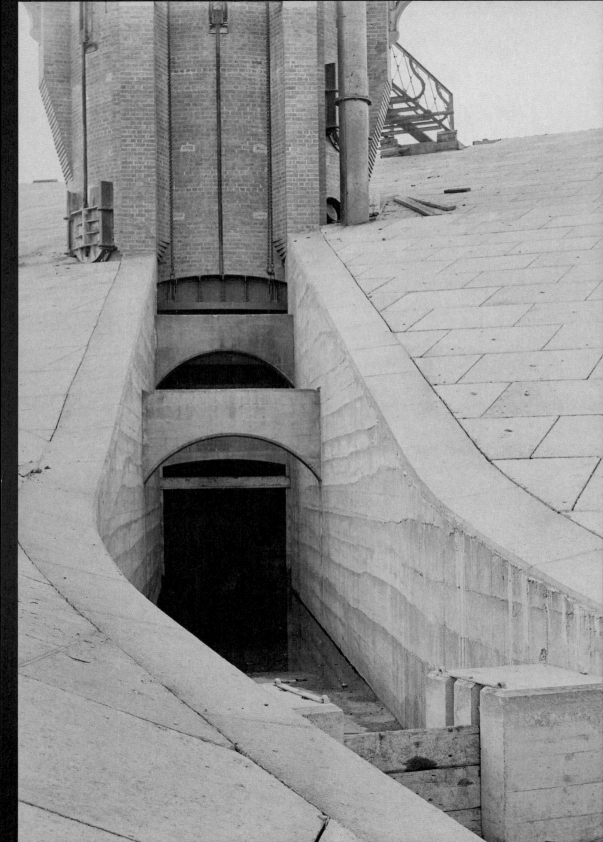

PROCESSING & TREATING SEWAGE

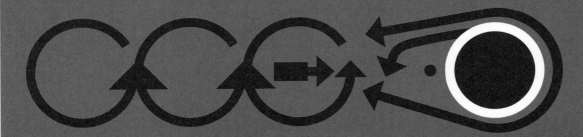

'THERE IS NO DOUBT THAT THE BACTERIAL PROCESS
OF SEWAGE TREATMENT HAS COME TO STAY.'

Scientific American, Volume 93, Number 24 (1905)

The treatment of sewage and the removal from it of harmful pathogens has undergone many changes since humans first settled in cities, but the process has always depended upon the existence of microbes that consume our waste as nutrients. In the cities of Mesopotamia, sewage was conveyed to fields where this task was performed by bacteria in the soil. They consumed the pathogens and turned sewage into plant nutrients and water, thus completing the cycle of harvesting, consumption, decay, fertilization and growth. The arrangement continues to persist in many developing countries and the writer Han Suyin (1916–2012) born in Xinyang, China, to Chinese and Flemish parents, wrote that in 1949, before the Communist takeover of China, the wealthiest families in some parts of China were those who owned the public sewers and sold excrement to the farmers. As the centuries passed, techniques have been developed to apply science to these processes in a systematic way, making this natural process more efficient and manageable. Each of these processes has led naturally to the next, though there were some strange deviations on the way.

Modern sewage treatment works are still commonly referred to as 'sewage farms', reflecting their origins in the work of the nightsoilmen. Yet the late 19th and 20th centuries saw the development

---

P. 207   **GROWTHS IN GELATINE TEST TUBES**. THE 20TH CENTURY
USHERED IN A NEW PERIOD OF CHEMICAL AND BIOLOGICAL
INVESTIGATIONS INTO SEWAGE TREATMENT.

FIG. 1 ←   1909 **OUTLET TOWER NUMBER ONE** — STAINES, ENGLAND.
OUTLET TOWERS LIFT WATER FROM RESERVOIRS SO THAT
IT MAY BE CONVEYED TO WATER TREATMENT PLANTS.

of sophisticated treatment systems that ensure a modern sewage treatment works harnesses the powers of physics, chemistry and biology to purify waste, create fertilizer and return clean water to the environment – similar to what the nightsoilmen were doing in earlier centuries but with a greater understanding of the science that is at work, and its more systematic application. The process is based upon the knowledge that if something can be eaten then something will eat it. It uses anaerobic (oxygen-free) and aerobic (oxygen-rich) conditions in conjunction with each other to treat different types of pollutant and render them harmless or useful by a process involving several distinct stages. The septic tank was the first step towards this scientific approach to sewage treatment.

The septic tank is an effective means of treating small quantities of sewage, sometimes from one building and sometimes from a small community. Wastewater enters the sealed tank from a WC, bath or similar facility. In these anaerobic conditions the solids are digested and reduced in volume, the residue sinking to the bottom of the tank, while a layer of scum forms on the surface until this is itself digested and sinks to the bottom, forming sludge. The water in the intermediate layer between the scum and the sludge will flow out through a pipe into the septic drain field through perforated pipes to allow the liquid to spread evenly into the gravel or similar material surrounding the pipes. From there it will find its way into the soil where microbes, now in aerobic conditions, will consume further harmful impurities, producing fertilizer in liquid form that will be taken up by the roots of plants. The solids will be removed from the tank at intervals. The process is in some respects similar to the biochemistry of a compost heap, which also breaks down organic waste and harmful pathogens into nutrient-rich compost.

The precise origins of the septic tank are unclear. In 1876, in Worcester, Massachusetts, a 'sedimentation' tank was installed to serve the state insane asylum. This featured many characteristics of systems that were later patented. It was designed to facilitate the decomposition of solid wastes from the hospital in conditions free of oxygen. In 1895, the term 'septic system' was coined and a patent obtained by English scientist Donald Cameron (dates unknown), based in Exeter, who designed a sealed container to treat sewage by anaerobic digestion. However, in 1860 a very similar mechanism had been devised by a

---

FIGS. 2–7   1905 **THE DESIGN OF A SEPTIC TANK**.
THESE SIMPLE DEVICES ARE DESIGNED TO TREAT
SEWAGE IN SMALL QUANTITIES.

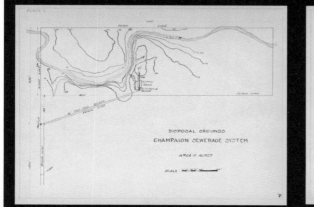
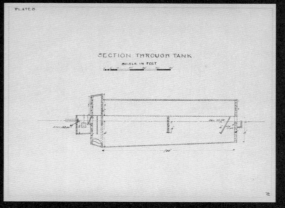

Frenchman called Jean-Louis Mouras (dates unknown) who appears to have discovered its properties as a means of sewage treatment by accident. He came from Pontarlier, near the French border with Switzerland, and ran a small engineering business in Vesoul, north-east of Dijon. In about 1860, he built a concrete, airtight container to hold the sewage from his business, fed by a clay pipe. Some ten years later, he decided to clean out the container and was surprised to learn that it now contained only a relatively small quantity of sludge. He sought the advice of Abbé François-Napoléon-Marie Moigno (1804–84), a Jesuit priest who had devoted his life to scientific enquiries, who advised him to apply for a patent for the '*Fosse Mouras*' ('*fosse*' = 'ditch'), which was duly granted in the 1880s. It appears that the liquid contents of the tank were intended to be emptied into public sewers in accordance with Haussmann's ideas, leaving the solids ('sludge') to be collected by vidangeurs (nightsoilmen) as in the past, though less frequently. In contrast, Donald Cameron's septic tank emptied the liquid into soil.

Some septic tanks have two chambers. The first chamber allows some solids to settle and scum to form in anaerobic conditions, releasing liquid to the second chamber for similar treatment before the relatively clear liquid is released into the leach field. A later development of the septic tank, the Imhoff Tank, was developed by the German engineer Karl Imhoff (1876–1965) and patented in 1906. This is essentially a tank within a tank, the heavier solids being discharged from an upper, cone-shaped

> ## 'FILTERS HAVE BEEN INVENTED AND PUT INTO OPERATION WHICH HAVE THE POWER TO CONVERT THE MOST FOUL AND TURBID SEWAGE INTO CLEAR, SPARKING WATER.'
> *Scientific American*, Volume 93, Number 24 (1905)

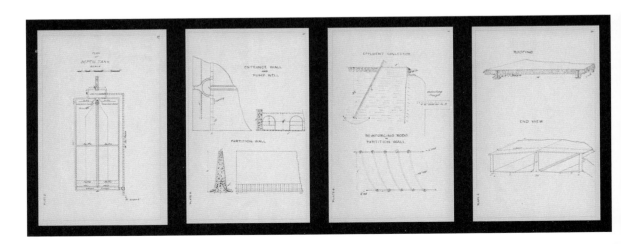

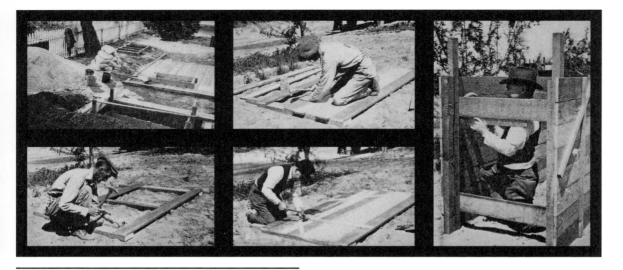

FIGS. 8–16   1923 **A SEPTIC TANK ON AN AMERICAN FARM**.
MANY US CITIZENS DEPEND UPON PERSONAL SEPTIC
TANKS FOR SEWAGE TREATMENT.

tank, to a lower chamber where they can be subjected to more prolonged anaerobic treatment, while the relatively clear liquid in the upper chamber can be discharged more quickly into the 'septic drain field' or 'leach field'.

Modern septic tanks, with a capacity of 3,800–7,700 litres (1,000–2,000 gallons), are often used in isolated buildings or small communities, unconnected to public sewers or treatment works. They depend upon the availability of plenty of land free of buildings, which can be used as the leach field for the contents of the septic tanks. Licences have to be obtained for their installation to ensure that the soil is sufficiently porous and that they do not endanger local sources of drinking water or supplies of fish for human consumption. Such tanks are usually made of concrete, fibreglass or, more recently, tough plastics, and will last about fifty years. In municipal and larger treatment plants, septic-tank systems can also be combined with more advanced forms of secondary treatment such as trickling filters, reed beds and other aerobic systems to provide enhanced treatment and effluent quality. The sludge in the bottom of the tank will be removed by a vacuum lorry at intervals ranging from two years to twenty years, dependent upon the usage of the system by the community. A certain amount of residual sludge is left behind to ensure that some microorganisms remain to continue their essential work. The use of septic tanks is more common in rural areas, especially in developing countries, but about 20% of the population of France uses such systems (4 million households); the figure for the Irish Republic is 27%; and for the USA 25%, this including parts of some surprisingly large cities such as Indianapolis.

The anaerobic conditions that prevail in septic tanks may lead to gas and other fumes being released. In May 2014, there were reports that a Chinese woman had dropped her mobile phone into a septic tank in Xinxiang. To retrieve it, her husband jumped into the tank through a 1-m-sq (11-ft-sq) hole and was overcome by fumes; in an effort to help, his elderly mother followed him, with the same results. They were then joined by the wife, the husband's father and two villagers, in a desperate rescue attempt. All six were eventually pulled out on ropes by other villagers, but the husband and his mother died.

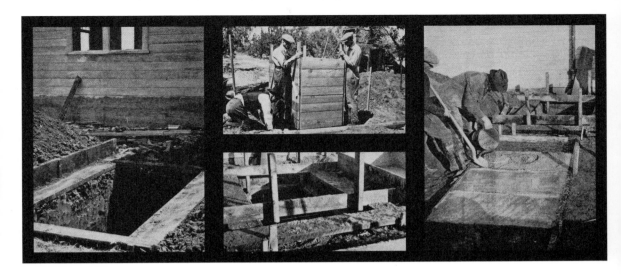

A septic tank is sometimes used in conjunction with a reed bed – some natural and others artificially created – to supplement the process of purification. They are used for the further purification of wastewater from which the greatest pollutants such as solid excrement have been removed. The common reed (*Phragmites australis*) can help transfer oxygen from its leaves through the stem and roots to the septic tank field, accelerating the process by which microbes break down the pollutants in sewage. Other types of vegetation are found in these natural waste units including gipsywort, water plantains and yellow iris. They also provide a habitat for many animals, some of them endangered species, including grass snakes, water voles, otters and even beavers, together with birds such as the bittern, heron, marsh harrier and reed bunting. However, they also attract mosquitoes and flies, which provide food for birds and irritation for humans. Small reed beds are called 'treatment ponds' and may serve a single dwelling. Horizontal-flow systems in reed beds are sometimes built to treat the outflow from small sewage treatment plants, while vertical-flow reed beds are built in a series of steps, following the same principle as a double-chamber septic tank, with wastewater flowing from one level to the next through a process of gradual purification. They are often used in rural areas and not only in developing countries. Anglian Water and Severn Trent Water have many such installations in the rural areas they serve. Septic tanks and reed beds are now commonly used in conjunction with filters of various kinds.

The purification of water, including wastewater, by means of filters may be said to have begun with its application to soil as fertilizer, though in the early 17th century Sir Francis Bacon (1561–1626) tried without success to remove the salt from seawater by filtering it through sand. It was not until the 19th century that the mechanism by which the process of purification worked was understood and its use became widespread. From the 17th century onwards, the application of microscopy, among other techniques, to the examination of water enabled scientists to understand both the means by which water could transmit diseases such as dysentery, typhoid and cholera, and the ways by which it could be purified. The systematic analysis of London's drinking water by Sir Edward Frankland in the 19th century, using microscopes and other methods of analysis, proved decisive both in 216

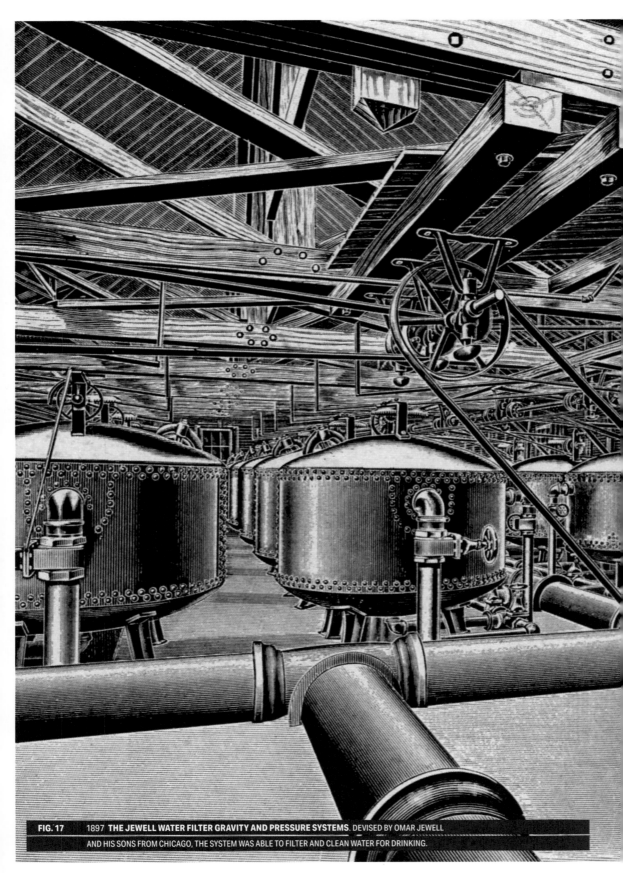

FIG. 17 1897 **THE JEWELL WATER FILTER GRAVITY AND PRESSURE SYSTEMS**. DEVISED BY OMAR JEWELL AND HIS SONS FROM CHICAGO, THE SYSTEM WAS ABLE TO FILTER AND CLEAN WATER FOR DRINKING.

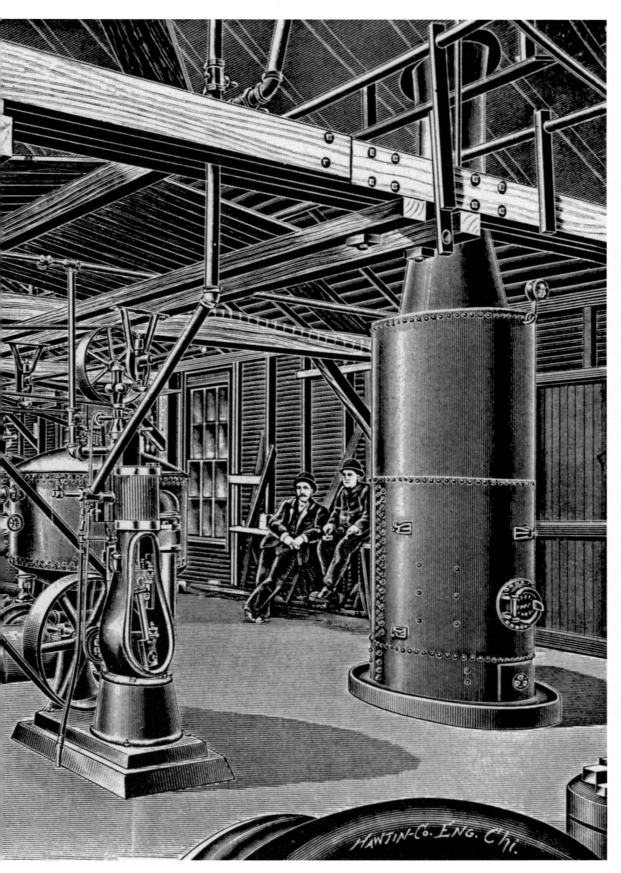

HAWTIN-Co. ENG. CHI.

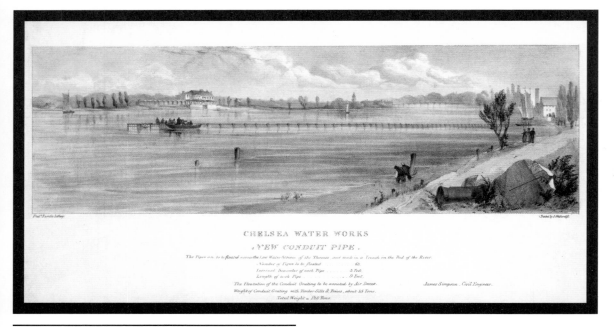

FIG. 18   1850 **A NEW CONDUIT PIPE BUILT BY THE CHELSEA
WATERWORKS COMPANY** — LONDON, UK. UNFORTUNATELY
BY 1850 THE WATER FROM THE THAMES THAT THE COMPANY
DELIVERED TO LONDON HOMES WAS HEAVILY POLLUTED.

identifying pathogens and eliminating them, effectively disposing of the widely held belief that foul
air, not polluted water, caused epidemics of cholera and typhoid. Frankland became an enemy of the
London water companies, who were carrying waterborne diseases into the homes of the population,
but he won his case.

In the meantime, engineers such as James Simpson (1799–1869) were applying what seemed like
common sense to the process of purification without fully understanding the science behind it. In
1823, Simpson became engineer to the Chelsea Water Company and constructed the first 'slow sand
filter bed'. This was a 61 cm (2 ft) deep layer of fine sand above further layers of sea shells, gravel and
bricks. Beneath these were clay pipes in which holes had been pierced. The water passed through the
sand, gravel and shells and entered the pipes, from which it passed to reservoirs. The top inch of sand
filtered out 95% of impurities. Simpson regarded his sand as a physical barrier to impurities, which it
was, but it wasn't until many years later that Sir Edward Frankland demonstrated that microbes in the
sand also acted as a biological barrier by consuming the pathogens. Simpson's methods were adopted
by his fellow engineer Thomas Hawksley (1807–93) in bringing water to Liverpool, Nottingham and
London, where he has a visible monument in the Le Petit Trianon pumping station at the head of the
Serpentine in Hyde Park.

By the 1890s, it was becoming more widely understood that biology as well as physical filtration
and chemistry were involved in the purification of wastewater. Experiments in Germany in the 1880s
showed that, by spraying surfaces with wastewater at intervals, a slimy 'biofilm' of microorganisms
formed that played a part in removing some organic substances. It became clear that both aerobic

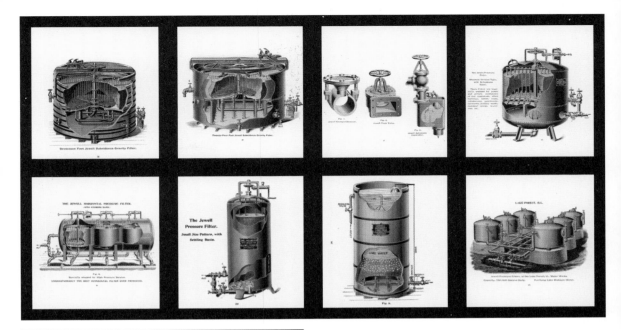

FIGS. 19–26 1897 **THE JEWELL WATER FILTER GRAVITY AND PRESSURE SYSTEMS.** VARIOUS FILTERS AND VALVES FROM THE JEWELL WATER FILTER SYSTEM, TAKEN FROM A HANDBOOK CREATED BY THE COMPANY.

and anaerobic bacteria were involved in the process. In 1887, in Lawrence, Massachusetts, the Lawrence Experimental Station was established to investigate methods of purifying water and treating sewage and revealed that such intermittent treatment of waste enabled both aerobic and anaerobic bacteria to digest pollutants.

These discoveries were incorporated in the trickling filter, which is commonly found in sewage treatment works for small and medium-sized towns. In 1912, the city of Madison, Wisconsin, became an early adopter. Trickling filters combine anaerobic and aerobic treatment to remove impurities in a series of processes. Wastewater is first delivered to a primary settlement tank to which chemicals can be added to speed up the process by which solids are deposited at the bottom of the tank in anaerobic conditions for removal and further treatment. The liquid above the settled solids, known as supernatant, then passes to the filter tank itself. This is typically circular, about 10–20 m (33–66 ft) in diameter, enclosed by a wall of brick or cement and 2–3 m (7–10 ft) deep. It is filled with 'filter media', which consists of materials with generous internal as well as external surface areas to permit maximum exposure of the wastewater to air; clinker, coke from furnaces and lava have all been used for this. The wastewater is sprayed over the media via rotating arms to which the water is delivered, the arms being hydraulically moved by the entry of the water itself so that they distribute the waste evenly over the media. On larger filters, the arms are sometimes mechanically driven along rails. A biofilm layer of microbial slime forms on the media, which gradually thickens as it consumes the food source in the waste before delivering the remaining water to drains that lie at the bottom of the tank. The partially treated effluent passes to a final clarifier similar in design to a primary settlement tank and is settled until the liquid is pure enough to be delivered to a river or canal. Within the media of the trickling filter, the growing biofilm is continuously scoured and ○———————➤ 221

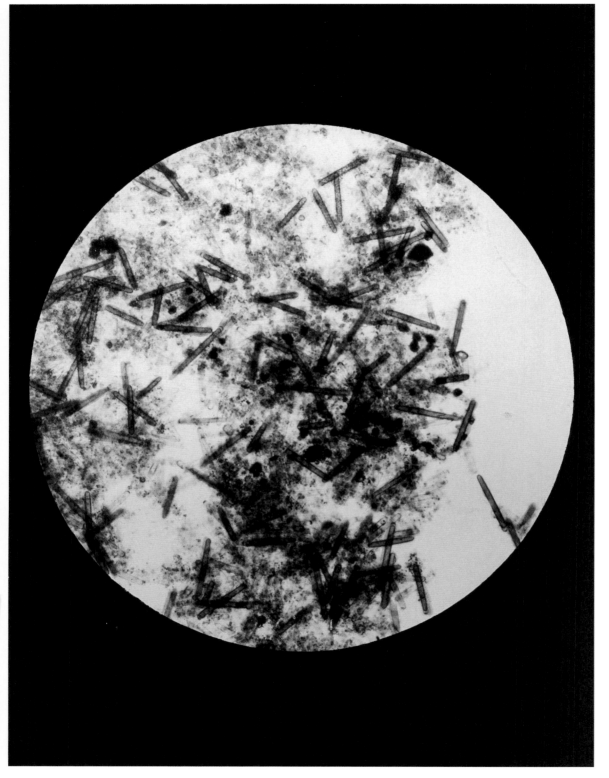

FIG. 27 ↑ **SPORES OF APHANIZOMENON**. THIS IS A TYPE OF
CYANOBACTERIA, WHICH LIVES IN FRESH WATER AND PRODUCES
MULTIPLE TOXINS, MAKING IT HARMFUL TO CONSUME.

FIGS. 1888–90 **INVESTIGATIONS INTO THE PURIFICATION**
28–31 → **OF SEWAGE** — MASSACHUSETTS, USA. SAMPLES OF BACTERIA
OBSERVED DURING INVESTIGATION INTO SEWAGE PURIFICATION.

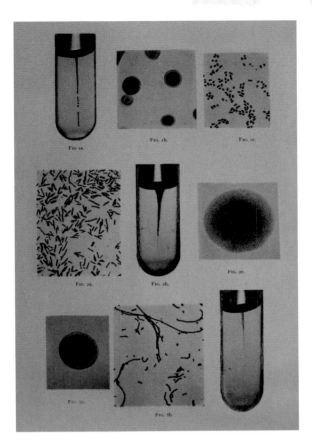

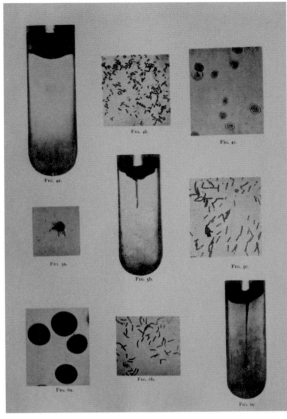

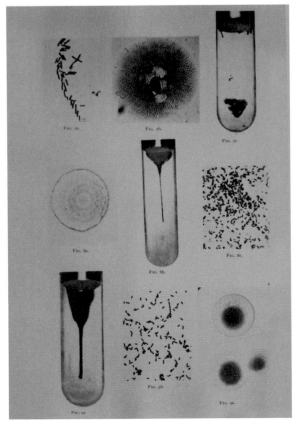

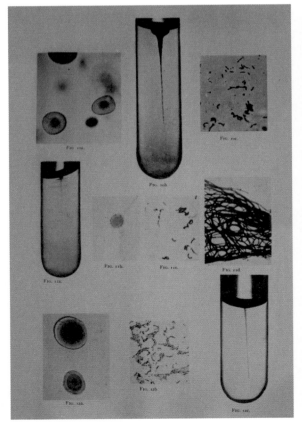

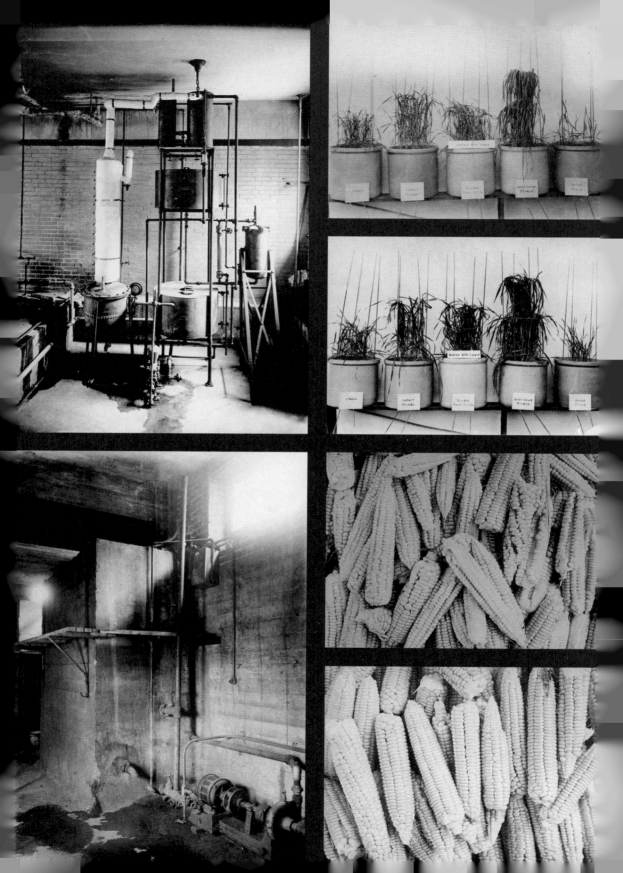

is delivered to the final clarifier for the separation of solids. Some sewage-treatment works operate a vertical process whereby the water, gradually purified, passes from one tank down to the next, the liquid being treated further at each stage as it becomes gradually clearer before being released. The next major step towards sewage treatment – the 'activated sludge process' – occurred in the late 19th century.

In 1887, William Dibdin (1850–1925), Chief Chemist to the Metropolitan Board of Works and later to its successor the London County Council, wrote:

> *The true way of purifying sewage will be first to separate the sludge and then turn into neutral effluent a charge of the proper organism, whatever that may be, specially cultivated for the purpose; return it for a sufficient period, during which it should be fully aerated and finally discharge it into the stream in a purified condition. This is indeed what is aimed at and imperfectly accomplished on a sewage farm.*

This statement is a rather clumsy description of what came to be known as the activated sludge process, by which microbes within the sewage can be stimulated and harnessed to purify the effluent. The process was developed by two chemists who worked for the Manchester Corporation rivers department in the early 20th century. Its origins lay in a visit to the Lawrence Experimental Station in Massachusetts by Dr Gilbert Fowler (1868–1953) of the University of Manchester in his capacity as consultant to the Manchester Corporation. During his stay, he observed a series of experiments into the aeration of municipal wastewater. He passed on his observations to two chemists at Manchester's Davyhulme wastewater treatment plant – William Lockett (c. 1887–1960) and Edward Ardern (dates unknown) – who, in a series of experiments, exposed sewage from different areas of Manchester to air in glass bottles, covering the bottles with brown paper to exclude sunlight and thus preventing the growth of algae. After a few days the water, now reasonably clear, was poured from the bottles but the sediment remained in the bottle, the digested molecules having stuck together in a process known as 'flocculation'. As more aerated water was added the process of clarification accelerated, while the quantity of sediment increased. Lockett and Ardern called this sediment 'activated sludge' in recognition of the fact that the suspensions in the aerated wastewater promoted the process of digestion of pollutants. In 1914, the process was tested on a larger scale in a pilot plant ○————▶ 224

FIG. 32 ⬉ **EXTRACTION OF GREASE FROM DRIED ACTIVATED SLUDGE.**
A CHEMICAL ENGINEERING THESIS CONDUCTED IN 1920 AT THE UNIVERSITY OF ILLINOIS INVESTIGATED HOW GREASE FROM ACTIVATED SLUDGE MAY BE EXTRACTED AND USED.

FIG. 33 ⬊⬊ **THE ACTIVATED SLUDGE METHOD OF SEWAGE TREATMENT.**
A CHEMISTRY PhD THESIS CONDUCTED IN 1916 AT THE UNIVERSITY OF ILLINOIS RESEARCHED THE ACTIVATED SLUDGE PROCESS OF SEWAGE TREATMENT.

FIGS. 34–37 ← **THE FERTILIZER VALUE OF ACTIVATED SLUDGE.**
TAKEN FROM A CHEMISTY PhD THESIS CONDUCTED IN 1918 AT THE UNIVERSITY OF ILLINOIS BY WILLIAM DURRELL HATFIELD, THESE EXAMPLES ILLUSTRATE THE BENEFICIAL EFFECTS ON PLANTS OF FERTILIZER EXTRACTED FROM SLUDGE. SEWAGE HAD BEEN USED AS FERTILIZER SINCE ANCIENT TIMES, AND SCIENTIFIC RESEARCH INTO THE PROCESS CONFIRMED ITS POSITIVE EFFECTS. DEDICATED AND METHODICAL LABORATORY WORK SUCH AS THIS WAS FUNDAMENTAL TO THE DEVELOPMENT AND REALIZATION OF THE ACTIVATED SLUDGE PROCESS.

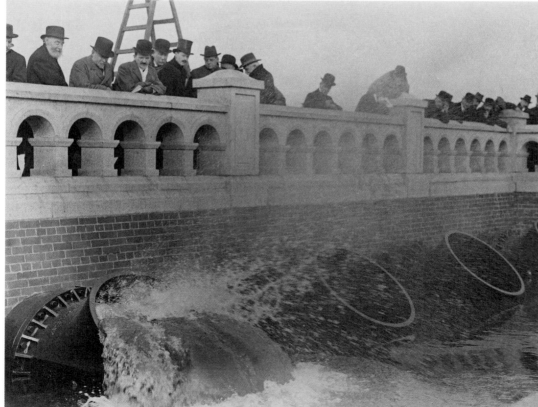

FIGS. 38–41 1913 OPENING OF THE KING GEORGE V RESERVOIR AT CHINGFORD — LONDON, UK. OPENED BY KING GEORGE V IN 1913 THE RESERVOIR. BECAME PART OF A CHAIN

OF RESERVOIRS IN THE LEE VALLEY THAT CONTINUE TO SUPPLY WATER TO LONDON VIA THE RING MAIN, A MAJOR ELEMENT OF LONDON'S WATER SUPPLY INFRASTRUCTURE.

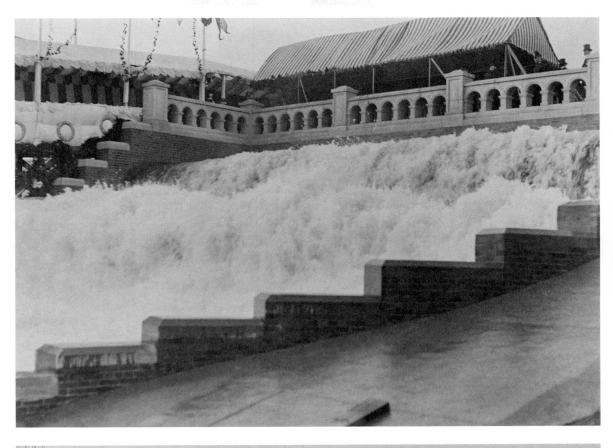

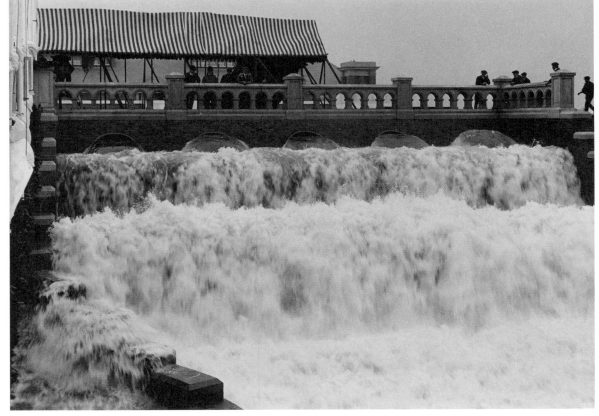

consisting of a wooden box on a horse-drawn wagon and finally on a full-scale plant at Salford; another, constructed in 1916 at Sheffield, employed paddles in the wastewater to ensure adequate circulation of air. In 1915, an activated sludge plant was built at Milwaukee, Wisconsin, with Dr Gilbert Fowler acting as consultant. Oxygen can be added to the mix to promote the process in heavily loaded plants when the wastewater is very heavily polluted.

The activated sludge process is now commonly used for medium-sized and large urban communities. It typically involves two stages. Initially, liquid is pumped to large, open tanks into which air is pumped at high pressure, the turbulence in these aerobic conditions ensuring that the solids remained suspended in the water where microorganisms, their appetites stimulated by the oxygen in the liquid, consume the pathogens in the waste. When an appropriate level of purity is achieved, the liquid is released into settlement tanks, the solids sinking to the bottom from which they are removed for sale as fertilizer or to re-seed the biological process.

The above processes, and others, are now combined in the operations of the sewage treatment facilities found throughout the world. They are more like oil refineries or factories than the farms that received the nightsoilmen's waste, though with one major difference. Oil refineries and factories control their inputs. Sewage treatment works have to deal with whatever we pour into the sewers (and some of the more troublesome intruders are described below).

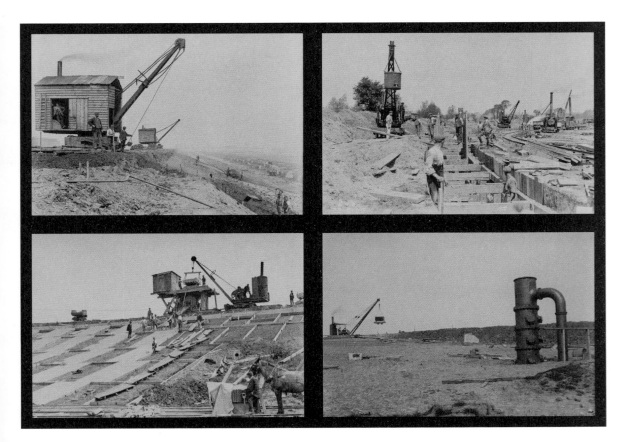

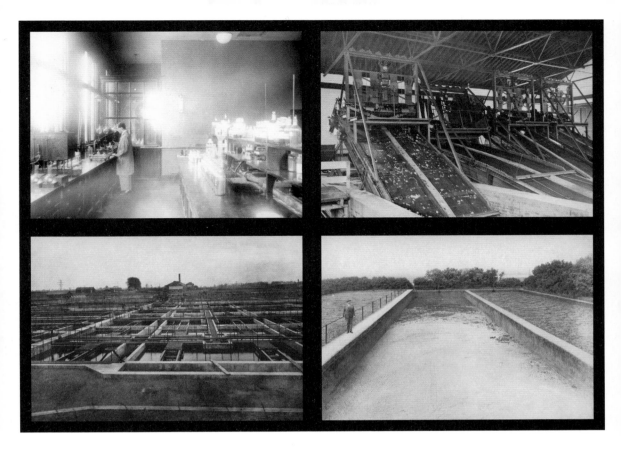

The great majority of the waste that enters a treatment process is water, from WCs, baths, washing machines and other domestic appliances. In combined systems, which also collect surface water, the volume of water is further swollen by rain. So much of the treatment process is devoted to 'dewatering' the waste. Preliminary treatment makes use of 'screens' (mechanical filters) to remove substances such as rags, condoms, tampons, corks, branches and larger objects including, on one occasion at Bazalgette's Abbey Mills pumping station in east London, a motorbike! These residues are collected and incinerated or taken to landfill. The effluent then proceeds to primary treatment in sedimentation tanks, where the laws of physics ensure that heavier solids, including grit and faeces, sink to the bottom of the tanks, sometimes helped by the addition of chemicals, while grease and oils float on the surface and are removed by skimming: a sophisticated septic tank. The sludge that has sunk to the bottom is propelled by mechanical scrapers, rotating slowly around the bottom of the tank, to hoppers in the base of the tanks, whence it is dispatched for further treatment. At this point more than half of the pollutants will have been removed from the wastewater and will have been concentrated in the sludge, which will then be subjected to further treatment in anaerobic tanks ○————————▶ 228

FIGS.
42–45 ←

THE CONSTRUCTION OF CHINGFORD RESERVOIR.
IN THE EARLY 20TH CENTURY THE CONSTRUCTION OF RESERVOIRS GATHERED PACE AS LONDON'S POPULATION EXPANDED.

FIGS.
46–49 ↑

DAVYHULME SEWAGE TREATMENT WORKS — MANCHESTER, ENGLAND. IT WAS THROUGH EXPERIMENTATION HERE THAT ARDERN AND LOCKETT FINE-TUNED THE ACTIVATED SLUDGE PROCESS.

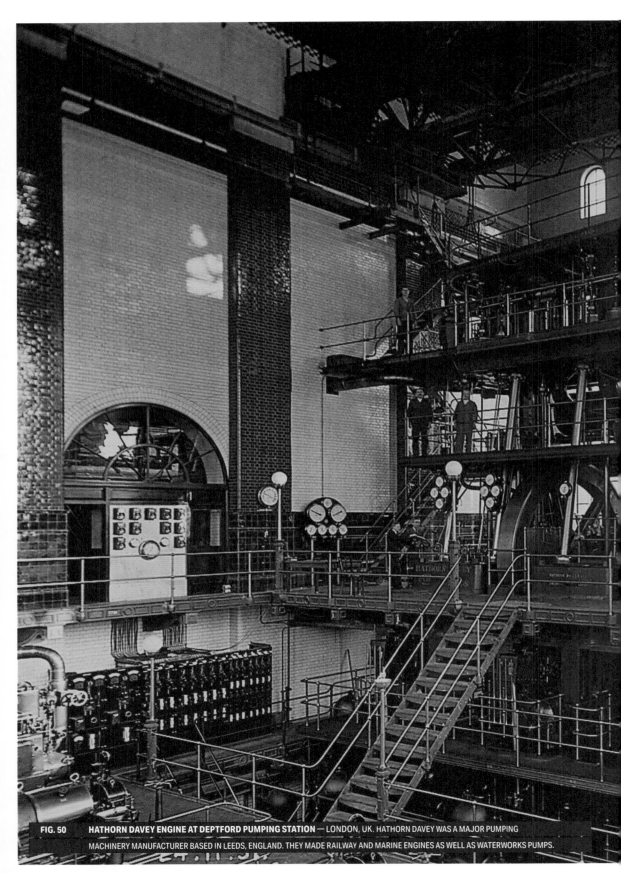

FIG. 50   **HATHORN DAVEY ENGINE AT DEPTFORD PUMPING STATION** — LONDON, UK. HATHORN DAVEY WAS A MAJOR PUMPING
MACHINERY MANUFACTURER BASED IN LEEDS, ENGLAND. THEY MADE RAILWAY AND MARINE ENGINES AS WELL AS WATERWORKS PUMPS.

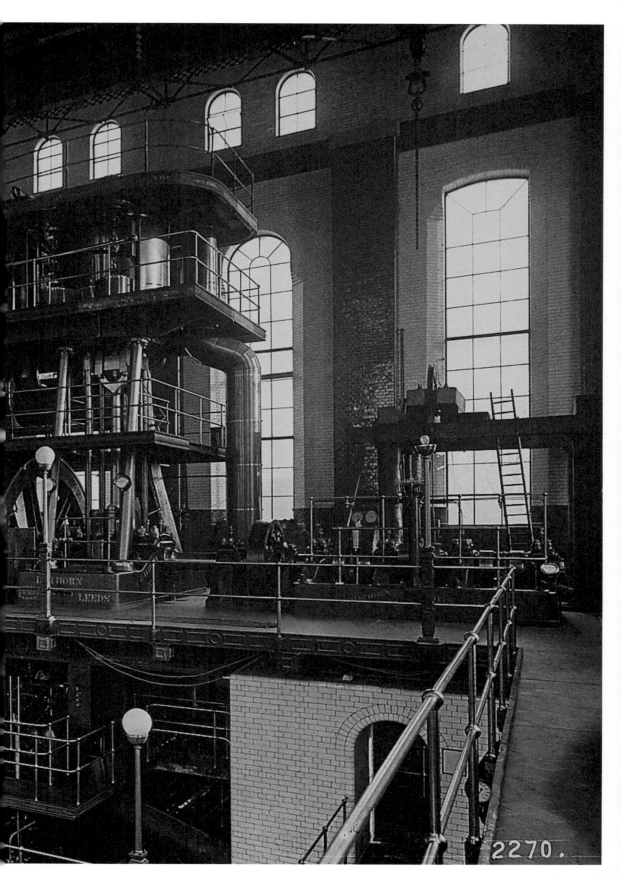

2270.

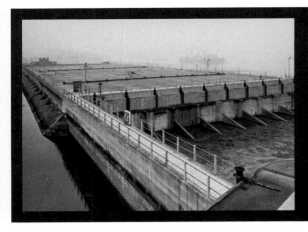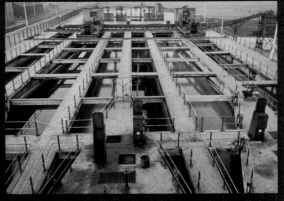

FIG. 51 **BECKTON SLUDGE DIGESTION** — LONDON, UK. WASTE ENTERS SETTLEMENT TANKS TO ENABLE SOLIDS TO SETTLE AND THEN BE SCRAPED AWAY.

FIG. 52 **BECKTON DETRITUS PITS** — LONDON, UK. THESE PITS ARE USED FOR STORING ASH AND OTHER WASTE PRODUCTS GENERATED BY THE SYSTEM.

> ## 'SCIENCE, AFTER LONG EXPERIMENT, NOW KNOWS THAT THE MOST FERTILIZING AND THE MOST EFFECTIVE OF MANURES IS THAT OF MAN.'
>
> **Victor Hugo, *Les Misérables* (1862)**

and aerobic tanks to enable microorganisms that flourish in those conditions to consume many of the remaining pathogens. One of the processes now used at this stage of treatment is thermal hydrolysis, which involves boiling the sludge under pressure (think of the way a pressure cooker works). This kills pathogens, boils off water and breaks down organic molecules into more easily biodegradable substances before being converted into methane gas during the anaerobic digestion stage itself. The flammable methane is captured and used as a source of energy to generate electricity. This is used to power the treatment process and surplus energy is exported to the National Grid as 'green' electricity. The sludge is then further 'dewatered' using such techniques as centrifuges or Archimedes screws and emerges as 'cakes' of treated sewage that are automatically deposited in skips and sold to farmers as fertilizer or, in urban areas with little farmland, taken to landfill.

The liquid from the primary sedimentation tanks, now freed of the sludge, is piped to secondary treatment, which uses a variety of methods, such as trickling filters and the aerobic activated sludge process, described above. These aerobic processes involve the introduction of oxygen to stimulate the appetites of microorganisms, which feed on the remaining pollutants and thereby remove them from the effluent, leaving sedimentary deposits that are either returned to the process to provide more microorganisms or disposed of and mixed with the sludge from the primary treatment to be sold as

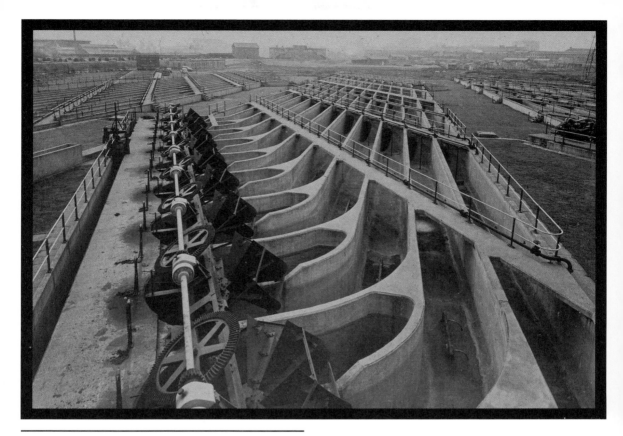

FIG. 53   **BECKTON AERATION PADDLES** — LONDON, UK.
THESE PADDLES INTRODUCE OXYGEN TO THE SLUDGE WHICH
ALLOWS MICROBES TO DIGEST PATHOGENS IN THE SEWAGE.

fertilizer. The condition of the effluent is monitored by measuring the level of oxygen it contains
to ensure that the aerobic process is sustained. When the required level of purity is reached, the
effluent may be released into rivers, lakes or the sea.

This is illustrated by the treatment works at Beckton on the north bank of the Thames and Crossness
on the south, both created by Sir Joseph Bazalgette. He bequeathed to London a system by which
solid waste, including faeces, was separated from liquid waste and the solids dumped by sludge
boats in the North Sea where they would be dispersed, settled and consumed by microbes aided
by fish. That system continued until 1998, when it was replaced by a new method that purifies or
consumes the waste instead of dumping it. Waste is deposited in settlement tanks, the liquid running
off into activated sludge treatment pools, where oxygen is used to stimulate the appetites of microbes
that consume the pollutants until the liquid can, after settlement, safely be released to the Thames.
Some of the activated sludge is reused while the surplus sludge (still, of course, containing much
liquid) is pumped into huge chambers, which are then squeezed like a concertina, discharging more
liquid for further and more prolonged purification treatment before release. Finally, the remaining
solids, still wet, are pumped into incinerators, known as 'sludge-powered generators'. Human waste
contains organic matter, which enables it to be incinerated at a temperature of 850°C (1,562°F). ⊶——————⟶ 236

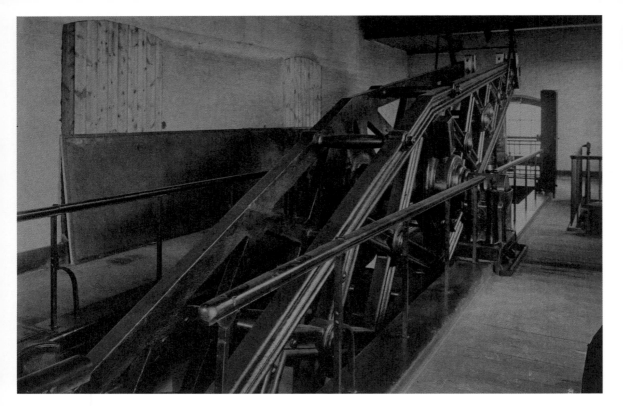

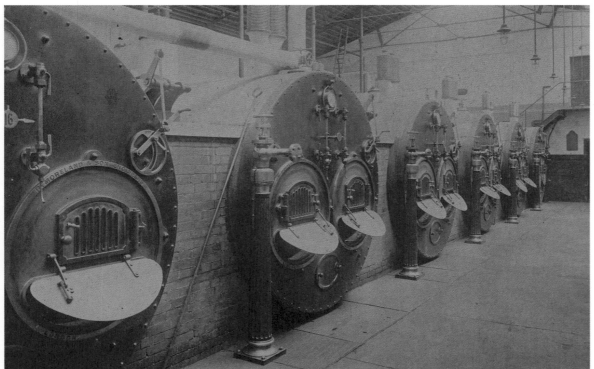

FIG. 54 ↑   1914 **BATTERSEA WORKS BEAM ENGINE** — LONDON, UK.
BEAM ENGINES SUCH AS THIS WERE USED IN THE MAJORITY
OF PUMPING STATIONS IN THE UK.

FIG. 55 ↓   **HAMPTON WORKS BOILERS** — LONDON, UK.
BOILERS PROVIDED THE STEAM FOR THE STEAM-DRIVEN
PUMPS AT PUMPING STATIONS.

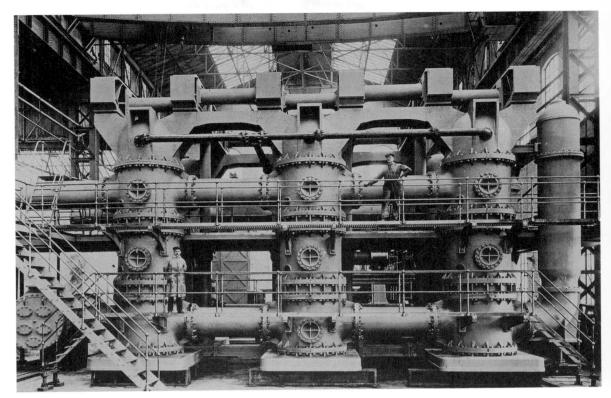

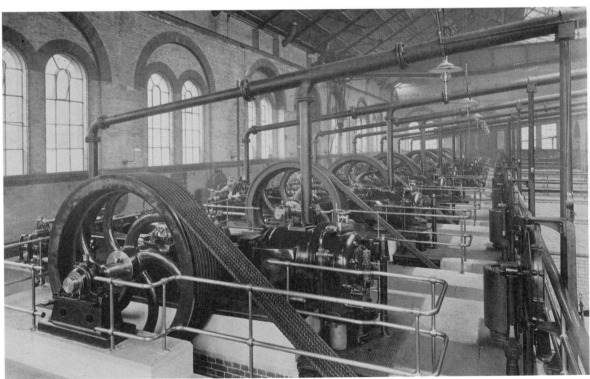

FIG. 56 ↑   **KEMPTON PARK WORKS PUMP** — LONDON, UK.

THE WATERWORKS AT KEMPTON WERE FOUNDED IN 1897

BY THE NEW RIVER COMPANY.

FIG. 57 ↓   **LOTS ROAD STORM SEWAGE PUMPING STATION** — LONDON, UK.

THIS WAS CONSTRUCTED IN 1904 TO RELIEVE LONDON'S DRAINAGE

SYSTEM BY PUMPING STORM WATER INTO THE THAMES.

THE WASTEWATER TREATMENT PROCESS

TIMELINE BASED ON TYPICAL OPERATING REGIME AND AVERAGE INCOMING FLOW.

1 PRIMARY [3 HOURS]

WHEN THE CRUDE SEWAGE ARRIVES AT THE TREATMENT PLANT, PRELIMINARY TREATMENT SIFTS OUT LARGE SOLIDS, RAGS AND DEBRIS FROM THE WASTEWATER USING A COMBINATION OF COARSE AND FINE SCREENS. GRIT – WHICH INCLUDES SAND, CINDER AND SMALL FOOD PARTICLES – IS ALSO REMOVED. PRIMARY SETTLEMENT TANKS THEN ALLOW HEAVIER ORGANIC SOLIDS TO SETTLE AND BE REMOVED TO SLUDGE TREATMENT.

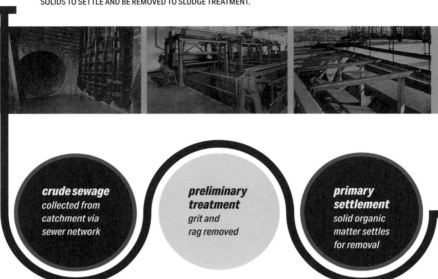

crude sewage
collected from catchment via sewer network

preliminary treatment
grit and rag removed

primary settlement
solid organic matter settles for removal

SOLID/SLUDGE

THE FIRST PART OF SLUDGE TREATMENT IS THICKENING, WHICH MAKES THE SLUDGE MORE MANAGEABLE AS IT DRASTICALLY REDUCES THE VOLUME. SECONDLY, DIGESTION REDUCES THE TOTAL MASS OF SOLIDS FURTHER, DESTROYS PATHOGENS AND RENDERS THE SLUDGE HARMLESS AND INOFFENSIVE. THIS PROCESS ALSO PRODUCES BIOGAS, WHICH CAN BE USED AS A RENEWABLE ENERGY SOURCE. THE DIGESTED SEWAGE IS THEN DEWATERED, WHICH IS ACHIEVED EITHER BY SPREADING IT OVER SAND BEDS AND ALLOWING IT TO DRY NATURALLY, OR BY USING MECHANICAL SYSTEMS. THE TREATED SLUDGE CAN ALSO BE USED AS A FERTILIZER.

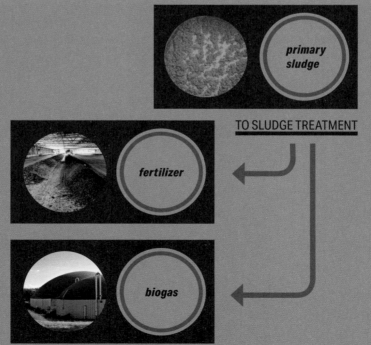

primary sludge

TO SLUDGE TREATMENT

fertilizer

biogas

SECONDARY [10 HOURS]

TERTIARY [3 HOURS]

WASTEWATER IS ADDED TO AN AERATION TANK AND ACTIVATED THROUGH THE ADDITION OF MICROBES AND EXPOSURE TO OXYGEN. THE MICROBES CONSUME ANY HARMFUL PATHOGENS IN THE ACTIVATED SLUDGE. THE EFFLUENT IS THEN SETTLED AGAIN, ALLOWING REMAINING SLUDGE TO BE REMOVED.

WHETHER THIS FINAL STAGE IS CARRIED OUT DEPENDS ON LOCAL WATER REGULATIONS. A VARIETY OF TECHNIQUES MAY BE USED TO ACHIEVE THIS 'EFFLUENT POLISHING', INCLUDING UV DISINFECTION, ULTRA-FILTRATION AND ADDING CHEMICALS SUCH AS CHLORINE.

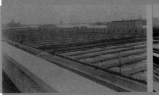

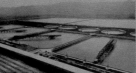

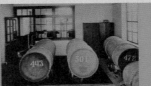

activated sludge treatment
exposure to microbes and oxygen

final settlement
separation of treated water from sludge

tertiary treatment
optional polishing depending on local requirements

final effluent
clean water returned to water system

AIR (OXYGEN)

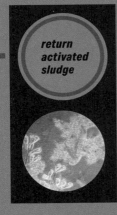

return activated sludge

surplus activated sludge

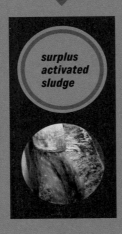

THE CLEAN, RECLAIMED WATER MAY NOW BE USED FOR INDUSTRY, IRRIGATION OR RECREATION.

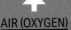

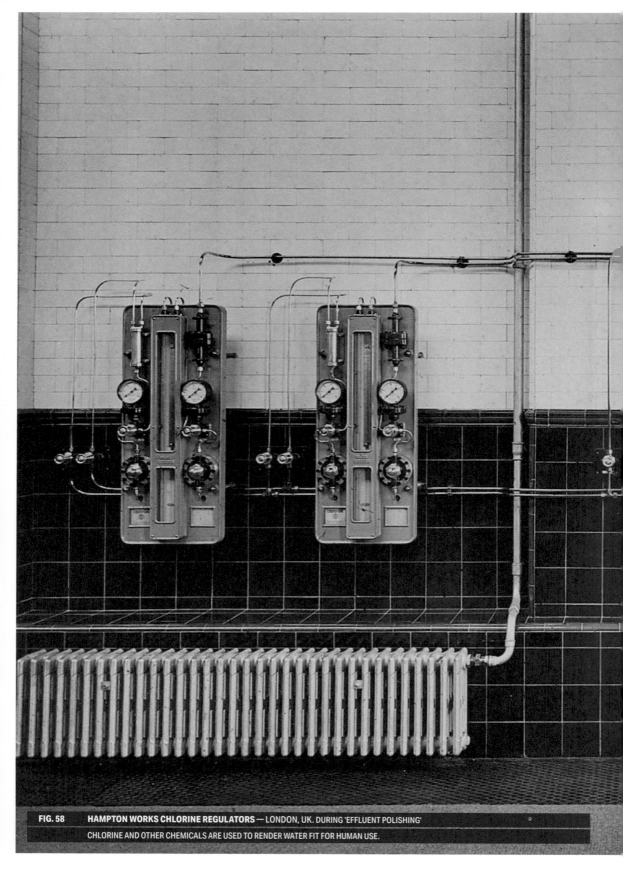

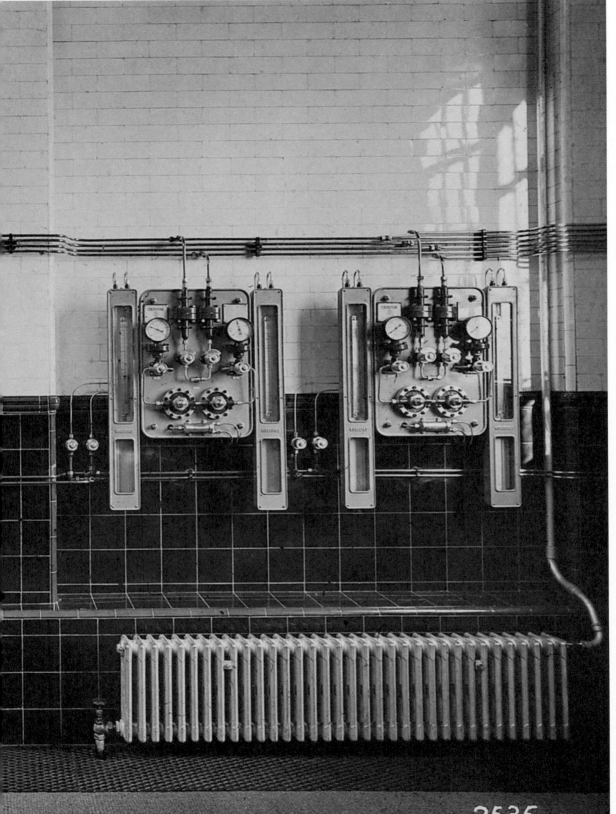

2535.

The heat thus generated drives a steam turbine, which provides electricity to run the treatments works and exports the remainder, as 'green energy', to the National Grid. Ash is removed from the incinerators at intervals, and taken to landfill sites.

In some cases, tertiary treatment methods (known as 'effluent polishing') are applied in areas where natural habitats (rivers, lakes) are particularly sensitive. At this stage, chemicals such as chlorine may be used to remove or neutralize remaining pathogens where bathing or recreational waters are involved; ultraviolet light is also used and sometimes further biological treatments are applied for nutrient removal or more natural processes are used such as lagoons and reed beds, which capture solids and further purify the water. And so we have come full circle from the nightsoilmen. They recycled waste as fertilizer to improve crop yields. Today's engineers use chemistry, biology and physics to turn our waste into electricity, pathogen-free solids for agriculture and clean water.

Unwelcome deposits constantly find their way into sewers and treatment works. The most troublesome are heavy oils and grease for cooking, which block the pipework. More recently, the use of non-biodegradable waste such as cigarette ends, cotton buds and, worst of all, rags and wet wipes have been causing blockages or failure of the collection and treatment systems. Brine from water softeners can also compromise the effectiveness of the treatment, but a far greater problem is the excessive use of powerful disinfectant agents, especially bleach, which can kill the microorganisms upon which the whole process depends, with fatal consequences for the system and hence pollution of the environment. Attempts to persuade the manufacturers of wet wipes to make them of biodegradable materials have so far been in vain. Such abuses of the systems lead to accumulation of FOGs (Fats, Oils and Grease), which can form into fatbergs that regularly block public sewers and sometimes cause flooding in urban areas or individual properties. The 'Whitechapel Fatberg' discovered in 2017 in London was a particularly horrifying example, reaching 250 m (820 ft) in length and weighing 130 tonnes. A forensic examination of the berg revealed its contents as condoms, sanitary towels, wet wipes and cotton buds, encased within solidified cooking oil and skin products. The Museum of London deemed the fatberg such an important part of London's history that since 2018 they have had a chunk of it on display. Moreover, a livestream can be tuned into online to watch it slowly decompose, or one can buy 'don't feed the fatberg' slogan t-shirts in the museum shop.

'ONE OF THE MOST FASCINATING AND DISGUSTING OBJECTS WE HAVE EVER HAD ON DISPLAY.'

Curator Vyki Sparkes commenting on the Museum of London's display of the Whitechapel fatberg (2018)

FIGS. 59–61 1950s **SEWAGE TREATMENT AND WATER SUPPLY —**
LONDON, UK. THESE LANTERN SLIDES FROM THE 1950s
SHOW THE OPERATION OF LONDON'S WATER SUPPLY SYSTEM.

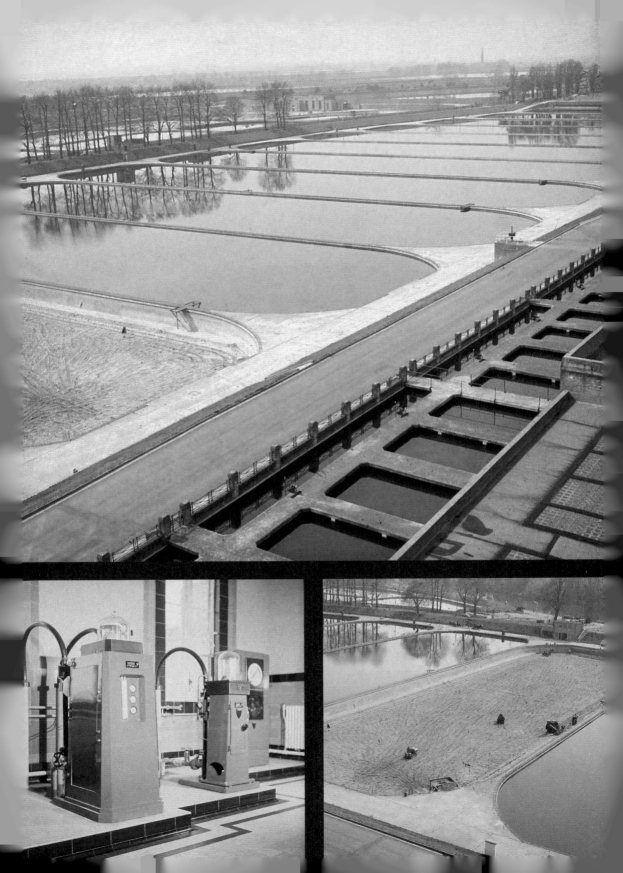

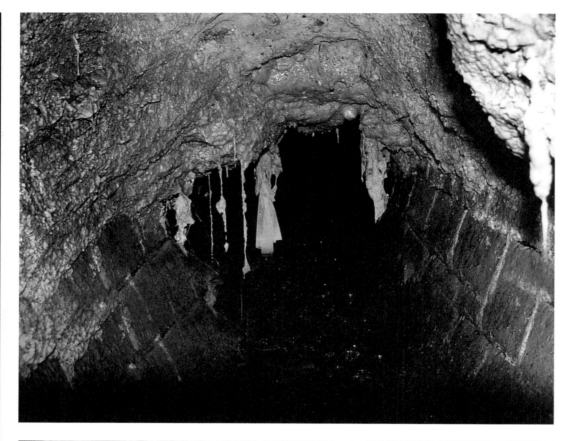

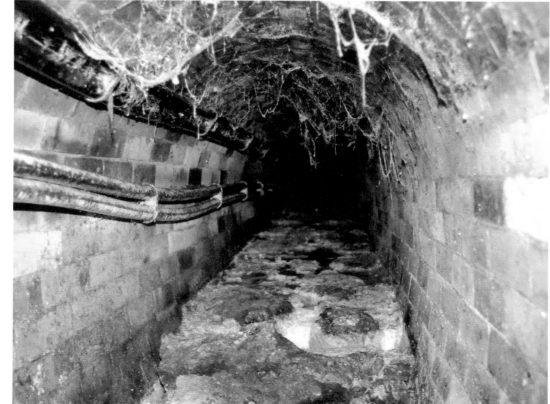

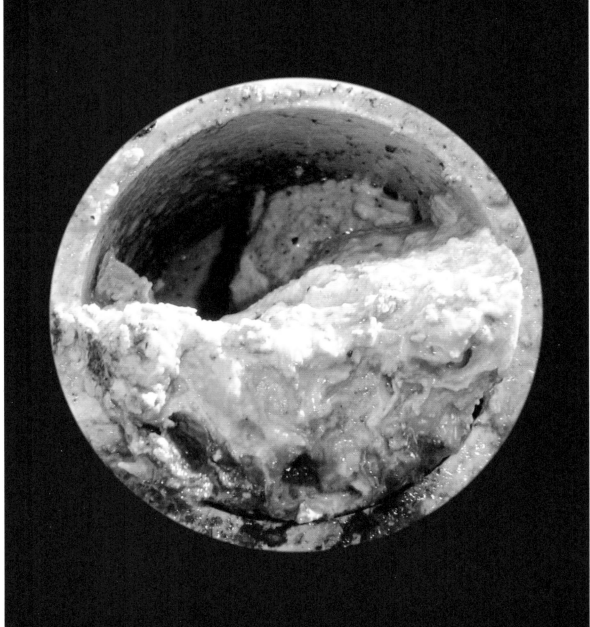

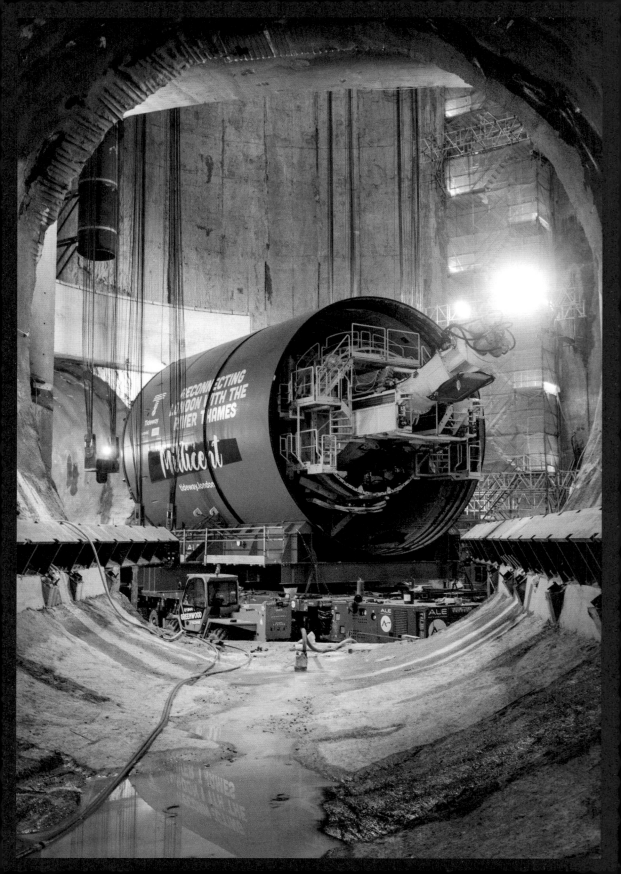

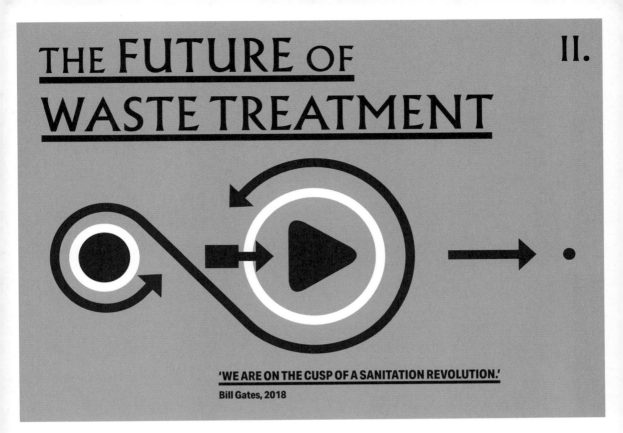

THE FUTURE OF WASTE TREATMENT

'WE ARE ON THE CUSP OF A SANITATION REVOLUTION.'

Bill Gates, 2018

It has been estimated that in the early 21st century about 3.3 billion people (of a total population of 7.8 billion) lack adequate sanitation and about 3 million die each year of diseases related to diarrhoea, most of those being due to the ingestion of pathogens in polluted water. Cholera and typhoid remain threats in developing nations. The majority of sewage is untreated, even in rapidly developing nations such as China and India, and this is also true of Taiwan with its well-developed economy. And as these nations develop, more of their citizens will move from the countryside to towns and cities, where heavy expenditure is required to deal with the problems of sanitation that the concentration of population brings. Three approaches may already be discerned in dealing with the problems of the 21st century: civil engineering for large cities; more natural processes in rural areas with plenty of available land; and the combination of technology and urban design.

London has chosen the civil engineering solution in combination with its existing technology, described in the previous section. Reference has been made to the extension of London's sewerage system as the population expanded in the 1920s and 1930s (see page 136). The later 20th century has brought other problems, which will require different solutions. One of these is climate change. Although some disagreement still exists about the precise cause and likely effects of global 244

FIG. 1   2018 **'MILLICENT' THE TUNNEL BORING MACHINE** —
LONDON, UK. NAMED AFTER SUFFRAGIST MILLICENT
FAWCETT, THE MACHINE IS CURRENTLY EMPLOYED
IN BORING THE THAMES TIDEWAY TUNNEL.

FIG. 2 2018 **UNDERGROUND DISCHARGE CHANNEL OF GREATER TOKYO** — TOKYO, JAPAN. THE LARGEST STORM DRAIN ON EARTH, 99 KM (62 MILES) LONG, PROTECTS TOKYO FROM FLOODING DURING THE TYPHOON SEASON.

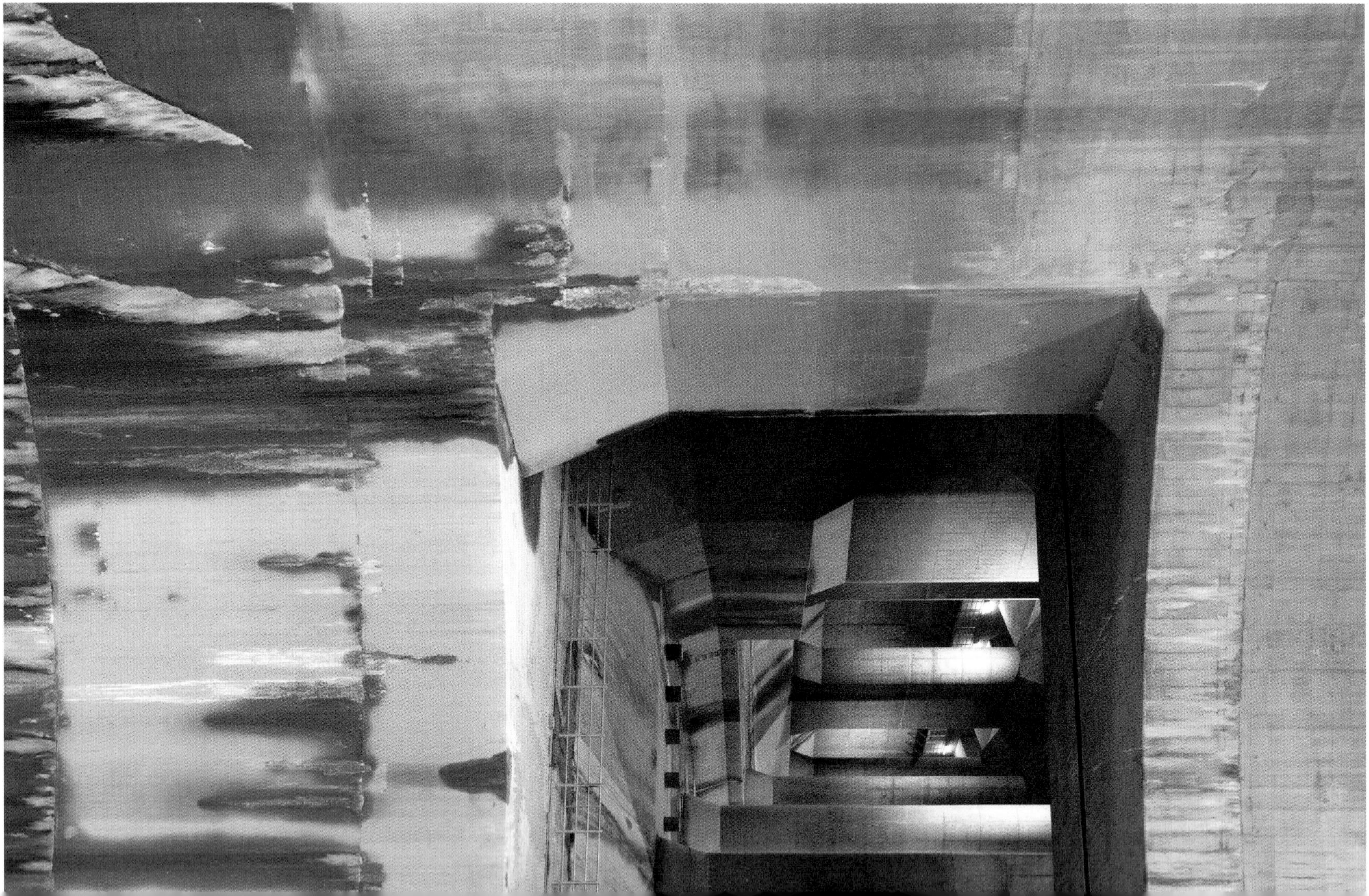

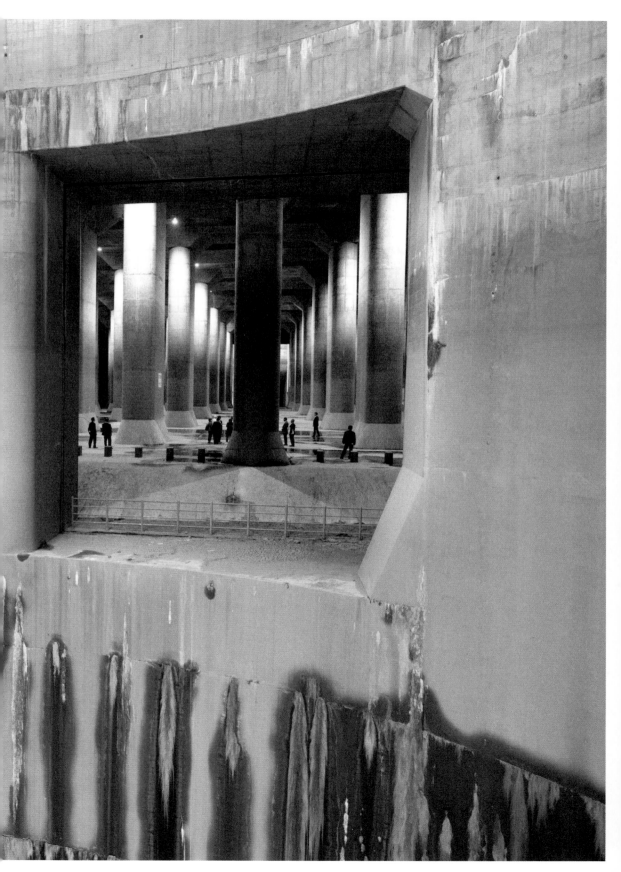

warming, most experts agree that 'extreme weather events', however defined, are a growing feature of our lives, with records for temperature and rainfall broken at shorter intervals than ever before. This has affected London, and other cities, in ways that Sir Joseph Bazalgette could not have anticipated. Storms, generating huge amounts of rain in a short period, are becoming more frequent. The Japanese have combatted this problem with a remarkable feat of engineering – the largest storm drain on earth that lies beneath the ground 31 km (19 miles) north of Toyko, and protects the city from flooding during the typhoon season. Construction begun in 1992 and took 17 years and 2 billion dollars to complete. The system includes tunnels that run to over 100 km (62 miles) in length, and drainage pumps that can remove 200 tonnes of water per second. The main hall – or water tank – is held up by 59 columns, each 25 m (82 ft) high, which is such an awesome sight that it has been nicknamed the 'underground temple'.

In London, increasing storms have meant that sewage overflows directly into the Thames are no longer a rare occurrence. The gradual disappearance of green spaces in the face of advancing concrete makes the situation worse. When rain falls on grass, trees or other vegetation, much of it will come to rest on them and evaporate. Some will be taken up by the roots and the rest will filter through the soil before finding its way gradually into underground streams or reservoirs. As more housing estates are built and more garden areas are converted into dwellings – or as lawns are turned into hard standing for cars, or concrete advances farther as roads are built to serve the houses – rain runs immediately into drains and overburdens the sewers, causing sewage overflows. Bazalgette estimated that overflows would occur twelve times a year. That figure has now reached sixty times a year, depositing 39 million tonnes of rainwater containing sewage into the Thames annually.

Thames Water's answer to this is the traditional civil engineering solution. It is officially called the 'Thames Tideway Tunnel', although in the title of three documentaries broadcast by BBC2 in July 2018 it was described as 'The Five Billion Pound Super Sewer'. It is being constructed under the supervision of a company specially created for the purpose and appropriately called Bazalgette Tunnel Ltd. And the engineering is of a scale that Bazalgette would have recognized. In anticipation of the population of the capital rising to 9 million within the next few years, and possibly 13 million by 2030, the supersewer will run beneath the course of the Thames for 26 km (16 miles), from Acton in the west to Thames Water's Abbey Mills, Beckton and Crossness in the east. It is 7.2 m (23 ft 7 in.) in diameter (compared with 3.5 m (11 ft 5 in.) for the Tube railway and 6.2 m (20 ft 4 in.) for the Crossrail tunnels), lies 30–70 m (99–230 ft) beneath the surface and passes beneath the existing sewers and Underground railway lines. The supersewer will collect the outfall of thirty-four sewer overflows. In addition the separate River Lee tunnel will run from Abbey Mills to Beckton, capturing sewage overflows that would otherwise run into the Lee or Thames. At Beckton six huge pumps will lift the overflow from the tunnels to Beckton for processing in Europe's largest treatment works. The construction cost is estimated as £4.2 billion, which, given the inflation of the past 150 years, bears comparison with Bazalgette's expenditure on sewers of £4.2 million.

The first shafts, 30 m (99 ft) in diameter, were sunk 70 m (230 ft) beneath the surface at Battersea in 2016 and near Tower Bridge in 2017 and the tunnel boring machines (TBMs) were loaded into them.

FIG. 3 ↑   **OVERVIEW OF THAMES WATER'S BECKTON TREATMENT PLANT** — LONDON, UK. BAZALGETTE'S TREATMENT WORKS IS THE LARGEST TREATMENT PLANT IN EUROPE.

FIG. 4 ↓   2018 **THE THAMES TIDEWAY TUNNEL** — LONDON, UK. WHEN COMPLETED IN 2024 THE TUNNEL WILL COLLECT SEWAGE OVERFLOWS DURING STORMS AND CONDUCT IT TO BECKTON.

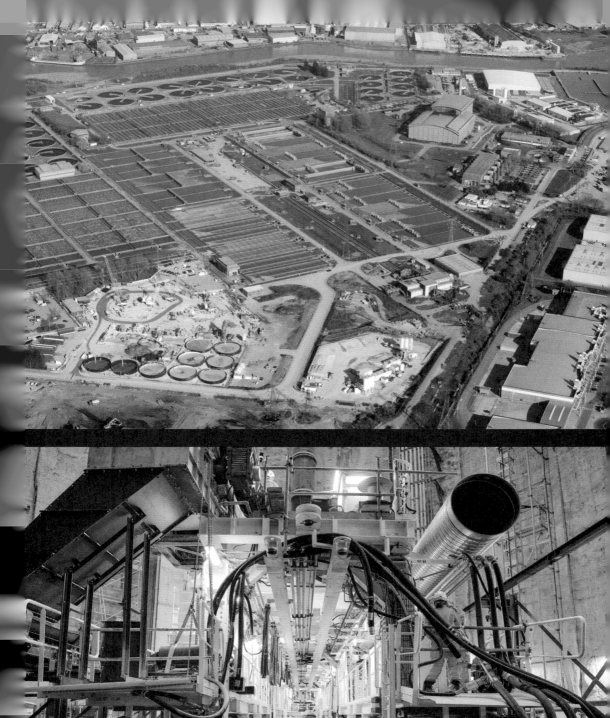

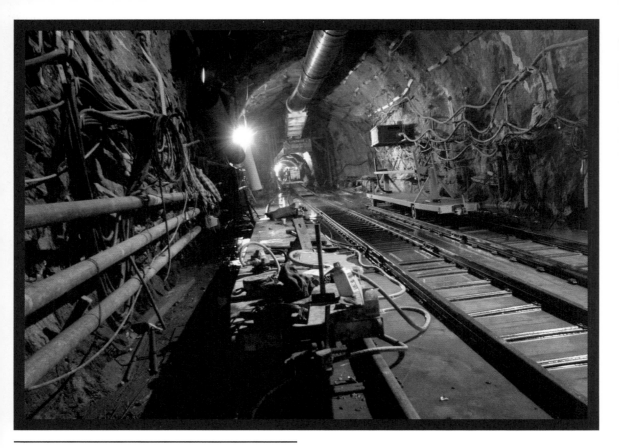

FIG. 5 2003 **CONSTRUCTING TUNNEL NO. 3** — NEW YORK, USA.
NEW YORK CITY'S WATER SUPPLY HAS BEEN UPGRADED WITH
THE CONSTRUCTION OF A 97-KM (60-MILE) LONG TUNNEL.

When reassembled they weigh 900 tonnes each. They are similar to those used to create the Crossrail tunnels, each of them 110 m (361 ft) long and resembling a factory: cutting the tunnel with a 9-m (30-ft) diameter cutting head, installing concrete lining panels and conveying away the waste from the newly bored tunnel. Each has a crew of 350, who enable the machines to run 24 hours a day. There are six TBMs, all named after notable women. The first two to enter service were named 'Millicent' in memory of Millicent Fawcett (1847–1929), a suffragist who is the first woman to be commemorated in Parliament Square; and 'Ursula' after Ursula Smith (1915–81), whose discoveries enabled red blood cells to be preserved during medical procedures. The other four are named 'Charlotte', after suffragette Charlotte Despard (1844–1939); 'Annie' (Russell, 1868–1947), the first woman to work at the Royal Observatory, Greenwich; 'Selina' (Fox, 1871–1958) founder of the Bermondsey Medical Mission; and 'Rachel' (Parsons, 1885–1956), one of the first women to study engineering at Cambridge and who later entered the profession. And another woman is present, apart from the female engineers among the tunnellers. This is St Barbara, the Patron Saint of miners and, by extension, tunnellers, whose image was also to be found in the Crossrail tunnels.

But the massive investment in civil engineering required for the London supersewer, or New York City's 96.5 km (60 mile) long 'Tunnel No. 3' designed to improve the adequacy and dependability of the city's water supply, are beyond the means of the smaller, often rural communities in which most

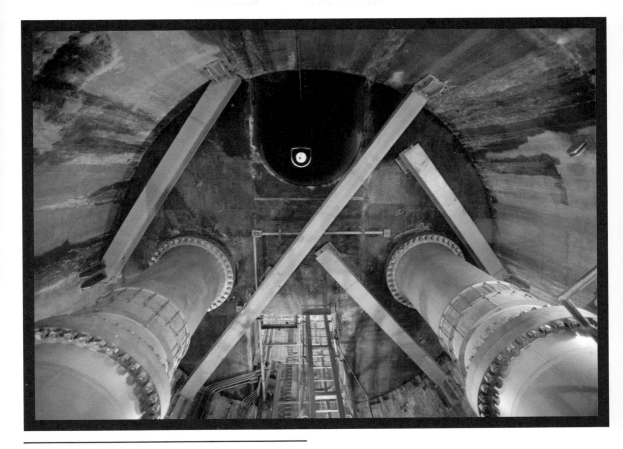

FIG. 6   2013 **TUNNEL NO. 3** — NEW YORK, USA. THE LOWER MANHATTAN
DISTRIBUTION SHAFT TERMINUS OF NEW YORK CITY'S NEW WATER
SUPPLY TUNNEL.

of the world's population still live. For that reason many of them are adopting more natural solutions
for sewage treatment. One method is the waste stabilization pond, which bears some resemblance to the
activated sludge process discussed earlier and to the treatment lagoons used to treat Melbourne's waste.
The ponds consist of man-made pools with earth embankments into which the wastewater enters. Like
activated sludge tanks, they depend upon natural organisms to consume the pathogens in the waste. Since
they are not subjected to artificial stimuli, as in activated sludge treatment, the process takes much longer
than in a modern treatment works and often involves the waste travelling through several ponds before
being released to a river or lake. This method of treatment is well suited to small towns with warm climates
and plenty of available land, though it is employed in Agadir, Morocco, with a population of over 400,000.

Innovative solutions to sewerage problems around the world have also been provided through the
application of cutting edge technology and design. In Antananarivo, the capital city of Madagascar
– with a large population of about 1.3 million – this ingenuity comes in the form of the products of the
Loowatt company. The company's mobile toilets are more often encountered at fairs and festivals, but
in Antananarivo it is installing toilets that dispatch the waste to an anaerobic digester, which extracts
methane for the generation of electricity and turns the remaining waste into fertilizer. This requires
no major civil engineering works and may be a way forward for some larger communities in developing

nations. They are certainly preferable to the 'flying toilets' found in some cities, notably Nairobi in Kenya, where the expression is applied to the practice of defecating in a plastic bag and throwing it as far as possible into a neighbouring street.

Technology has also been successfully applied in other areas. For instance, in regions where water is in very short supply or where freezing temperatures are commonplace, the transport of waste by gravity, using water as the medium, can be problematic. Vacuum sewers, tentatively introduced to Prague by captain Charles Liernur (see page 160), are in use in Norway and Sweden and also in the small French town of Flavigny-sur-Ozerain, north-west of Dijon, while a vacuum toilet (which doesn't use water to flush away the waste), similar to those used on aircraft, has been installed as a public facility in Hong Kong. On a small estate of 117 dwellings at Flintenbreite, to the west of Lübeck in Germany, the waste from toilets is fed direct to an anaerobic digester, which generates gas for power generation for the community while rainwater from roofs is distributed to the groundwater rather than being dispatched to drains. The project is being monitored by the Technical University, Hamburg and it is estimated that construction costs for the project are 40% more than conventional methods but running costs are 25% lower. Another glimpse of the future may also be found at the Eddington community to the north-west of Cambridge. Named after the scientist Sir Arthur Eddington (1882–1944), this 150-hectare (370-acre) site has been developed

FIG. 7 ↓   **ANAEROBIC DIGESTER TANKS IN A WATER TREATMENT PLANT**. ANAEROBIC DIGESTION REDUCES THE VOLUME OF EXCESS SLUDGE THAT NEEDS TO BE ELIMINATED.

FIG. 8 →   **THE JANICKI OMNI PROCESSOR**. PHYSICAL, CHEMICAL AND BIOLOGICAL TREATMENT ALLOWS THE PROCESSOR TO TURN SEWAGE INTO DRINKABLE WATER.

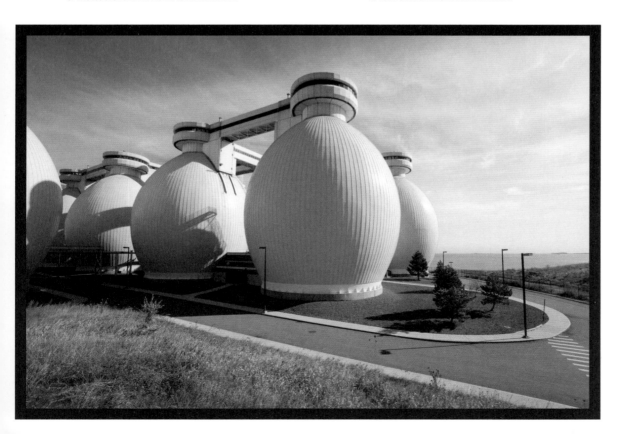

by Cambridge University to provide 3,000 dwellings and 2,000 student bedrooms with a primary school, community centre and superstore. A district heating system is partly powered by solar energy and rainwater is collected and recycled for flushing toilets and other purposes.

A particularly promising innovation is Sedron Technologies's Janicki Omini Processor, funded by the Bill and Melinda Gates Foundation. The steam-engine-powered device is able to convert human waste into clean, drinkable water in just minutes, as well as producing the energy to incinerate the remaining waste solids and leave 250 kilowatts spare. The installation of this technology in third world countries clearly has great potential in the provision of clean water and thus the prevention of disease. It was first trialled in Senegal in 2015, and in its first year converted 700 tonnes of excreta into energy and water.

At the other end of sewerage innovation, the Japanese have given the world the Toto Toilet, offering heated seats, a stream of warm water directed at the rear to eliminate the need for anything as crude as loo paper, an automatic seat-closing system (eliminating domestic friction on that sensitive subject) and an air de-odorizing process. They are very popular in Japan and catching on in the USA, though with prices approaching £7,000 each it is likely that they may take time to become widespread. And in 2018, the unlikely combination of researchers at the European Space Agency, the Massachusetts Institute of Technology and sanitation engineers have designed the Fitloo, which will screen human waste for signs of incipient diseases, such as cancer and diabetes, and pass the data to the user's mobile phone or GP for early treatment.

However, as developed and refined as our processes of waste removal become, and as luxurious the experience, one fact remains the same: the need for good sewers.

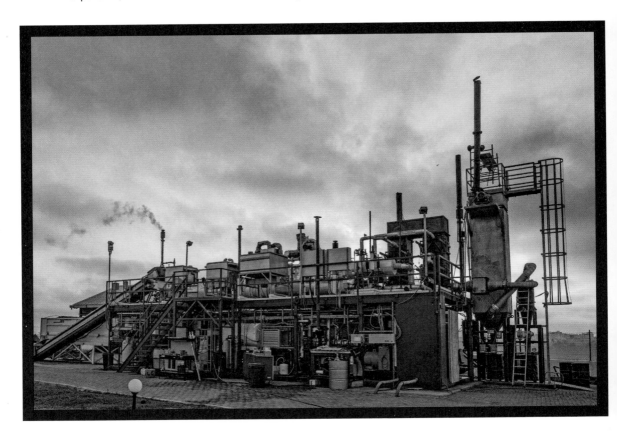

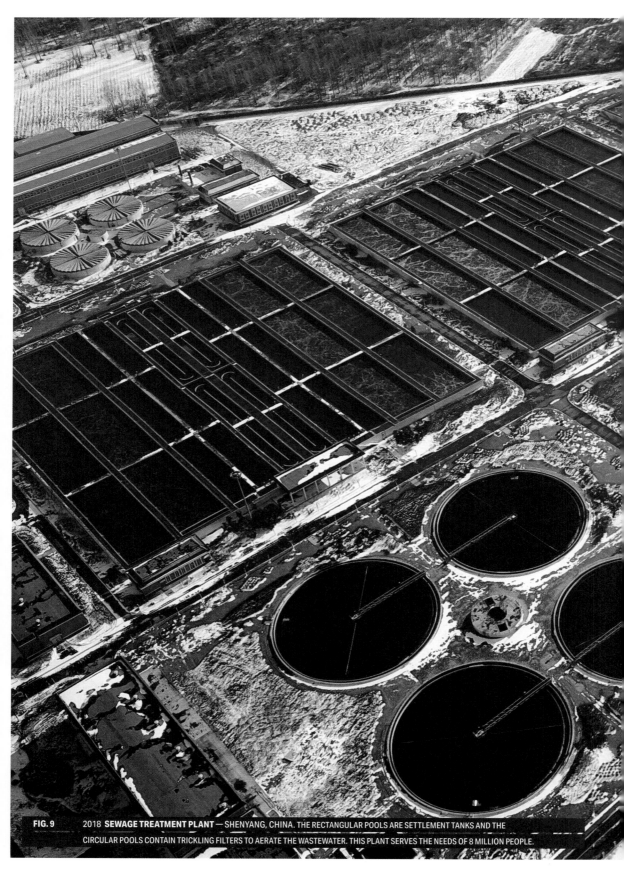

FIG. 9   2018 **SEWAGE TREATMENT PLANT** — SHENYANG, CHINA. THE RECTANGULAR POOLS ARE SETTLEMENT TANKS AND THE CIRCULAR POOLS CONTAIN TRICKLING FILTERS TO AERATE THE WASTEWATER. THIS PLANT SERVES THE NEEDS OF 8 MILLION PEOPLE.

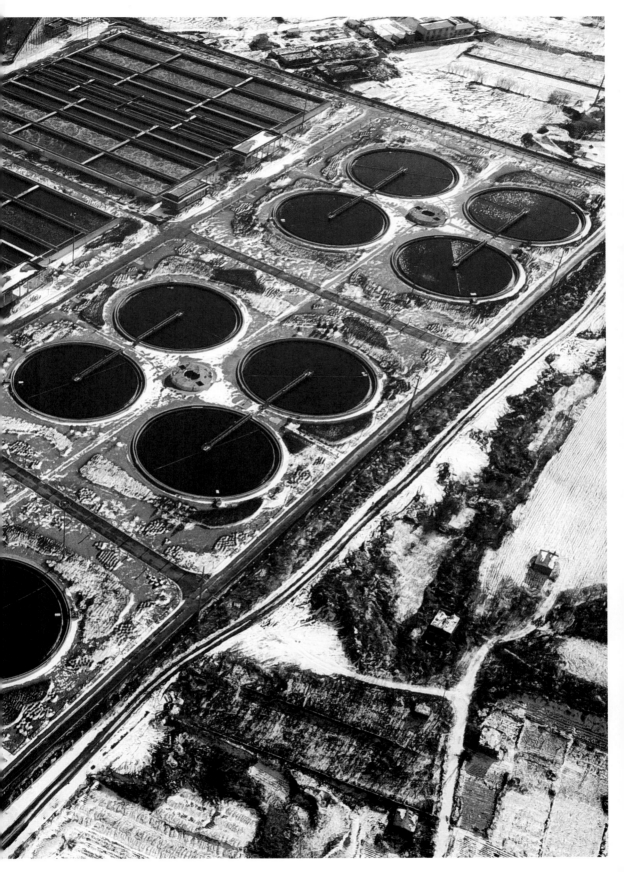

PRELUDE: CHOLERA IN THE CITY

P. 10. Joseph Bazalgette, 'On the main drainage of London and the interception of the sewage from the River Thames', *Minutes of the Proceedings of the Institution of Civil Engineers*, Vol. 24 (1864–65), p. 285.

P. 10. *The Lancet* (22 October 1853) pp. 393–4.

P. 10. Heinrich Heine, 'The cholera in Paris' (April 19 1832).

P.11. 'The cholera', *Preston Chronicle* (28 April 1832).

P. 21. Edwin Chadwick, *Metropolitan Sewage Committee Proceedings* (1846), p. 10.

P. 22. Michael Faraday, 'Observations on the filth of the Thames, contained in a letter addressed to the editor of *The Times* newspaper', *The Times* (7 July 1855).

P. 22. Charles Dickens, *Little Dorrit* (1857).

P. 23. William Farr, *Report on the Cholera Epidemic of 1866* (1867), p. 53.

P. 24. Antony van Leeuwenhoek, *Letter to the Royal Society* (September 17 1683).

P. 24. *Hamburger Fremdenblatt* (1892).

P.24. Johannes Versmann, cited in Stephen Halliday, *The Great Stink of London* (Stroud: The History Press, 1999), p. 187

P. 24. Robert Koch, *Hamburger Freie Presse* (26 November 1892) cited in Richard J. Evans, *Death in Hamburg: Society and Politics in the Cholera Years 1830–1910* (Oxford: Oxford University Press, 1987), p. 313.

SANITATION IN THE ANCIENT WORLD

P. 29. *The Bible*, Deuteronomy 23: 12–13.

P. 31. Herodotus, *Histories, Book II* (440 BC).

P. 33. Victor Hugo, *Les Misérables* (1862).

P. 36. Dionysius of Halicarnassus, *Roman Antiquities*, 3.67.5.

SEWAGE IN THE STREETS

P. 41. Samuel Pepys, *The Diary of Samuel Pepys* (20 October 1660).

P. 49. *Ordnance Gazetteer of Scotland*, Vol. 2, (Edinburgh: Thomas C. Jack, Grange Publishing Works, 1884), p. 294.

P. 49. Nathaniel Wanley, *The Wonders of the Little World* (1678), p. 42.

P. 49. 'Building by-laws, London, 1189', in Douglas, D. C. (ed.), *English Historical Documents, 1189–1327*, (London: Eyre and Spottiswoode, 1975), p. 879.

P. 49. 'Petition to parliament, 1290' in *Report on an Inquiry into the Sanitary Condition of the Labouring Population of Great Britain* (London, 1842), p. 292.

P. 49. Jonathan Swift, 'A description of a city shower' (1711).

P. 52. Edward III, 'Royal order for cleansing the streets of the City and the banks of the Thames' (1357).

THE CLEANSING OF PARIS

P. 59. Victor Hugo, *Les Misérables* (1862).

P. 62. Edwin Chadwick, quoted in G. M Young, *Victorian England: Portrait of an Age* (Oxford: Oxford University Press, 1936), p. 11.

P. 63. Victor de Persigny, *Memoires* (1890).

P. 63. Léon Halévy, *Carnets 1862–69*, cited in Hervé Maneglier, *Paris Impérial: La Vie Quotidienne sous le Second Empire* (Paris: Armand Colin, 1990), p. 263.

P. 67. Georges-Eugène Haussmann, *Mémoires du Baron Haussmann* (1890–93).

P. 67. Victor Hugo, *Les Misérables* (1862).

P. 68. Émile Zola, *La Terre* (1887).

P. 69. Georges-Eugène Haussmann, *Mémoire sur les Eaux de Paris Présenté à la Commission Municipale Par M. Le Préfet de la Seine* (4 August 1854)

P. 82. Henry Haynie, *Paris Past & Present*, Vol. 2 (New York: Frederick A. Stokes, 1902), p. 292

P. 83. J. J. Waller, 'Under the streets of Paris', *Good Words*, Vol. 35 (1894), p. 494

P. 83. J. J. Waller, 'Under the streets of Paris', *Good Words*, Vol. 35 (1894), p. 494

P. 83. Karl Baedeker, *Paris and Environs*, 13th edition (1898), p. 64.

P. 83. Francis White, 'A visit to the Paris sewers', *Harper's Weekly*, Vol. 37 (29 April 1893), p. 395.

P. 83. Thomas W. Knox, *The Underground World* (Hartford, C.T.: J. B. Burr, 1882), p. 528.

P. 83. Louis Veuillot, *Les Odeurs de Paris*, (Paris: Georges Crès, 1914), pp.1–2.

LONDON & THE GREAT STINK

P. 99. Charles Dickens, *Little Dorrit* (1857).

P. 101. 'Obituary. Sir Joseph William Bazalgette.', *Minutes of the Proceedings of the Institution of Civil Engineers*, Vol. 105 (1891), pp. 302–303.

P. 107. Florence Nightingale (1820–1910) writing to the Liverpool council in appreciation of James Newland's work in Crimea in 1855.

P. 111. *Hansard* (7 June 1858).

P. 111. Benjamin Disraeli, *Hansard* (15 July 1858).

P. 122. Joseph Bazalgette, 'Narrative of proceedings of the General Register Office during the cholera epidemic of 1866', *Parliamentary Papers*, Vol. 37, 95 (1867–68).

P. 131. *Farmers Magazine* (1860).

P. 140. 'Death of Sir Joseph Bazalgette', *The Times* (16 March 1891).

P. 140. 'Norman Foster: Interview', *Time Out* (18 September 2008).

WORLD WIDE ADAPTIONS

P. 143. Bernard Lee as Sergeant Paine in *The Third Man* (1949).

P. 153. Obituary. William Lindley.', *Minutes of the Proceedings of the Institution of Civil Engineers*, Vol. 142 (1900), pp. 363–370.

P. 160. Robert Więckiewicz as Leopold Socha in *In Darkness* (2011).

P. 161. Extract from a speech made by Dr Kühn, second secretary to the mayor of Prague (1896).

RAISING STREETS

P. 177. *The Great Chicago Lake Tunnel* (Chicago: Jack Wing, 1867).

P. 204. Captain John Smith, 1608. Reported in *The Generall Historie of Virginia, New England & The Summer Isles*, Vol. 2 (1907), pp. 44–45.

P. 204. *Report of the Sewerage Commission of the City of Baltimore* (1897).

PROCESSING & TREATING SEWAGE

P. 209. *Scientific American*, Vol. 93, 24 (1905).

P. 221. William Dibdin, *Chief Chemist's Annual Report to the Metropolitan Board of Works* (1887), p. 23

P. 228. Victor Hugo, *Les Misérables* (1862).

P. 237. Vyki Sparkes, 'Fatberg! The Museum of London's most disgusting exhibit goes on display', *Museums + Heritage Advisor* (8 February, 2018).

THE FUTURE OF WASTE TREATMENT

P. 241. Address by Bill Gates, The Reinvented Toilet Expo, Beijing (6 November, 2018).

Addis, F., *Rome: Eternal City* (London: Head of Zeus, 2018)

Angelakis, A. N. and Rose, J. B. (eds.), *Evolution of Sanitation and Wastewater Technologies through the Centuries* (London: IWA Publishing, 2014)

Angelakis, A. N. et al., 'The Historical Development of Sewers Worldwide', *Sustainability*, Vol. 6, 6 (2014), 3936–74

Christiansen, R., *City of Light: the Reinvention of Paris* (London: Head of Zeus, 2018)

Eyles, D., *Royal Doulton, 1815–1905* (London: Hutchinson, 1965)

Halliday, S., *The Great Stink of London: Sir Joseph Bazalgette and the Cleansing of the Victorian Metropolis* (Stroud: History Press, 1999)

Lofrano, G. and Brown, J., 'Wastewater Management Through the Ages: A History of Mankind', *Science of the Total Environment*, Vol. 408, 22 (2010), 5254–64

Markham, A., *A Brief History of Pollution* (London: Earthscan Publications, 1994)

Marshall, R., *In the Sewers of Lvov* (London: Collins, 1990)

Pinkney, D. H., *Napoleon III and the Rebuilding of Paris* (Princeton, N.J.: Princeton University Press, 1972)

Reid, D., *Paris Sewers and Sewermen: Realities and Representations* (Cambridge, M.A.: Harvard University Press, 1991)

Saalman, H., *Haussmann: Paris Transformed* (New York, N.Y.: Braziller, 1971)

Seeger, H., 'The History of German Wastewater Treatment', *European Water Management*, Vol. 2, 5 (1999), 51–6

Wiesmann, U., Choi I. S. and Dombrowski E., 'Historical Development of Wastewater Collection and Treatment', in *Fundamentals of Biological Wastewater Treatment* (Weinheim: Wiley 2006) 1–20

[PICTURE CREDITS]

Every effort has been made to locate and credit copyright holders of the material reproduced in this book. The author and publisher apologise for any omissions or errors, which can be corrected in future editions

Key: t: top, b: below, c: centre, l: left, r: right

1 Joe Belanger / Shutterstock; **2** Adam Powell; **3t** Courtesy Thames Water Utilities Limited; **3tr** Library of Congress, Washington, D.C.; **3cr** Courtesy Thames Water Utilities Limited; **3br** Courtesy Thames Water Utilities Limited; **3b** Library of Congress, Washington, D.C.; **3bl** Courtesy Thames Water Utilities Limited; **3cl** Boston Public Library, Edgar Sutton Dorr Photograph Collection; **3tl** Commonwealth of Massachusetts State Archives, Massachusetts Archives & Commonwealth Museum, Boston, MA; **4–5** London Metropolitan Archives (City of London) / Collage – The London Picture Archive 218521; **6** Bibliothèque nationale de France, Paris; **8** Institution of Civil Engineers Library and Archives; **9** Universal History Archive / Getty Images; **11** Stu Haats, ebay-nls. Antique Engravings, Prints, Maps and Newspapers; **12tl**, tr *Du choléra-morbus en Russie, en Prusse et en Autriche, pendant les années 1831 et 1832*, by Auguste Nicolas Vincent Gérardin, Paul Gaimard, 1832; **12bl**, **br**, **13** Wellcome Collection, London; **14–15** *A treatise on epidemic cholera; including an historical account of its origin and progress,to the present period. Comp. from the most authentic sources*, by Amariah Brigham, 1832. Library of Congress, Washington, D.C.; **16tl** De Agostini / Biblioteca Ambrosiana / Getty Images; **16tr** "The Cholera and Fever Nests of New York City", 1866. Illustrations from the Healy Collection; **16bl** De Agostini / Getty Images; **16br** Granger Historical Picture Archive / Alamy Stock Photo; **17tl** Wellcome Collection, London; **17tr**, bl De Agostini / Biblioteca Ambrosiana / Getty Images; **17br** Private Collection / Look and Learn / Illustrated Papers Collection / Bridgeman Images; **18–19** *Appendix to report of the committee for scientific inquiries in relation to the cholera-epidemic of 1854*, 1855. Printed by George E. Eyre and William Spottiswoode for H.M.S.O.; **20** Wellcome Collection, London; **22l** This image was reproduced by kind permission of London Borough of Lambeth, Archives Department, 11135; **22r** Wellcome Collection, London; **23** Wellcome Collection, London; **25** Bibliothèque nationale de France, Paris; **27** Courtesy of the Oriental Institute of the University of Chicago; **28** From *Early India and Pakistan to Ashoka*, by Sir Mortimer Wheeler, Thames & Hudson Ltd., 1959; **30l** Satellite photograph courtesy Douglas Comer. Illustration courtesy Ueli Bellwald; **30r** Courtesy Guido Camici; **31l** Raveesh Vyas; **31c** Bernard Gagnon; **31r** De Agostini / Getty Images; **32l** akg-images / Rabatti & Domingie; **32bc**, **br** View of China; **33l** Leonid Serebrennikov / Alamy Stock Photo; **33r** forumancientcoins.com; **34–35** American School of Classical Studies at Athens: Agora Excavations; **36l** Rijksmuseum, The Netherlands; **36r** The J. Paul Getty Museum, Los Angeles; **37l** © Herbert List / Magnum Photos; **37r** The Metropolitan Museum of Art, New York. Gilman Collection, Gift of The Howard Gilman Foundation, 2005; **39** Victor Fraile / Corbis / Getty Images; **40** Roger-Viollet / TopFoto; **42l** New York Public Library; **42c** Library of Congress, Washington, D.C.; **42r** The Trustees of the British Museum, London; **43l** Courtesy Alexa Helsell; **43r** Anthony Majanlahti; **44l** francesco de marco / Shutterstock.com; **44r** Courtesy Fabrice Mrugala; **45l** akg-images; **45r** Gemäldegalerie, Berlin; **46–47** National Maritime Museum, Greenwich, London; **48tl** Mary Evans Picture Library; **48tr** The Trustees of the British Museum, London; **48bl** The Trustees of the British Museum, London; **48br** Wellcome Collection, London; **50** The Metropolitan Museum of Art, New York. Gilman Collection, Purchase, Mr. and Mrs. Henry R. Kravis Gift, 2005; **51** Roger-Viollet / Topfoto; **52l** Erddig, Clwyd, North Wales / National Trust Photographic Library / Bridgeman Images; **52r** *The metamorphosis of Ajax, a Cloacinean satire: with the Anatomy and Apology ... To which is added Ulysses upon Ajax*, by Sir John Harington, 1814; **53l** Fisher Library at the University of Toronto; **53r** Wellcome Collection, London; **54** The Trustees of the British Museum, London; **55tl**, **tr**, **cl**, br The Trustees of the British Museum, London; **55 tc** Heritage Image Partnership Ltd / Alamy Stock Photo; **55c** Library of Congress, Washington, D.C.; **55cr**, **bl**, **bc** Heritage Image Partnership Ltd / Alamy Stock Photo; **57** Boston Public Library, Norman B. Leventhal Map Center; **58** Bibliothèque nationale de France, Paris, département Société de Géographie, SG W-58; **60–61** *Les Travaux de Paris. 1789-1889*, sous la direction de M. A. Alphand par les soins de M. Huet, M. Humblot, M. Bechmann, M. Fauve, M. F. de Mallevoue, 1889; **62–65** Ville de Paris / BHVP; **66** Centre Pompidou, MNAM-CCI, Dist. RMN-Grand Palais / image Centre Pompidou, MNAM-CCI. © Estate Brassaï – RMN-Grand Palais; **68–69** Ville de Paris / BHVP; **70–71** Bibliothèque nationale de France, Paris; **72–73** Ville de Paris / BHdV; **74–77** Roger-Viollet / Topfoto; **78–81** Bibliothèque nationale de France, Paris; **82** Design Pics Inc / Shutterstock; **83l** Roger-Viollet / Topfoto; **83r** Private Collection; **84t**, **cl** Bibliothèque nationale de France, Paris; **84cr**, **br**, **bl** Lebrecht Music & Arts / Alamy Stock Photo; **85tl**, br Private Collection; **85cl**, **cr** Collection BIU Santé Médecine; **85bl** Roger-Viollet / Shutterstock; **86** Bibliothèque nationale de France, Paris; **87tl** The Print Collector / Alamy Stock Photo; **87tr**, **cl**, **cr**, **clb**, **crb**, **br** Roger-Viollet / Topfoto; **87bl** Courtesy sewerhistory.org; **88–93** Bibliothèque nationale de France, Paris; **94–97** Roger-Viollet / Topfoto; **98** Courtesy Thames Water Utilities Limited; **100** Science and Society Picture Library; **101l** Private Collection; **101r** Twyford; **102** Wellcome Collection, London; **103** Twyford; **104** London Metropolitan Archives (City of London) / Collage – The London Picture Archive 2364; **105** London Metropolitan Archives (City of London) / Collage – The London Picture Archive 2359; **106** *Mayhew's London; being selections from 'London labour and the London poor'*, by Henry Mayhew, 1851; **107** London Metropolitan Archives (City of London) / Collage – The London Picture Archive 2743; **110** London Metropolitan Archives (City of London) / Collage – The London Picture Archive 3092; **111l** *Punch Magazine*, 10 July 1858; **111r** *Punch Magazine*, 3 July 1858; **112–113** *A record of the progress of modern engineering 1865: comprising civil, mechanical, marine, hydraulic, railway, bridge, and other engineering works, with essays and reviews*, by William Humber, 1866; 114t London Metropolitan Archives (City of London) / Collage – The London Picture Archive 3092; **114b** London Metropolitan Archives (City of London) / Collage – The London Picture Archive 28213; **115t** London Metropolitan Archives (City of London) / Collage – The London Picture Archive 28218; **115b** London Metropolitan Archives (City of London) / Collage – The London Picture Archive 28217; **116t** SSPL / Getty Images; **116b** The Print Collector / Print Collector / Getty Images; **118–119** By permission of Historic England Archive; **120–121** London Metropolitan Archives (City of London) / Collage – The London Picture Archive 228416; **122** *The Engineer*, 1867; **123** Courtesy Frontispiece, www.mapsandantiqueprints.com; **124t** Hulton-Deutsch Collection / Corbis / Getty Images; **124b**, **125** Otto Herschan Collection / Hulton Archive / Getty Images; **126–127** Adam Powell; **128** Courtesy Thames Water Utilities Limited; **129** *A record of the progress of modern engineering 1865: comprising civil, mechanical, marine, hydraulic, railway, bridge, and other engineering works, with essays and reviews*, by William Humber, 1866; **130** SSPL / Getty Images; **132–133** Courtesy Thames Water Utilities Limited; **134–135** Library of Congress, Washington, D.C.; **136** Courtesy Thames Water Utilities Limited; **137l** Courtesy Susan Eacret; **137tr** Courtesy Andy Mabbett; **137br** Courtesy sewerhistory.org; **138–141** Courtesy Thames Water Utilities Limited; **142** Mitchell Library, State Library of New South Wales, Sydney; **144–145** The Trustees of The Brunel Museum, London; **146** *Stadt-Wasserkunst, Hamburg, Entworfen & Ausgeführt von W. Lindley in den Jahren 1844-1861 (Fortgesetzt bis 1863)*, 1864. State and University Library Hamburg; **147l** PA Images; **147r** Hamburger Stadtentwässerung; **148–149** Institution of Civil Engineers Library and Archives; 150–151 Collection Christian Terstegge; **152** Historic Archive Berliner Wasserbetriebe, photographer unknown; **153l** Studio Canal / Shutterstock; **153r** London Films / Kobal / REX / Shutterstock; **154–155** Historic Archive Berliner Wasserbetriebe, photographer unknown; **156–157** National Library of Poland, Warsaw; **158**, **159tr**, cr Mazovian Digital Library, Poland; **159br** *Marta Sapała Dla dobra publicznego : 120 lat Wodociągów Warszawskich 1886–2006*, Miejskie Przedsiębiorstwo Wodociągów i Kanalizacji, Warszawa 2006; **160** Cit. Archive of Prague Waterworks and Sewerage (APVK), fund Archive of Photography, box 9, signature OK-34/9, OK-34/10; **161** National Library of Poland, Warsaw; **162–163** *The shone hydro-pneumatic system of sewerage*, by Urban H. Broughton, 1887; **164–165** Mitchell Library, State Library of New South Wales, Sydney; **166l** National Library of Australia, Canberra; **166r** *Illustrations from Progress in Public Works & Roads in NSW, 1827-1855*, by Sir Thomas Mitchell. State Library of New South Wales, Sydney; **167** *Sydney City and Suburban Sewage and Health Board: photographs, with excerpts from the final report of the committee appointed "To inquire into the state of crowded dwellings and areas in the city of Sydney and suburbs, so far as it affects public health"*, 1875. State Library of New South Wales, Sydney; **168–169** Mitchell Library, State Library of New South Wales, Sydney; **170–171** Kew Historical Society, Melbourne; **172–173** Melbourne Water Archives; **174l** Courtesy the National Archives of Australia. NAA: A3560, 1724; **174r** Courtesy the National Archives of Australia. NAA: A3560, 1725; **175tl**, **bl** Bureau of Sewerage, Tokyo Metropolitan Government; **175tr**, br National Diet Library, Tokyo; **176**, **178** Boston Public Library, Edgar Sutton Dorr Photograph Collection; **179** Lawrence Public Library, Massachusetts; **180** Harvard Map Collection, Harvard Library, Cambridge, MA; **181** Boston Public Library, Norman B. Leventhal Map Center Collection; **182–183** Boston Public Library, Edgar Sutton Dorr Photograph Collection; **184–185** *Sanitary and social chart of the Fourth Ward of the City of New York, to accompany a report of the 4th Sanitary Inspection District, made to the Council of Hygiene of the Citizens' Association*, by E.R. Pulling, M.D. assisted by F.J. Randall, New York Public Library; **186–187** The David Rumsey Map Collection, www.davidrumsey.com; **190–191** New York Public Library; **188–189** Science, Industry & Business Library, The New York Public Library; **192–193** Courtesy of the Passaic Valley Sewerage Commission, Newark, New Jersey; **194** *Sewers and drains*, by Anson Marston, 1912; **196tl** *Design of a combined sewer system for the village of Peotone Will County Illinois*, by Henry F. Israel and George L. Opper, 1913; **196tr**, **cl**, **cr** *Design of a separate sewer system and disposal plant for the town of Arlington Heights*, Illinois, by J. G. Chandler; R. S. Claar, R. Neufeld, 1912; **196clb** *Design of a sanitary sewer system for the town of Glen Ellyn Illinois*, by John J. Fieldseth, Bernard Phillips, F. A. Trujillo, 1913; **196crb**, **br** *Design of water works and sewer system for St.Charles, Kane co. Il*, by F. T. Pierce, E. F. Hiller, C. O. Johnson, 1906; **196bl** *Design of a sanitary sewer system and a septic tank for the city of Rushville, Illinois*, by F. J. Munoz, E. Vynne, 1910; **197** *Sewers and drains*, by Anson Marston, 1912; **198** Courtesy sewerhistory.org; **199** California Historical Society. University of Southern California Libraries, L. A.; **200–201** *Progress report of the engineers in charge to devise and provide a system of sewerage for the city and county of San Francisco: for the fiscal year ending June 30, 1893*, by Marsden Manson, Carl Ewald Grunsky, San Francisco (Calif.). Board of Supervisors, 1893; **202–203** The David Rumsey Map Collection, www.davidrumsey.com; **205** New York Public Library; **207–208** Courtesy Thames Water Utilities Limited; **210–211** *The design of a septic tank*, by George Rockwell Bascom, 1905; **212–213** *A farm septic tank*, by William B. Herms, H. L. Belton, 1923; **214–215** *The Jewell water filter gravity and pressure systems*, by O.H. Jewell Filter Company; **216** SSPL / Getty Images; **217** *The Jewell water filter gravity and pressure systems*, by O.H. Jewell Filter Company; **218** Courtesy Thames Water Utilities Limited; **219** *Experimental investigations by the State Board of Health of Massachusetts upon the purification of sewage by filtration and by chemical precipitation and upon the intermittent filtration of water. Made at Lawrence, Mass.*, 1888-1890 by Massachusetts. State Board of Health, 1890; **220** *Extraction and utilization of grease from dried activated sludge*, by Robert Joseph Gnaedinger, 1920; **220** *The activated sludge method of sewage treatment*, by Floyd William Mohlman, 1916; **220** *The fertilizer value of activated sludge*, by William Durrell Hatfield, 1918; **222–224** Courtesy Thames Water Utilities Limited; **225** United Utilities, Warrington, UK; **226–231** Courtesy Thames Water Utilities Limited; **232tl**, **tc**, **tr** Courtesy Thames Water Utilities Limited; **232clb** James King-Holmes / Alamy Stock Photo; **232crb** LusoEnvironment / Alamy Stock Photo; **232b** Lena Wurm / Alamy Stock Photo; **233tl** US National Archives and Records Administration; **233tc** *Modern sanitary engineering practice: the applications of Dorr equipment to modern sewage treatment and water purification plants*, by Dorr Company, 1930; **233tr** Courtesy Thames Water Utilities Limited; **233bl** Jeff Kalmes; **233bc** Michael Fritzen / Alamy Stock Photo; **233r** Courtesy Thames Water Utilities Limited; **234–237** Courtesy Thames Water Utilities Limited; **238t** Thames Water; **238b** AP / Rex / Shutterstock; **239** Courtesy Thames Water Utilities Limited; **240** Tideway; **242–243** Carl Court / Getty Images; **245t** Courtesy Tideway; **245b** Tideway; **246** Richard Levine / Alamy Stock Photo; **247** ZUMA Press, Inc. / Alamy Stock Photo; **248** Huntstock / Getty Images; **249** © 2016 Shimon Mor; **250–251** VCG / Getty Images; **256** Courtesy Thames Water Utilities Limited

Illustrations are in **bold**.

A

Abbey Mills, London 117, 122, 123, 225, 244
accidents 45, 49, 131, 166–7, **192, 201,** 212
activated sludge **220,** 221, 224, **225,** 228, 229, **233**
Adelaide 167, 170
Agadir, Morroco 247
Agrippa, Marcus 37
Aigues-Mortes, France 44
Al-Andalus 42
Algeciras, Spain 42
alligators 198
Altona, Germany 16–17
America *see* USA
anaerobic digesters **248**
Antananarivo, Madagascar 247
Antwerp 49
aquadoros 41–2
aqueducts
  Mayan 41
  Melbourne **173**
  New York 187
  Paris **96–7**
  Roman 36, **37,** 43
  Washington, DC 198
Ardern, Edward 9, 221
Asnières, Paris 68–9
assassination attempts 83
assassinations 36–7
Athens **34–5,** 36
Aubriot, Hugues 49
Australia *see also specific cities*
  dams **142,** 167, **168–9**
  population growth 143
  toilets **164–5**
  treatment plants 166, 167, 171, **173,** 174, 247

B

Bacon, Francis 213
bacteria
  cyanobacteria **218**
  Robert Koch's discovery in water 9
  sewage treatment **207,** 210, 216–17, **219,** 221, 224, 228
Baltimore 204, **205**
bateaux-vannes 69, 82, **82,** 83, **88–9**
Bazalgette, Joseph
  appointed Chief Engineer 106–7
  background 106
  bridges 140
  on cholera 10
  family **9**
  obituary 101
  sewers 23–4, 69, **108–9,** 110–11, **112–13,** 117, 122–3, **129,** 131, 140
Bazalgette Tunnel Ltd 244
Beausire, Jean 62
Beckton, London 110, 111, 117, 122, **123,** 131, 136, **228,** 229, 244, **245**
Belgrand, Eugène 67, 68, 90
Berlin 21, 45, 152–3, **154–5**
Bible 29
biofilms 216, 217
biogas **232**
Boccaccio **45**
Bondi Beach 166, 167
Boston, USA **57, 176,** 177, **178–83,** 186
Bramah, Joseph 100
bricks/brickmaking 32, 36, 42–3, **126–7,** 136, **137**
Broad Street pump 21–2, **22**
Brueghel, Peter, the Elder **45**
Brunel, Isambard Kingdom 106, 146
Brunel, Marc Isambard **144–5,** 146

C

Cameron, Donald 210, 211
Canberra 171, 174
Carracci, Ludovico 37
Celje, Slovenia 38
cesspits/cesspools
  19th century Italy 42
  accidents 49

ancient civilizations 30, **31,** 37, 38
  Australia 167
  Baltimore 204
  Croatia 44
  floors collapsing 49
  London 45
  Paris 45, **66,** 90
  San Francisco **200**
  St Petersburg 161
  water closet problems 106
Chadwick, Edwin 21, 62, 136
chamber pots 52, **54**
Chang'an, China 32
Chavín de Huántar, Peru 41
Chesborough, Ellis 195
Chicago **194,** 195, **197, 214–15**
Chiger family 160
China 32, 33, 209, 241, **250–1**
chlorine **234–5,** 236
cholera
  bacillus identification 24
  epidemics and pandemics 10–11, **14–15,** 16, **20,** 24, **25,** 122–3, 147, 161, 166, 177, 186
  John Snow 9, 21–2, **22,** 23
  miasma 9, 17, 21, 67
  modern threat 241
  symptoms and effects 10, **12, 13,** 23
  water samples **18–19,** 216
cisterns
  ancient civilizations **30,** 33, 38, **39**
  water samples **18–19**
Cîteaux, France 43
cities
  21st century growth 241
  battlement toilets 44
  importance of sewers 9
Clark, William 167, 170
climate change 241, 244
Cloaca Maxima, Rome 33, 36, 37
Cloacina 33
Cluny, France 43
Committee for Scientific Enquiry 21, 23
composting 32–3, 210
Constantinople 38, **39**
Copenhagen 11
Craigentinny Meadows, Edinburgh 46, 49
Crapper, Thomas 100, **101**
Creighton, Charles 24
Crete 32, 33
Croatia 44
Crossness pumping station, London **4–5, 8,** 110, 117, **118–21,** 131, 229, 244
Cruickshank, Isaac **55**
Crystal Palace 106
Cummings, Alexander 100
cyanobacteria **218**

D

dams, Australia **142,** 167, **168–9**
de Gaulle, Charles, assassination attempts 83
Decameron (Boccaccio) **45**
'dewatering' 225, 228, **232**
Dibdin, Willam 221
Dickens, Charles 22, 99
Diocletian 44
Dionysius of Halicarnassus 36
disinfectants 236
Disraeli, Benjamin 111
Doulton and Watt 136, **137**
drains
  ancient civilizations **27, 28,** 31, 32
  Romney Marsh **46–7**
Dubrovnik, Croatia 44
Duncan, William Henry 107, 110
'dunny carts' 166, 170
Dusseldorf 152
Dutch Proverbs (Breughel) **45**
dysentery 167, 170, 186

E

earth closets 67, 166, 170
East London Water Company **18,** 23
Eaton, Fred 199

Eddington community, Cambridge 248–9
Edinburgh 46, 49, **54**
'effluent polishing' **233, 234–5,** 236
Egypt, ancient 30–1
electricity generation 229, 236, 247, 249
Elizabeth I 49, 53
embankments 43, **114–16,** 117, 122, 140
Evans, Arthur 32

F

Faraday, Michael 22, 106
farming 46, 49, 67, 131, 171, 174, 209
Farr, William 21, 23
fatbergs 236, **238–9**
'The Fauna of the Hamburg Water Main' 24
fertilizer 32–3, 42, 45, 67, 90, 99, 131, 167, 209, 224, 228, **232**
films 38, 143, 152, **153,** 160, 204
filters
  Jewell water filter **214–15, 217**
  sand 143, 147, 213, 216
  sand filters 152
  trickling 212, 217, 221, 228, **250–1**
filtration beds 24
Fitzalwyn, Henry 49
floods 43
Florence, Italy 42
FOGs (Fats, Oils and Grease) 236, **238–9**
Foster, Norman 140
Fountains Abbey, Yorkshire 44
Fowler, Gilbert 221, 224
France 43–4, 160, 212, 248 *see also* Paris
Frankfurt 147, 152
Frankland, Edward 213, 216
Frederick I 49

G

Galton, Douglas 111
garbage disposal 52, 99
'Gardy Loo' 44, **54**
Germany
  17th century 45
  19th century 42, 143, 146–7, 152–3
  cholera 11, 16–17, **17,** 147
  monasteries 44
  population growth 21
  smuggling 153
  toilets 248
Gibbs family 99
Gillray, James **55**
gong-fermors 45
Grand Junction Canal Company 45
Great Exhibition 1851 106
'Great Stink' 21, 111
Greece, ancient 32, **34–5,** 36
Greenway route, London 137
guano 99
gunpowder 49

H

Halévy, Léon 63
Hall, Benjamin 110–11
Hamburg
  cholera 16, **17,** 24, 123
  population growth 21
  sewers 147, **150–1**
  water main organisms 24
  water supply **146,** 147, **150**
Hamburger Fremdenblatt 24
Harington, John **52,** 53, 100
Harper's Weekly 83
Haussmann, Georges-Eugène 9, 37, 62–3, **64–5,** 67, 83, 90
Hawksley, Thomas 216
Heine, Heinrich 10–11
Heliogabalus 36–7
Herculaneum, Italy 37
Herodotus 31
Hippocrates 17, 36
  History of Epidemics in Britain (Creighton) 24
Hobrecht, James 153
Hong Kong 143, 248

Hope, William 131
Hugo, Victor 59, 67, 228
hydraulic house-sewage ejector **162–3**
hydrolysis, thermal 198, 228
Hyperion treatment plant 199, 204

I

Illinois **196**
Illustrated London News 24
Imhoff, Karl 211–12
India 31, 241
Indus Valley 31, 33
The Invisible Man (Parks) 198
Ireland 212
Istanbul 38, **39**
Italy *see also* Romans, ancient
  19th century 42
  ancient civilizations 33
  cholera **17**

J

James Bond 38
James, Clive 167
Jamestown 204
Japan 16, 143, 174–5, **242–3,** 244, 249
Jennings, George **100,** 101, **102,** 106
Jervis, John 177, 187
Jewell, Omar **214–15, 217**
Jews in World War II 160

K

Kast, Alfred **13**
Kelston, Bath 53
kennels 38, **40,** 44, 49, 52, 99
Kenya 248
Khorasabad, Iraq **27**
Knossos, Crete 32
Koch, Robert 9, 24

L

La Villette, Paris 90
The Lancet 10, 17
latrines *see* toilets
Latrobe, Benjamin 177
lavatories *see* toilets
Lawrence Experimental Station 217, 221
laystalls 38, 52–3
Le Petit Journal **25**
Lea (river) 23
leather tanning 38
Leeuwenhoek, Antony van 24
legends 198
legislation
  cesspits/cesspools 42, 49
  sewers 45, 111, 170, 174–5, 186, 187
  waste disposal 52
Leipzig 152
Leroux, Pierre 67
Les Misérables (Hugo) 59, 67, 228
Liebig, Justus von 67
Liernur, Charles 160, 248
Lima, Peru 41–2
Lindley, William 143, 146–7, **148–9,** 152, 153, 160–1
Lindley, William Heerlein 143, **148–9,** 152
Little Dorrit (Dickens) 22, 99
Liverpool 107, 110, 216
Livy, Titus 33
Lockett, William 9, 221
London *see also* Thames
  cholera 11, **20,** 21–2, 23, 122–3
  embankments **114–16,** 117, 122, 140
  Fleet River **107**
  'Great Stink' 21
  medieval legislation 49, 52
  population growth 21, 99, 136–7
  public toilets **100,** 106
  pumping stations **4–5, 8, 98,** 110, 117, **118–21,** 123, **128,** 225, **226–7, 230–1,** 244
  Romans 38
  sewers 4, 23–4, 99, **104–5,** 106, **108–9, 112–13,** 117, 122–3, **124–7, 129–30,** 131, **132–5,** 137, **139,** 244, **245**

'Shiteburne Lane' 49
stormwater 244
treatment plants **228**, 229, **237**, **245**
water supply 53, 216, **222–4**, **237**
Loowatt 247
Los Angeles **198**, 199
Lothal, India 31
Lvov, Poland 160

M
MacNeill, John 106
Madagascar 247
Madison, USA 217
malaria 198
Manchester 221, 224
manholes
ancient civilizations **31**
Japan 175
Mansergh, James 170
Marat, Jean-Paul 59
marijuana 198
Marseilles 10
martyrs 37
Mayans 41
McRedie, George **164–5**
Medusa **39**
Melbourne 170–1, **172–3**, 247
Men At Arms (Waugh) 170
Mesopotamia **27**, 30, 33, 209
The Metamorphosis of Ajax:
A Cloacinean Satire (Harington) 53
methane gas 167, 171, 228, 247, 248
Metropolitan Board of Works 106, 110
miasma 9, 17, 21, 67, 111
Milan, Italy 42
Mille, Adolphe 90
Minoans 32
Minotaur 32
On the Mode of Communication of
Cholera (Snow) 21
Mohenjo-daro, Pakistan **28**, 31
Moigno, François-Napoléon-Marie 211
monasteries 43–4
Morocco 247
Mosley, Charles **55**
Moule, Henry 67
Mouras, Jean-Louis 211
movies 38, 143, 152, **153**, 160, 204
Murcia, Spain 42
Murgia Timone, Italy 33
Mutant Ninja Turtles 198
myths 198

N
Nadar **70–1**, **80–1**, **84**, **91**
Nairobi, Kenya 248
Napier, William 131
Napoleon III 59, 62, 90
Nazareth, Israel 30
Netherlands 160
New River, London 53
New York 11, **16**, **184–5**, **186**, 187,
188–94, 198, **245–6**
Newgate prison 45
Newlands, James 107
Nightingale, Florence 9, 21, 107
nightsoilmen 45, **48**, 49, **66**, 67, 90, 99
Nobel Prize 24
Norway 143, 248
Notes on Nursing (Nightingale) 21
Nottingham 216

O
Old Ford reservoir 23
Omini Processor 249
Orkney Islands 33
Ostia, Rome 38

P
Palenque, Mexico 41
The Parcel Yard, King's Cross 100
Paris
cesspits/cesspools 45, **66**, 90
cholera 10–11, **16**
garbage disposal **50**
Haussmann reconstruction **60–1**,
62–3, **64–5**, 67, 68–9, 83, 90
métro station and line construction
74–5, **94–5**

population growth 21
sewers **58**, 59, **60–1**, 62, **64–5**, 68–9,
70–81, 82–3, **84–9**, 90, **91–7**
survey maps **6**
water supply **60–1**, 62, **64–5**, 67, 68
wells **51**, 90
Parks, Gordon 198
Pepys, Samuel 41
Pergamon, ancient Greece 36
Peru 41–2
Petra, Jordan 30
Pettenkofer, Max Joseph von 17
Philadelphia 177, 186
Philip, Arthur 166
Pingliangtai, China 32
pipes
ancient civilizations 30, 31, **32**,
33, 36, 37
Doulton and Watt **137**, **138**
Lima, Peru 41
monasteries 43–4
New River, London 53
Paris **78–9**, 83, **96–7**
sand filters 216
wood **160**, 177, 186
Piranesi, Giovanni 36
Poland 152, **156–9**, 160
Pompeii, Italy 37
Pont du Gard, France 37
population growth 21, 99, 136–7
Prague 160–1, 248
Pullman, George 195
pumping stations
Chicago **197**
Japan 174
London **4–5**, **8**, **98**, 110, 117,
118–21, 123, **128**, 225, **226–7**,
230–1, 244
Melbourne **172**
New York **193**
Punch 22, **111**
purification
development of 213, 216–17, **219**,
221, 224, 225, 236
future developments 249
tertiary treatment **233**, **234–5**, 236

R
raykers 38, 45, 49, 52
reed beds 212, 213, 236
reservoirs
sewage 110, **180**, 187, **208**
water supply 167, **173**, **222–4**
Richmond Palace 53
River Lee tunnel 244
Romans, ancient 33, 36, 38
Rome
6th century 43
floods 43
Mouth of Truth **37**, 38
Romney Marsh **46–7**
Russia 11, 101, 161
From Russia With Love (film) 38

S
Saint Sebastian 37
saltpetre 49
San Francisco **200–3**
sand filters 143, 147, 152, 213, 216
Santorini, Greece 32
scavengers **42**
Scientific American 209, 211
sedimentation tanks 225, 228
Sedron Technologies 249
Senegal 249
septic tanks 210–13
settlement tanks 136, 217, 224, **228**,
229, **250–1**
sewage ejector **162–3**
sewage farms *see* treatment plants
sewer hunters **106**
sewers
ancient civilizations 30, 32, 33,
36, 38
Baltimore 204
Berlin **152**, 153, **154–5**
Boston, USA **57**, **176**, 177, **178–83**,
186
Canberra 171, 174

Chicago **194**, 195
cleaning 69, 82–3, **84–9**, **141**
'collectors' 68–9, **70–1**, **78–9**, 82
construction overview **172–3**
Croatia 44
Frankfurt 147, 152
goddesses 33
Hamburg 147, **150–1**
Illinois **196**
Islamic Spain 42
Japan 174–5
London **2**, 23–4, 99, **104–5**, 106,
108–9, **112–13**, 117, 122–3, **124–7**,
129–30, 131, **132–5**, 137, **139**,
244, **245**
Los Angeles 199
Melbourne 170–1, **172–3**
New York 187, **188–93**, 198
Paris 45, 49, **58**, 59, **60–1**, 62, **64–5**,
68–9, **70–81**, 82–3, **84–9**, 90, **91–7**
Prague 160–1
San Francisco **200–3**
shapes **72–3**, 107, **108–9**, **161**,
183
St Petersburg 161, 166
Sydney 166, **168–9**
tourist visits 9, **82**, 83
vacuum 248
Warsaw **157–9**, 160
Washington, DC 198
Simpson, James 9, 111, 216
sink holes **201**
Skara Brae, Orkney Islands 33
sludge vessels **136**, 229
Smith, John, Captain 204
smuggling 153
Snow, John 9, 21–2, **22**, 23
Socha, Leopold 160
South America 16, 41
Spain **17**, 42
'spend a penny' 106
Split, Croatia 44
Sprot, William 49
St Petersburg 161, 166
Stephenson, Robert 106, 146
stormwater 131, **199**, 204, **231**,
242–3, 244
Strachey, Lytton 9
street level raising 195
Šulak 29
sumps, Indus Valley civilizations 31
Sunderland 10, **23**
Suyin, Han 209
Sweden 143, 248
Swift, Jonathan 49
Sydney **164–5**, 166–7, **168–9**

T
Taiwan 241
tanning industry 38
Tchaikovsky, Pyotr Ilyich 161
telephone cables **91–3**
Tell Asmar, Iraq 30
Thames 22, **23**, 99, **111**
Thames Tideway Tunnel 244, **245**
Thames Tunnel **144–5**, 146
thermal hydrolysis 198, 228
The Third Man (film) 143, 152, **153**
Thwaites, William **172**
The Times 17, 22, 140
toilets
18th century **55**
anaerobic digesters 247
ancient civilizations 30, 31, 32, **33**,
37, 38, 248
Australia **164–5**, 166, 170
demons 29
earth closets 67, 166, 170
floors collapsing 49
'flying' 248
future developments 249
Islamic Spain 42
Japan 175, 249
medieval **44**, **45**
monasteries 44
USA **184–5**
vacuum 248
water closet development 100–1,
102–3, 106

water closet invention **52**, 53
tours of sewers 9, **82**, 83
treatment plants
Australia 166, 167, 171, **173**,
174, 247
Britain 131, **208**
China **250–1**
Czech Republic **160**
Japan **175**
London **228**, 229, **237**, **245**
modern method 225, 228–9, **232–5**,
236
modern method, development of
210, 217, **219**, 221, 224
USA 186, 187, 195, 198, 199, 204
waste stabilization ponds 247
trickling filters 212, 217, 221, 228,
250–1
Trouville, France 160
Tumbes, Peru 42
tunnel boring machines (TBMs) **240**,
244, 246
Turkey **33**
Twyford, Thomas 101, **103**
Tyntesfield, Somerset 99
typhoid 152, 170, 177, 186, 198,
216, 241

U
ultraviolet light 236
'unitas' 101
Ur and Uruk, Babylonia 30
urine, leather tanning 38
USA *see also specific cities*
aqueducts 187, 198
cholera 11, 16, **16**, 177
septic tanks 212
sewers **57**
toilets **184–5**
treatment plants 187, 195, 198, 199,
204, 221
water supply 177, 186

V
vacuums 143, 160, 248
Venice 44
Veuillot, Louis 83
Vienna 10, 152, **153**

W
Warsaw 152, **156–9**, 160
Washington, DC 198
waste, non-biodegradable 236
water carriers 41–2
water closet **52**, 53, 100–1, **102–3**
water conservation 171
water pollution 199, 204
water supply
Adelaide 167
ancient civilizations 30–1, 32, 36, 37
Chicago **214–15**
Hamburg **146**, 147, **150**
London 53, 216, **222–4**, **237**
monasteries 43–4
New York **245–6**
Paris **60–1**, 62, **64–5**, 67, 68
Philadelphia 177, 186
St Petersburg 161
Sydney 166, 167, **168–9**
Warsaw 152, **156**, **158–9**
Waugh, Evelyn 170
wells
ancient civilizations 30, **34–5**
New York 187
Paris **51**, 90
water samples **18–19**
wet wipes 236
Whitechapel
cholera 23
Fatberg 236
Wilhelm II 24
Williams, Charles **55**
World War II **122**, 160

X
Xi'an, China 32

Y
Yongchuan, China **32**

ACKNOWLEDGMENTS

I owe many debts to people who have helped me with the research for this book: Debbie Francis, the librarian at the Institution of Civil Engineers, and those at Cambridge University Library who delved deep into their records and archives to find sources that are unlikely to command a great following among modern engineers or undergraduates; my editors at Thames & Hudson, Jane Laing and Isabel Jessop, and their colleagues, creative director Tristan de Lancey and picture editor Phoebe Lindsley; Sir Peter Bazalgette, who recommended me for the task and whose great-great-grandfather features prominently in the preceding chapters; Dina Gillespie, the Site Performance Manager at Beckton Sewage Treatment Works, who updated me on the latest developments in the largest treatment works in Europe; Sadia Kashem of Thames Water, who went to great lengths to answer my awkward and unfamiliar enquiries concerning the operations of treatment works and the availability of illustrations; and above all, Dr Wilfrid Bourgeois, Process Scientist at Anglian Water, who escorted me around the Cambridge Water Recycling Centre, patiently explaining how the processes worked, and who corrected my first feeble attempts to explain it all to the reader. Any remaining errors are mine. Curiously, Wilf's family comes from the small town of Vesoul, near Dijon in France, one of whose former residents occupies an honoured place in our story.

Thames & Hudson would like to thank Pavan Badesha at Thames Water, Debra Francis at the Institution of Civil Engineers, Kryštof Drnek at Prague Water Supply and Sewerage and Stephan Natz at Berlin Water Utilities for generously sharing their archives with us.

ABOUT THE AUTHOR

Dr Stephen Halliday is a writer, lecturer and broadcaster with a particular interest in Victorian London and in the engineers who made nineteenth-century cities safe and habitable. He has written for BBC History, the *Observer*, the *Guardian*, the *Financial Times* and the *Daily Telegraph*. He has also made several radio and television programmes based on his books.

Front cover image: Joe Belanger / Shutterstock

Back cover image: Adam Powell

Published by arrangement with Thames & Hudson Ltd., London, by the MIT Press

An Underground Guide to Sewers
© 2019 Thames & Hudson Ltd, London

Text © 2019 Stephen Halliday

Foreword © 2019 Sir Peter Bazalgette

For image copyright information, see p.253

Designed by Anıl Aykan at Barnbrook

ISBN 978-0-262-04334-2

Library of Congress Control Number: 2019933593

Printed and bound in China by
C&C Offset Printing Co. Ltd

The MIT Press
Massachusetts Institute of Technology
Cambridge, Massachusetts 02142
http://mitpress.mit.edu

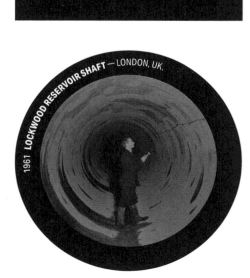

1961 LOCKWOOD RESERVOIR SHAFT — LONDON, UK.

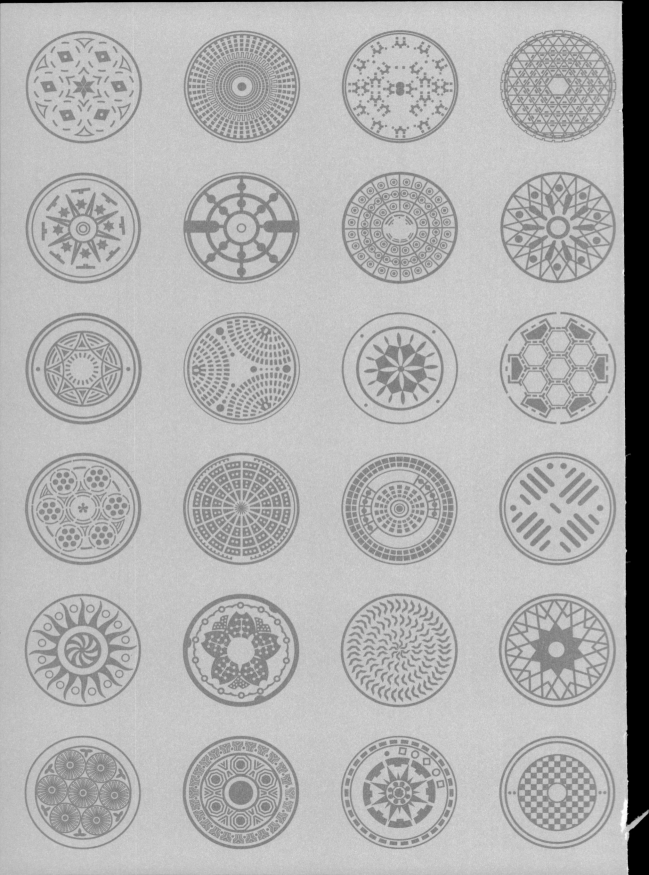